Inflammatory and Thrombotic Problems in Vascular Surgery

Edited by

R. M. GREENHALGH MA MD MChir FRCS

Professor of Surgery and Chairman,
Department of Surgery,
Charing Cross and Westminster Medical School,
London

J. T. POWELL PhD MD

Professor of Vascular Biology,
Department of Surgery,
Charing Cross and Westminster Medical School,
London

W. B. SAUNDERS COMPANY LTD
London · Philadelphia · Toronto · Sydney · Tokyo

W. B. Saunders Company Ltd 24–28 Oval Road
London NW1 7DX

The Curtis Center
Independence Square West
Philadelphia, PA 19106-3399, USA

Harcourt Brace & Company
55 Horner Avenue
Toronto, Ontario M8Z 4X6, Canada

Harcourt Brace & Company, Australia
30-52 Smidmore Street
Marrickville, NSW 2204, Australia

Harcourt Brace & Company, Japan
Ichibancho Central Building, 22-1 Ichibancho
Chiyoda-ku, Tokyo, 102, Japan

A catalogue record for this book is available from the British Library.

ISBN 0-7020-2336-1

Editorial and Production Services by Jane Duncan
10 Barley Mow Passage, London W4 4PH

Typeset by Phoenix Photosetting, Chatham, Kent
Printed in Great Britain at the University Press, Cambridge

Contents

INTRODUCTION

AORTIC ANEURYSMS

PERIPHERAL VASCULATURE

VEIN GRAFT STENOSIS

VENOUS THROMBOSIS

Contributors

M. D'ADDATO, MD
Professor of Vascular Surgery University of
  Bologna
Policlinico S Orsola
Via Massarenti 9
40138 Bologna
Italy

R.N. BAIRD, ChM FRCS
Consultant Surgeon
Directorate of Surgery
Bristol Royal Infirmary
Bristol BS2 8HW, UK

A.A.B. BARROS D'SA, MD FRCS FRCEd
Consultant Vascular Surgeon
Royal Victoria Hospital
The Royal Group of Hospitals
Health and Social Services Trust
Grosvenor Road
Belfast BT12 6BA
Northern Ireland

J.D. BEARD, ChM FRCS MB BS BSc
Consultant, Sheffield Vascular Institute
Northern General Hospital
Herries Road
Sheffield S5 7AU, UK

D.K. BEATTIE, FRCS FRCSI
Lecturer and Honorary Registrar
Department of Surgery
Charing Cross and Westminster Medical
  School
Fulham Palace Road
London W6 8RF, UK

M. BELKIN, MD
Associate Professor of Surgery
Harvard Medical School
Department of Vascular Surgery
Brigham and Women's Hospital
75 Francis Street
Boston MA 02115
USA

P.R.F. BELL, MB ChB MD FRCS
Professor of Surgery
Department of Surgery
University of Leicester
Faculty of Medicine
Robert Kilpatrick Building
Leicester Royal Infirmary
PO Box 65
Leicester LE2 7LX, UK

D. BERGQVIST, MD PhD
Professor of Vascular Surgery
Department of Surgery
University Hospital
S-751 85 Uppsala
Sweden

S.D. BLAIR, MS FRCS
Consultant Surgeon
Arrowe Park Hospital
Arrowe Park Road
Upton
Wirral
Merseyside
L49 5PE, UK

A.W. BRADBURY, BSc MD FRCSEd
Senior Lecturer in Vascular Surgery
Vascular Surgery Unit
University Department of Surgery
Royal Infirmary
Edinburgh EH3 9YW, UK

N. BRINDLE PhD
Lecturer in Vascular Cell Biology
Department of Surgery
University of Leicester
Robert Kilpatrick Building
Leicester Royal Infirmary
Leicester LE2 7LX, UK

SIR NORMAN BROWSE, MD FRCS
Professor of Surgery
Surgical Unit
St Thomas' Hospital UMDS
Lambeth Palace Road
London SE1 7EH, UK

C.B. BUNKER, MA MD FRCP
Consultant Dermatologist
Charing Cross and Chelsea & Westminster
    Hospitals
Honorary Senior Lecturer
Charing Cross and Westminster Medical
    School
Fulham Palace Road
London W6 8RF, UK

K.G. BURNAND, MS FRCS
Professor of Vascular Surgery
Surgical Unit
St Thomas' Hospital UMDS
Lambeth Palace Road
London SE1 7EH, UK

W. BRUCE CAMPBELL, MS MRCP FRCS
Consultant in Vascular and General Surgery
Royal Devon and Exeter Hospital
Exeter EX2 5DW, UK

N.J. CHESHIRE, MD FRCS
Lecturer in Surgery and Senior Registrar
Academic Surgical Unit and Regional
    Vascular Unit
Imperial College of Science, Technology
    and Medicine School of Medicine
St Mary's Hospital NHS Trust
Praed Street
Paddington, London W2 1NY, UK

A.W. CLOWES, MD
Department of Surgery
University of Washington
Box 356410
1959 NE Pacific Street
Seattle
WA 98195-6410, USA

P.D. COLERIDGE SMITH, DM FRCS
Senior Lecturer
Department of Surgery
University College London Medical School
The Middlesex Hospital
Mortimer Street
London W1N 8AA, UK

A.H. DAVIES, MA DM FRCS
Senior Lecturer and Honorary Consultant
    Surgeon
Department of Surgery
Charing Cross and Westminster Medical
    School
Fulham Palace Road
London W6 8RF, UK

C.B. ERNST, MD
Clinical Professor of Surgery
University of Michigan Medical School
Vascular Surgery Program Director
Henry Ford Hospital
Detroit, Michigan, USA

P. FIORANI, MD
Professor and Head of Vascular Surgery
University of Rome 'La Sapienza'
Policlinico Umberto I
00161 Rome, Italy

M. GARGIULO, MD
Department of Vascular Surgery
University of Bologna
Policlinico S Orsola
Via Massarenti 9
40138 Bologna
Italy

J. GOLLEDGE, MA FRCS
Lecturer in Surgery
Department of Surgery
Charing Cross and Westminster Medical
    School
Fulham Palace Road
London W6 8RF, UK

K. GRABITZ, MD
Professor of Surgery
Department of Vascular Surgery and
    Kidney Transplantation
Heinrich-Heine University
Moorenstrasse 5
D-4000 Dusseldorf
Germany

G. HAMILTON, FRCS
Consultant General and Vascular Surgeon
Department of Surgery
Royal Free Hospital
The Royal Free Hampstead NHS Trust
Pond Street
London NW3 2QG, UK

A.I. HANDA, FRCS(Eng) FRCS(Ed)
Vascular Research Fellow
University Department of Surgery
Royal Free Hospital
The Royal Free Hampstead NHS Trust
Pond Street
London NW3 2QG, UK

D.O. HASKARD, DM FRCP
Sir John Michael Professor of
  Cardiovascular Medicine
Department of Medicine
Royal Postgraduate Medical School
Hammersmith Hospital
Du Cane Road
London W12 0NN, UK

D.J. HIGMAN, MS FRCS
Senior Registrar
Department of Surgery
Charing Cross and Westminster Medical
  School
Fulham Palace Road
London W6 8RF, UK

M. HORROCKS, MS FRCS
Compass Professor of Surgery
University Department of Surgery
Royal United Hospital Trust
Combe Park
Bath BA1 3NG, UK

K. HOUGH, MD
Department of Haematology
Charing Cross and Westminster Medical
  School
Fulham Palace Road
London W6 8RF, UK

R.D. KENAGY, PhD
Department of Surgery
University of Washington
Box 356410
1959 NE Pacific Street
Seattle
WA 98195-6410, USA

U.J. KIRKPATRICK, FRCS
Clinical Research Fellow
Department of Surgery
University Hospital of South Manchester
Nell Lane
West Didsbury
Manchester M20 8LR, UK

D.A. LANE, MD
Professor of Molecular Haematology
Department of Haematology
Charing Cross and Westminster Medical
  School
Fulham Palace Road
London W6 8RF, UK

L.J. LEVIEN, MB BCh PhD(Med) FCS(SA)
Professor and Head of Department of
  Surgery
University of the Witwatersrand
7 York Road
Parktown
Johannesburg 2193, South Africa

S.T.R. MACSWEENEY, MA MChir FRCS
Consultant Vascular and Endovascular
  Surgery
University Hospital
Queen's Medical Centre
Nottingham NG7 2UH, UK

C.N. McCOLLUM, MD FRCS
Professor of Surgery
Department of Surgery
University Hospital of South Manchester
Nell Lane
West Didsbury
Manchester M20 8LR, UK

C.L. McGUINNESS, FRCS
Lecturer in Surgery
Surgical Unit
St Thomas' Hospital UMDS
Lambeth Palace Road
London SE1 7EH, UK

J.A. MANNICK, MD
Moseley Distinguished Professor of Surgery
Harvard Medical School
Surgeon-in-Chief, Emeritus
Brigham and Women's Hospital
75 Francis Street
Boston MA 02115, USA

A.O. MANSFIELD, ChM FRCS
Professor of Surgery
Imperial College of Science, Technology
  and Medicine School of Medicine
St Mary's Hospital NHS Trust
Praed Street, Paddington
London W2 1NY, UK

M.L. MARIN, MD
Associate Professor of Surgery
Division of Vascular Surgery
Department of Surgery
Montefiore Medical Center
The University Hospital for the Albert
  Einstein College of Medicine
111 East 210th Street
New York, NY 10467, USA

A. MAURIELLO, MD
Department of Pathology
University of Rome 'Tor Vergata'
Rome, Italy

M. MIRESKANDARI, MD MB ChB
Research Fellow
Regional Vascular Unit
Imperial College of Science, Technology
   and Medicine School of Medicine
St Mary's Hospital NHS Trust
Praed Street
Paddington, London, W2 1NY, UK

H.O. MYHRE, MD PhD
Professor of Surgery
Department of Surgery
University Hospital of Trondheim
7006 Trondheim
Norway

L. NORGREN, MD PhD
Professor of Vascular Surgery
Department of Surgery
Lund University Hospital
S-221 85 Lund
Sweden

T. OHKI, MD
Director of Vascular Research Laboratory
Division of Vascular Surgery
Montefiore Medical Center
The University Hospital for the Albert
   Einstein College of Medicine
111 East 210th Street
New York, NY 10467, USA

R.E. PARSONS, MD
Assistant Professor of Surgery
Division of Vascular Surgery
Department of Surgery
Mount Sinai Medical Center
The University Hospital of the Mount Sinai
   College of Medicine
New York, NY, USA

A.M. PETERS, MD FRCR
Department of Imaging
Royal Postgraduate Medical School
Hammersmith Hospital
Du Cane Road
London W12 0NN, UK

M. PILLNY, MD
Fellow in Vascular Surgery
Department of Vascular Surgery and
   Kidney Transplantation
Heinrich-Heine University
Moorenstrasse 5
D-4000 Dusseldorf
Germany

A. PLATTS, FRCS FRCR
Consultant Radiologist
Department of Radiology
Royal Free Hospital
The Royal Free Hampstead NHS Trust
Pond Street
London NW3 2QG, UK

J.T. POWELL, MD PhD
Professor of Vascular Biology
Department of Surgery
Charing Cross and Westminster Medical
   School
Fulham Palace Road
London W6 8RF, UK

J.W. QUARMBY, FRCS
Lecturer in Surgery
Surgical Unit
St Thomas' Hospital UMDS
Lambeth Palace Road
London SE1 7EH, UK

R. RITTER, MD
Fellow in Vascular Surgery
Department of Vascular Surgery and
   Kidney Transplantation
Heinrich-Heine University
Moorenstrasse 5
D-4000 Dusseldorf
Germany

J.R. ROCHESTER, MD FRCS BM
Senior Registrar
Sheffield Vascular Institute
Northern General Hospital
Herries Road
Sheffield S5 7AU, UK

M.L. ROSE, BSC PhD
Reader in Transplant Immunology
Division of Cardiac Surgery
Imperial College of Medicine & National
   Heart and Lung Institute
Heart Science Centre
Harefield Hospital
Harefield
Middlesex UB9 6JH, UK

W.W. ROSE III, MD MPH
Vascular Surgery Research Fellow
Division of Vascular Surgery
Henry Ford Hospital
Detroit, Michigan, USA

C.V. RUCKLEY, ChM FRCSEd
Professor of Vascular Surgery
Vascular Surgery Unit
University Department of Surgery
Royal Infirmary
Edinburgh EH3 9YW, UK

O.D. SAETHER, MD
Consultant Vascular Surgeon
Department of Surgery
University Hospital of Trondheim
7006 Trondheim
Norway

W. SANDMANN, MD
Professor and Chairman
Department of Surgery;
Director, Department of Vascular Surgery
    and Kidney Transplantation
Heinrich-Heine University
Moorenstrasse 5
D-4000 Dusseldorf
Germany

E. SBARIGIA, MD
Department of Vascular Surgery
University of Rome 'La Sapienza'
Policlinico Umberto I
00161 Rome
Italy

C.V. SOONG, MD FRCSI
Senior Registrar in Surgery
Royal Victoria Hospital
The Royal Group of Hospitals
Health and Social Services Trust
Grosvenor Road
Belfast BT12 6BA
Northern Ireland

F. SPEZIALE MD
Department of Vascular Surgery
University of Rome 'La Sapienza'
Policlinico Umberto I
00161 Rome
Italy

A. STELLA, MD
Associate Professor of Vascular Surgery
University of Bologna
Policlinico S Orsola
Via Massarenti 9
40138 Bologna
Italy

P. SWARTBOL, MD PhD
Department of Surgery
Lund University Hospital
S-221 85 Lund
Sweden

J. SWEDENBORG, MD PhD
Head, Division of Vascular Surgery
Karolinska Hospital
S-171 76 Stockholm
Sweden

M. TAURINO, MD
Department of Vascular Surgery
University of Rome 'La Sapienza'
Policlinico Umberto I
00161 Rome, Italy

W.G. TENNANT, BSc MD FRCSEd(Gen)
Consultant Surgeon
Department of Vascular and Endovascular
    Surgery
University Hospital
Queen's Medical Centre
Nottingham NG7 2UH, UK

J.E. THOMPSON, MD
Clinical Professor of Surgery
University of Texas Southwestern Medical
    Center at Dallas;
Former Chief of Surgery and Vascular Surgery
Baylor University Medical Center
Dallas, Texas, USA

S. TÖRNGREN, MD
Department of Surgery
South Hospital
Stockholm, Sweden

J. B. TOWNE, MD
Professor of Surgery
Department of Vascular Surgery
Medical College of Wisconsin
9200 West Wisconsin Avenue
Milwaukee, WI 53226, USA

F.J. VEITH, MD
Professor and Chief, Vascular Surgical
  Service
Montefiore Medical Center
The University Hospital for the Albert
  Einstein College of Medicine
111 East 210th Street
New York, NY 10467, USA

J. WESCHE, MD PhD
Senior Registrar
Department of Surgery
University Hospital of Trondheim
7006 Trondheim
Norway

A.D. WHITTEMORE, MD
Professor of Surgery
Harvard Medical School;
Chief, Vascular Surgery
Brigham and Women's Hospital
75 Francis Street
Boston MA 02115
USA

J.H.N. WOLFE, MS FRCS
Consultant Surgeon
Regional Vascular Unit
Imperial College of Science, Technology
  and Medicine School of Medicine
St Mary's Hospital NHS Trust
Praed Street, Paddington
London W2 1NY, UK

Preface

In health and youth, endothelium lines the entire cardiovascular system, providing a non-thrombogenic boundary of selective permeability between the flowing blood and structural elements of the blood vessel and extravascular space. When the endothelium is damaged or activated the anti-thrombotic properties are attenuated and the activated endothelium becomes the site for recruitment of inflammatory cells into the vessel wall. In turn, the behaviour of these inflammatory cells in the vessel wall depends on their interaction with resident cells and plasma components which permeate the endothelium. This provides a focus for complex interactions generating cytokines which fuel the inflammatory process and, depending on the precise circumstances, provoke atherosclerosis, intimal hyperplasia or an inflammatory vasculitis. Dissection and understanding of these complex inflammatory reactions in the vessel wall provides the prospect of generating new reagents with which to treat vascular disease. Currently the best examples come from outside vascular surgery. The recognition that tumour necrosis factor was the key inflammatory cytokine in rheumatoid arthritis preceded the successful use of monoclonal antibodies to this cytokine to treat refractory rheumatoid arthritis. Similarly interleukin 10, an anti-inflammatory cytokine is in clinical trials to treat Crohn's disease.

Whilst inflammation of the vessel wall is intrinsic to the symptomatic vascular lesions delineated by radiologists and vascular technologists, thrombosis often is the cause of the acute vascular emergency. The inadequate treatment of venous thrombosis can result in an inflammatory response which underlies many of the chronic venous problems seen by vascular surgeons. For these reasons it is particularly important that we understand the inflammatory and thrombotic causes of vascular disease and harness the rapid advances in biology to advances in imaging and patient management. For instance the recognition of the role of selectins in leukocyte adhesion to endothelium has pointed the way to new sensitive and specific methods of imaging inflammation (see pp. 31 to 42). Understanding the properties and kinetics of low molecular weight heparin has opened possibilities for the ambulant, outpatient treatment of deep venous thrombosis (see pp. 357 to 372). As new minimally invasive treatments are developed, including endovascular stenting, it is important to remember that these may induce unwanted inflammatory responses at the vessel wall. The surgical treatment of vasculitis or inflammatory aneurysms is technically demanding and disease recurrence frustrating. Surgery after patients have been treated with corticosteroids provides new problems and the development of more selective anti-inflammatory treatments before the resection of inflammatory aortic aneurysms is needed urgently (see pp. 57 to 76).

Vascular surgeons are accustomed to seeing inflammation and thrombosis. Frequently when they see one, it is accompanied by the other. If a vessel is inflamed, the chances are that the blood in the lumen tends to thrombose, If, on the other hand the lumen has a thrombus within it, then inflammatory reaction in the vessel wall around the thrombus often occurs. Determining which is *the chicken* and which is *the egg* is quite taxing. The time has certainly come for the vascular biologist and vascular surgeon to work together to attempt to unravel the mechanisms of the disease process for the better management of our patients.

R.M. Greenhalgh   *J.T. Powell*

INTRODUCTION

The Cytokine Response to Operative and Accidental Trauma

John A. Mannick

Surgeons have believed for some time that serious injury, including operative trauma, can leave the patient more susceptible to infection and that infection in turn may be associated with mortality in such patients.[1] The hypothesis that serious injury leads paradoxically to decreased resistance to infection has now been established as fact by investigation of injured patients and relevant animal models. It is apparent that injured patients are often victims of the so-called 'two-hit' phenomenon[2] in that the initial injury (first hit) which does not in itself prove fatal, leaves the patient vulnerable to fatal sepsis following an infectious challenge (second hit) which would be easily overcome by a normal individual.[2,3]

Now that this phenomenon has been well described, a number of laboratories have turned their attention to the mechanisms underlying the susceptibility to sepsis after injury. Recent experimental evidence has shown that the septic syndrome can occur in the absence of detectable invasive infection and that this syndrome reflects a leakage into the systemic circulation of mediators ordinarily confined to the site of injury.[4,5] These include the pro-inflammatory cytokines, interleukin-1β (IL-1β), interleukin-6 (IL-6) and tumour necrosis factor alpha (TNF-α) along with a variety of eicosanoids and the products of complement activation. Possible triggers for this systemic inflammatory response include endotoxin leaked from the gut into the portal and systemic circulation or produced by bacteria translocated from the gut, a phenomenon well described in animal models of injury,[6] or circulating anaphyla-toxins from the activation of complement by injured tissue.[7]

Much investigative attention has been focused recently on increased pro-inflammatory cytokine production after injury and on possible methods of control-ling this phenomenon. Less attention has been paid to abnormalities of lymphocyte function long noted to accompany serious injury and the septic syndrome. These abnormalities include diminished antibody production to protein antigens, lack of delayed hypersensitivity response, and depression of T lymphocyte activation by antigens and mitogens.[8–10]

Our laboratory began investigating this problem 18 years ago by studying 31 patients undergoing abdominal aortic aneurysm repair or coronary artery bypass grafting and compared them with 15 patients of similar age and sex undergoing more minor surgical procedures under general anaesthesia.[11] All patients were skin tested 2 days prior to surgery for delayed hypersensitivity reactions to four recall antigens. The skin tests were repeated on the 3rd, 7th, and 28th postoperative days. As shown in Table 1, 13 of the 21 patients undergoing major cardiovascular surgery who had previously been reactive became anergic to the skin test antigens in the postoperative period. None of the patients undergoing more minor surgical procedures became anergic. All anergic patients became reactive again by the 28th postoperative day. It

Table 1.   Induction of anergy by major cardiovascular curgery

Surgery	Skin test positive	Skin test negative	Total
Minor	15	0	15
Major	18	13	31

was thus apparent that major cardiovascular surgery could induce a loss of delayed hypersensitivity responsiveness previously reported in patients suffering from advanced cancer, chronic nutritional depletion and severe traumatic injury.

Since delayed hypersensitivity is a T lymphocyte-driven phenomenon, our laboratory began to investigate the relationship between anergy and T lymphocyte function in injured patients. In a series of patients with serious burn injury we were able to demonstrate a close correlation between loss of delayed hypersensitivity and the ability of circulating lymphocytes to respond to a T lymphocyte mitogen, phytohaemagglutinin (PHA).[9] In studying a further series of patients with serious burn injury (>30% body surface area) and comparing them with normal individuals and with a group of patients with lesser burns we were able to show that loss of mitogen responsiveness of circulating T lymphocytes was associated with failure of production of the cytokine interleukin-2 (IL-2) by the same cell population from the major burn patients compared with similar cells from simultaneously studied normal control individuals.[12] As evident in Fig. 1, patients with lesser burns had a far less

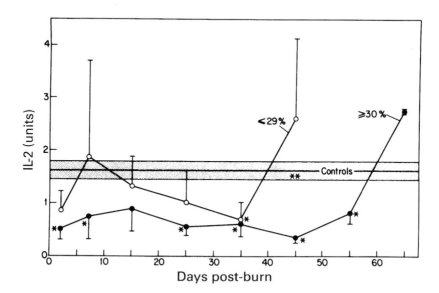

Fig. 1.   Mitogen-stimulated IL-2 production by PBMC from patients with large (>30%) and smaller (<29%) burns. It is apparent that in the larger burns IL-2 production was significantly depressed below the normal levels for a protracted period of time whereas IL-2 production by PBMC from patients with lesser burns was frequently not significantly different from normal. (Reprinted with the permission of the Editors of *Surgery*.)

serious defect in IL-2 production. It also appeared from this study that an impairment of IL-2 synthesis was correlated roughly with the occurrence of serious septic complications in the more seriously burned patient population. This is perhaps not surprising since the chief source of IL-2 is the T helper (Th) lymphocyte which orchestrates the adaptive immune response and therefore dysfunction of this cell type might be expected to have adverse consequences for the host.

Using an animal model of burn injury, we were able to show that the defect in IL-2 production after serious injury is at the level of messenger RNA expression (Fig. 2) and by applying transcription rate analysis ('nuclear run on') we found that the diminished messenger RNA expression results from decreased IL-2 gene transcription.[13,14] Using the same animal burn model we were able to show that serious injury was followed by a progressive increase in mortality from an infectious challenge administered by caecal ligation and puncture (CLP) reaching a peak (Fig. 3) at about 10 days following injury and declining thereafter to levels seen in control

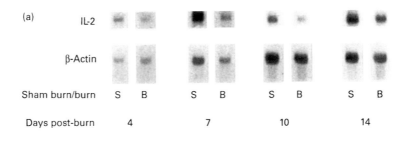

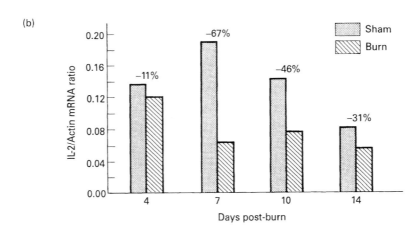

Fig. 2. (a) Northern blots of IL-2 messenger RNA expression in splenocytes from sham burn and burn mice at serial intervals following injury; β-actin message is also displayed as a control. It is apparent that IL-2 message was significantly decreased in burn splenocytes at days 7 and 10 after injury. (b) The depression of IL-2 mRNA expression by burn mouse splenocytes is confirmed by analysis of IL-2 to β-actin mRNA ratio as determined by laser densitometry. (Reprinted with the permission of the Editors of *Surgery*.)

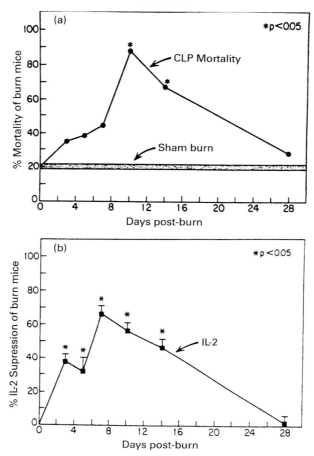

Fig. 3. (a) Mortality from caecal ligation and puncture performed in burn mice at serial intervals after burn injury. It is apparent that the mortality peaks at approximately 10 days following burn injury and thereafter returns slowly towards that seen in sham burn mice. (b) Percent suppression of IL-2 production by splenocytes from burn mice determined at serial intervals after injury. It is apparent that the maximum suppression of mitogen-stimulated IL-2 production occurs at approximately day 8 after burn injury and thereafter declines reaching normal levels by day 28. (Reprinted with the permission of the Editors of *Surgery*.)

animals by 3–4 weeks after injury.[3] This peak in mortality from CLP followed by only a day or two the nadir in IL-2 production in the same animals (Fig. 3). We and others were also able to show in experimental animals that treatment regimens designed to increase Th lymphocyte function including administration of cyclooxygenase inhibitors, to block the synthesis of inhibitory prostaglandins, and the systemic administration of IL-2 itself would lower the mortality from infectious challenge after injury[15-17] thus suggesting but not proving that Th lymphocyte dysfunction might play a role in lowered resistance to invading organisms following serious injury, both accidental and surgical.

It has become increasingly evident over the past 5 years that Th cells in animals can be converted by exposure to certain cytokines and antigens to one or two mature phenotypes.[18,19] T helper 1 (Th1) cells produce IL-2, interferon-γ (IFN-γ) and TNF-β and are principally responsible for cellular immune responses and activation of monocytes and macrophages. These cells also stimulate B cells to form complement fixing antibodies. T helper 2 (Th2) cells secrete IL-4, IL-5, IL-10 and IL-13, stimulate B cells to produce IgE and IgG1 antibodies and inhibit macrophage activation. In addition, Th2-like cells and the cytokines they produce are associated with and contribute to immune tolerance and suppression. It was at first believed that Th1 and Th2 polarization did not take place in man but Romagnani[20] and others have shown that under appropriate conditions it does occur clinically. Conversion to the production of Th2 cytokines has been shown to be inimical to the host in such human diseases as tuberculosis, leichmaniasis and leprosy.[21,22] Certainly the Th1–Th2 paradigm is a useful framework in which to consider alterations in cytokine production but because of uncertainty about the cells producing the cytokines in question many investigators preferentially refer to type 1 or type 2 cytokines rather than Th1 or Th2 cells when discussing this issue.

More recent evidence from our laboratory and others[23-27] suggests that there is increased production of the type 2 cytokines, IL-4 and IL-10 by circulating peripheral blood mononuclear cells (PBMC) in humans and by splenocytes in experimental animals after serious injury. These findings imply that there is not a generalized suppression of Th cytokine production or function after injury as had been previously supposed but a conversion from the production of predominantly type 1 cytokines, as seen in simultaneously studied normal controls, to production of predominantly type 2 cytokines. The cells responsible for the production of the type 2 cytokines have not been clearly identified and the reason for this shift in cytokine production is unknown.

However, studies of a series of patients following traumatic or thermal injury[23] have shown that in the first 2 weeks following injury there is increased production of IL-4 by PBMC along with diminished production of IFN-γ and IL-2 by the same cell populations (Fig. 4). In the animal burn model, we have also shown that at the time of maximal mortality from infectious challenge by CLP there is also diminished production of IFN-γ and IL-2 and increased production of IL-4 and IL-10 by the splenocytes from the injured animals (Fig. 5). The mechanisms underlying the altered T lymphocyte cytokine production following operative or traumatic injury are incompletely understood. One possible trigger for this phenomenon is prostaglandin E2 (PGE2) which has been repeatedly shown to be produced in increased quantities by cells of the monocyte/macrophage lineage following serious injury;[27] PGE2 is markedly inhibitory of IL-2 and IFN-γ production but does not inhibit IL-4 and IL-5 production.[28] Moreover, glucocorticoids which are often found in increased concentration in the plasma early after injury, are reportedly inhibitory of IL-2 production but stimulatory of IL-4 production.[29] Unfortunately, blocking PGE2 production by administration of cyclooxygenase inhibitors beginning early after injury has usually not induced a significant restoration of resistance to infection in animal models.[17] We have also been unable to correlate circulating corticosteroid

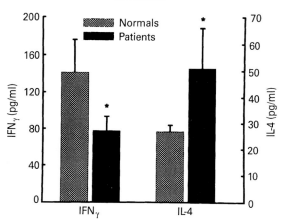

Fig 4. Mitogen stimulated IFN-γ and IL-4 production by PBMC from a series of burn and trauma patients and simultaneously studied age and sex matched normal controls. It is apparent that the patients' PBMC produced less IFN-γ and more IL-4 than PBMC from the normal individuals. (Reprinted with the permission of the Editors of *Annals of Surgery.*)

levels with abnormalities of cytokine production. Thus the explanation for the phenomena observed may very well prove to be a combination of factors including other cytokines for example, transforming growth factor β, which is strongly inhibitory of T lymphocyte activation.

It remains arguable whether or not increased type 2 cytokine production is beneficial or harmful after injury. In order to attempt to answer this question by an *in vivo* study, we used the animal burn model to determine the effect of interleukin-12 (IL-12) on survival of injured animals subjected to an infectious challenge (CLP) on day 10 after injury at the time of demonstrated maximal mortality in this system. The IL-12 therapy was chosen because this cytokine directs naive Th cells along the pathway to the Th1 phenotype.[21] As shown in Fig. 6, the administration of small dosages (25ng) of IL-12 to mice on days 3-7 following injury reduced the mortality from CLP performed on day 10 after injury to that of simultaneously studied uninjured control animals.[30] Saline-treated burn animals had the expected high mortality from CLP on day 10. Analysis of cytokine production by splenocytes of the three groups of animals showed that IL-12 treatment switched off IL-4 production by Th (CD4 enriched) cells in the spleens of injured animals and increased IFN-γ production.

These results suggest that lowering the production of type 2 cytokines after serious injury and/or increasing type 1 cytokine production may have beneficial effects for the injured host. Whether or not these initial findings will be in the future applicable to patients who have been subjected to serious accidental or operative trauma is unclear at present. Decisions as to clinical trials must await further animal experimentation and proof that the therapy is not harmful if administered after the onset of sepsis.

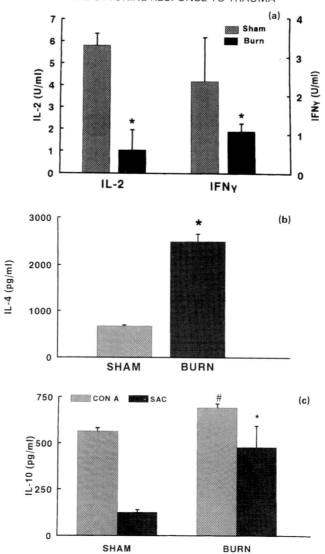

Fig. 5. (a) Mitogen stimulated IL-2 and IFN-γ production by splenocytes from burn and sham burn mice harvested on day 10 after injury. It is apparent that production of both IL-2 and IFN-γ was diminished by burn mouse splenocytes. (b) IL-4 production by burn and sham burn mouse splenocytes. It is apparent that the burn mouse splenocytes produced considerably more IL-4 than sham burn splenocytes at the 10-day interval. (c) IL-10 production by burn and sham burn splenocytes. It is apparent that burn splenocytes produce significantly more IL-10 than sham burn splenocytes at the 10-day interval when stimulated by both concanavalin-A and by bacteria (staphylococcus Cowan's strain A). (Reprinted with the permission of the Editors of *Annals of Surgery*.)

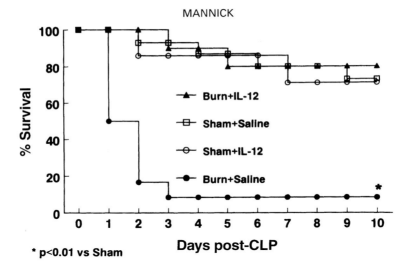

Fig. 6. Survival of burn and sham burn mice challenged with caecal ligation and puncture on day 10 after injury. It is apparent that IL-12 therapy restored the survival of burn mice to that of sham burn controls. IL-12 administered to sham burn mice had no apparent effect on survival. (Reprinted with the permission of the Editors of *Surgery*.)

REFERENCES

1. Baker CC, Oppenheimer L, Stephens B *et al*.: Epidemiology of trauma deaths. *Am J Surg* **140**: 144–150, 1980
2. Deitch EA: Multiple organ failure, pathophysiology and potential future therapy. *Ann Surg* **216**: 117–134, 1992
3. Moss NM, Gough DB, Jordan AL, *et al*.: Temporal correlation of impaired immune response after thermal injury with susceptibility to infection in a murine model. *Surgery* **104**: 882–887, 1988
4. Bone RC. Towards an epidemiology and natural history of SIRS (systemic inflammatory response syndrome). *J Am Med Assoc* **268**: 3452–3455, 1992
5. Goris RJA, teBoekhorst TPA, Nuytinck JKS, Gimbrere JSF: Multiple organ failure: Generalized autodestructive inflammation? *Arch Surg* **120**: 1109–1115, 1985
6. Maejima K, Deitch EA, Berg R: Promotion by burn stress of the translocation of bacteria from the gastrointestinal tracts of mice. *Arch Surg* **119**: 166–172, 1984
7. Davis CF, Moore FD Jr, Rodrick ML *et al*.: Neutrophil activation after burn injury: Contributions of the classic complement pathway and of endotoxin. *Surgery* **102**: 477–484, 1987
8. Wood JJ, O'Mahony JB, Rodrick ML *et al*.: Abnormalities of antibody production following thermal injury: An association with reduced interleukin 2 production. *Arch Surg* **121**: 1089–1115, 1986
9. Wolfe JHN, Wu AVO, O'Connor NE *et al*.: Anergy, immunosuppressive serum, and impaired lymphocyte blastogenesis in burn patients. *Arch Surg* **117**: 1266–1271, 1982
10. Antonacci AC, Calvano SE, Reaves LE *et al*.: Autologous and allogeneic mixed-lymphocyte responses following thermal injury in man: the immunomodulatory effects of interleukin-1, interleukin-2 and prostaglandin inhibitor, WY-18252. *Clin Immunol Immunopathol* **30**: 304–320, 1984

11. McLoughlin GA, Wu AV, Saporoschetz I, Nimberg R, Mannick JA: Correlation between anergy and a circulating immunosuppressive factor following major surgical trauma. *Ann Surg* **190**: 297–304, 1979
12. Wood JJ, Rodrick ML, O'Mahoney JB *et al.*: Inadequate interleukin 2 production: a fundamental immunologic deficiency in patients with major burns. *Ann Surg* **200**: 311–320, 1984
13. O'Riordain DDS, Mendez MV, O'Riordain MG *et al.*: Molecular mechanisms of decreased interleukin-2 production after thermal injury. *Surgery* **114**: 407–415, 1993
14. Horgan AF, Mendez MV, O'Riordain DS *et al.*: Altered gene transcription after burn injury results in depressed T lymphocyte activation. *Ann Surg* **220**: 342–352, 1994
15. Zapata-Sirvent RL, Hansbrough HF, Bender EM *et al.*: Postburn immunosuppression in an animal model. IV. Improved resistance to septic challenge with immunomodulating drugs. *Surgery* **99**: 53–58, 1986
16. Faist E, Ertel W, Cohnert. T. *et al.*: Immunoprotective effects of cyclooxygenase inhibition in patients with major surgical trauma. *J Trauma* **30**: 8–17, 1990
17. Horgan PG, Mannick JA, Dubravec DB, Rodrick ML: Effect of low dose recombinant interleukin-2 plus indomethacin on mortality after sepsis in a murine burn model. *Br J Surg* **77**: 401–404, 1990
18. Cherwinski HM, Schumacher JH, Brown KD, Mosmann TR: Two types of mouse helper T cell clone. III. Further differences in lymphokine synthesis between Th1 and Th2 clones revealed by RNA hybridization, functionally monospecific bioassays, and monoclonal antibodies. *J Exp Med* **166**: 1229–1244, 1987
19. Stevens TL, Bossie A, Sanders VM *et al.*: Regulation of antibody isotype secretion by subsets of antigen-specific helper T cells. *Nature* **334**: 255–258, 1988
20. Romagnani S: Lymphokine production by human T cells in disease states. *Ann Rev Immunol* **12**: 227–257, 1994
21. Trinchieri G: Interleukin-12 and its role in the generation of Th1 cells. *Immunol Today* **14**: 335–337, 1993
22. Sielin, PA, Wang X-H, Gately MK, Oliveros JL: IL-12 regulates T helper type 1 cytokine responses in human infectious disease. *J Immunol* 3639–3647, 1994
23. O'Sullivan ST, Lederer JA, Horgan AF: Major injury leads to predominance of the T helper-2 lymphocyte phenotype and diminished interleukin-12 production associated with decreased resistance to infection. *Ann Surg* **222**: 482–492, 1995
24. Ayala A, Lehman DL, Herdon CD, Chaudry IH: Mechanism of enhanced susceptibility to sepsis following hemorrhage. *Arch Surg* **129**: 1172–1178, 1994
25. DiPiro JT, Howdieshell TR, Goddard JK *et al.*: Association of interleukin-4 plasma levels with traumatic injury and clinical course. *Arch Surg* **130**: 1159–1163, 1995
26. Decker D, Schondorf M, Bidlingmaier F *et al.*: Surgical stress induces a shift in the type-1/type-2 T-helper cell balance, suggesting down- regulation of cell-mediated and up-regulation of antibody-mediated immunity commensurate to the trauma. *Surgery* **119**: 316–325, 1996
27. Grbic JT, Mannick JA, Gough DB, Rodrick ML: The role of prostaglandin E2 in immune suppression following injury. *Ann Surg* **214**: 253–263, 1991
28. Katamura K, Shintaku N, Yamauchi Y *et al.*: Prostaglandin E2 at priming of naive CD4+ T cells inhibit acquisition of ability to produce IFN-γ and IL-2, but not IL-4 and IL-5. *J Immunol* **155**: 4604–4612, 1995
29. Daynes RA, Araneo BA: Contrasting effects of glucocorticoids on the capacity of T cells to produce the growth factors interleukin 2 and interleukin 4. *Eur J Immunol* **19**: 2319–2325, 1989
30. O'Suilleabhain C, O'Sullivan ST, Kelly JL *et al.*: Interleukin-12 treatment restores normal resistance to bacterial challenge after burn injury. *Surgery* **120**: 290–296, 1996

Immune Responses to Endothelium Following Transplantation

Marlene L. Rose

INTRODUCTION

Approximately 36 000 transplants are performed throughout the world each year, of which the majority are kidney transplants. About 5000 hearts, 6500 livers and 1200 lung transplants are performed. Rejection remains the most common complication following transplantation and is the major source of morbidity and mortality. Endothelial cells forming the interface between donor and recipient are the first donor cells to be recognized by the host's immune system; this fact plus the observation that they express numerous molecules able to stimulate lymphocytes has stimulated much research into their precise role in transplant rejection. It is our view that endothelial cells are pivotal both in controlling the egress of inflammatory cells into the allografted organ but also as specific antigen presenting cells (APC), by presenting foreign molecules to the immune system (Fig. 1).

Rejection is mediated by both cell mediated and humoral mechanisms but the relative importance of these pathways differs in acute and chronic rejection. The aim of this chapter is to briefly describe the features of acute and chronic rejection and then to outline the role of endothelial cells in this process.

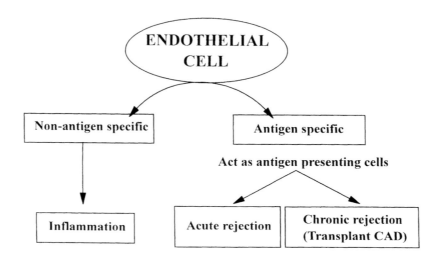

Fig. 1. Diagram to illustrate role of endothelial cells in transplant rejection. From ref. 29, with permission.

BASIC MECHANISM OF REJECTION

The major stimulus for rejection of allografted organs is recognition of foreign antigens coded by the major histocompatibilty complex (MHC). Class I (human leucocyte antigen: HLA-ABC) and Class II (HLA-DR, DP, DQ) antigens are highly polymorphic glycoproteins encoded by the MHC locus found on chromosome 6 in humans. The frequency of resting T cells which recognize foreign MHC molecules is very large (estimated at an astounding 0.1–1% of circulating T cells) – a fact which almost certainly accounts for the vigour of the anti-allograft response.

Rejection is initiated by the CD4+ T cell subset recognizing MHC class II antigens on APC within the graft (Fig. 2). Recognition of foreign MHC molecules results in CD4+ T cell activation and release of cytokines (IL-2, IL-4, IL-5, IL-6, IFN-γ, TNF-α, TNF-β) (IL: interleukin; TNF: tumour necrosis factor; IFN: interferon) which allow maturation of the effector mechanisms of rejection, namely maturation of CD8 + cytotoxic T cells, infiltration of macrophages, maturation of natural killer (NK) cells and lymphokine activated killer (LAK) cells and antibody formation (Fig. 2). These effector mechanisms have been listed for the sake of completeness, there is little evidence that NK or LAK cells are important in allograft rejection. Indeed, the precise mediators which cause graft dysfunction are unknown; although CD8+ cytotoxic T cells can cause graft destruction they are not essential for rejection, it is quite possible

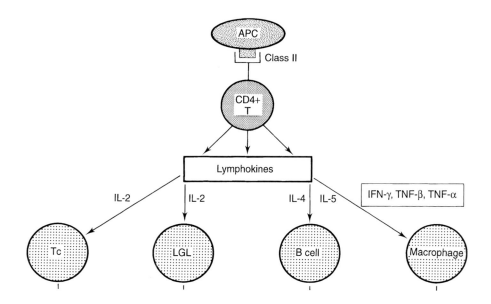

Fig. 2. Diagrammatic representation of T cell activation, illustrating the pivotal role of MHC class II antigens (presented by APC (antigen presenting cells) within the graft) in initiating rejection. Activation of CD4+ T cells results in a cascade of lymphokines causing the maturation of a number of possible effector mechanisms (in double lined boxes). Note that the cytokines IFN-γ, TNF-β and TNF-α may be directly damaging to tissues. From ref. 29, with permission.

that a direct effect of cytokines , in particular TNF-α and IFN-γ may be toxic to allografted cells. For example, TNF-α has a negative inotropic effect on cardiac myocytes. Similarly, induction of inducible nitric oxide synthase by activated macrophages may be an important effector mechanism.

Activation of CD4+ T cells is thus pivotal in initiating acute rejection (Fig. 2). In view of the fact that CD4+ T cells are activated by foreign MHC class II molecules, understanding the quantitative and qualitative distribution of these molecules on the allografted organ is of considerable importance. The advent of monoclonal anti-bodies, use of frozen sections and advances in immunocytochemical techniques have revolutionized knowledge about the normal distribution of MHC molecules in different tissues. Class II (HLA-DR and DP) antigens, originally thought to be restricted to macrophages, dendritic cells, monocytes and activated T cells have now been described on human endothelial cells and epithelial cells (reviewed in ref. 1). The expression of class II on human endothelial cells has been described in every organ[1] and it is particular striking on the microvessels i.e. capillaries , arterioles and venules. The large vessel endothelium (such as aorta, pulmonary artery, saphenous vein) are negative for MHC class II expression.

The expression of MHC antigens is not a constant feature of a cell; they can be upregulated or induced by cytokines.[2] After cardiac transplantation there is massive upregulation of MHC class I antigens (normally only on the interstitial cells) so that cardiac myocytes become MHC class I positive.[1] There is also upregulation of adhesion molecules during acute rejection (and see below).[3,4] The upregulation of these molecules is almost certainly mediated by local production of cytokines by infiltrating cells; thus some cytokines (such as TNF-α and IFN-γ) have been directly visualized in graft biopsies using immunocytochemical methods,[5] others (IL-2, IL-1, IL-4, IL-6, IL-10) have been detected using polymerase chain reaction to amplify cytokine mRNA.[6]

The consequences of T cell activation described above leads to infiltration of the graft with inflammatory cells (T cells and monocytes) – a process termed acute rejection. The majority of patients have one or two acute rejection episodes in the first 6 months following transplantation. Acute rejection may be suspected clinically but it is always confirmed by histological assessment of biopsies.

CHRONIC REJECTION

Chronic rejection, presenting as a rapidly progressing obliterative vascular disease occurring in the transplanted heart, is the major cause of late death and repeat transplantation after cardiac transplantation. This disease is variously termed cardiac allograft vasculopathy or transplant associated coronary artery disease (TxCAD). This same phenomenon is also present in renal, lung and liver allografts and has been designated chronic rejection, obliterative bronchiolitis and vanishing bile duct syndrome respectively. The reported incidence of TxCAD, detected by routine angiography varies greatly between cardiac transplant centres. Incidences of 18% at 1 year progressing to 44% at 3 years have been reported.[7] There are a number of reviews which describe the histological differences between TxCAD and spontaneous CAD and the various risk factors, both immunological and non-immunological have been described.[8] It is interesting that TxCAD is a much more diffuse disease, affecting the entire length of the epicardial vessels; the intimal proliferation is concentric as opposed to the eccentric plaque found in spontaneous CAD. These differences suggest the whole endothelium is the target of damage in TxCAD.

The occurrence of a vasculopathy, affecting the allografted organs, is almost certainly of multifactorial aetiology. It is useful to think of the disease in terms of the Ross hypothesis[9] – namely an initial damage to the endothelium resulting in release of growth factors and intimal proliferation. The latter process will be assisted by risk factors (circulating cholesterol, insulin resistance) common to both spontaneous atherosclerosis and TxCAD. Most investigators would acknowledge that the initial damage to the endothelium is mediated by the alloimmune response, athough it can also be argued that non-immunological damage such as ischaemia, surgical manipulation, and perfusion/reperfusion injury could also initially damage the endothelial cells.[10] Precisely which pathways of antigen presentation are involved, which endothelial antigens are recognized and the relative importance of cell mediated and humoral immunity in this process are unknown (see below for discussion of these topics).

PROPERTIES OF ENDOTHELIAL CELLS

The phenotypic properties of endothelial cells and their response to cytokines gives them a pivotal role in controlling rejection in three distinct ways:

1. they allow extravasation of inflammatory cells into the graft
2. they act as antigen presenting cells
3. they are the target of the alloimmune response.

Adhesion molecules and lymphocyte migration

There is currently extensive research on the role of endothelial adhesion molecules in controlling lymphocyte recirculation and extravasation of inflammatory cells. These processes are controlled by sequential interactions between different families of molecules on the endothelial cells (the selectins, $\beta1$ and $\beta2$ integrins and members of the immunoglobulin family) and their respective ligands on leukocytes. There are many excellent reviews of this subject[11] which is not within the remit of this chapter. Immunocytochemistry of frozen sections of human heart, coronary artery, aorta, pulmonary artery and endocardium have revealed differences with regard to basal expression of these molecules (Table 1). Many studies have demonstrated an upregu-lation of cell adhesion molecules (PECAM-1, ICAM-1, VCAM-1 and E-selectin) and other markers of endothelial cells (vWf) on endothelial cells during rejection,[4,12]

Endothelial cells as antigen presenting cells

Since MHC antigens initiate allograft rejection, it is of interest to describe the distribution of these molecules on endothelial cells of different origins (Table 1). All

Table 1. Distribution of adhesion molecules, MHC molecules and vWf in endothelial cells derived from microvessels and large vessels of the human cardiovascular system

	Myocardial Biopsies			Large vessels		
	capillaries	arterioles	venules	coronary	PA	aorta
CD31	++	++	++	++	++	++
ICAM-1	++	+	+	++	+	+
VCAM-1	neg	+/–	+/–	+	neg	neg
E-selectin	neg	neg	+/-	+	+/–	+/–
vWf	+/–	++	++	++	++	++
Class I	++	+	+	++	+	+
Class II	++	+/–	+/–	++	neg	neg

Summarized from refs 4,12.
++ Strong, even expression; + strong but patchy expression; +/– weak and patchy expression

endothelial cells constitutively express MHC class I molecules and many endothelial cells constitutively express MHC class II molecules (see ref. 1 for review). However, there is an interesting heterogeneity with regard to constitutive expression of class II antigens; the large vessels (aorta, pulmonary artery, endocardium, umbilical vein, umbilical artery) are negative but the capillaries within all organs examined are strongly positive (Table 1).[12,13] It was surprising to find that all pieces of coronary artery we examined expressed MHC class II molecules, as well as VCAM-1.[12] The coronary arteries were either obtained from heart donors deemed unsuitable for transplantation , or they were removed from the explanted heart of patients requiring transplantation (for diseases not involving the coronary artery). These molecules may therefore have been upregulated prior to harvest.

The term antigen presenting cell (APC) has a specific meaning to immunologists: it means the cell is able to present antigen to resting T cells: i.e. is able to cause activation of resting T cells. Only specialized cells (traditionally recognized as B cells, dendritic cells and monocytes) can perform this task. The T cells recognize nominal antigen as processed peptides presented by self-MHC molecules. An important step in the understanding of alloreactivity came with the discovery that T cells can engage and respond to allogeneic MHC molecules directly (Fig. 3). This form of antigen recognition, termed direct presentation or the direct pathway is responsible for the strong proliferative response to alloantigens seen *in vitro* and quite possibly the early acute rejection seen in non-immunosuppressed animals after transplantation of MHC mismatched organs. However, T cells can also recognize allogeneic peptides that have been processed and presented within self-MHC molecules by recipient APC in the same manner that T cells recognize nominal antigen (Fig. 3). This pathway is termed the indirect route or indirect pathway of T cell activation. Alloantigens shed from the graft are likely to be treated as exogenous antigen by recipient APC and will therefore be presented within MHC class II molecules to activate recipient CD4+ T cells.

Any graft cell expressing class II antigens will be able to activate the indirect pathway; it is likely that damaged endothelial cells are an important source of graft-derived MHC class II antigens – since these are the only parenchymal cells expressing class II in the heart. The contribution that the indirect pathway arising from

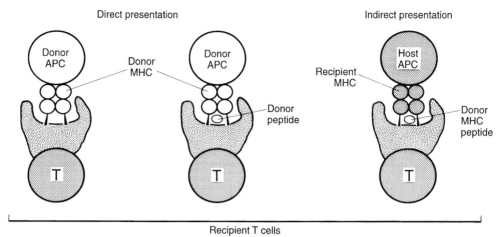

Fig. 3. Diagrammatic representation of mechanisms whereby recipient T cells recognize allo-class II determinants. Recipient T cells recognize donor MHC determinants on donor APC (direct presentation) or they recognize donor MHC peptides which have been released from donor cells and processed and presented by host APC within self-MHC molecules (indirect presentation). Drawing modified from ref. 14, with permission.

recognition of endothelial MHC class II makes to cellular rejection currently is unknown. However, the question which has received much attention of a number of groups in recent years is whether endothelial cells can cause direct allostimulation of resting T lymphocytes (see ref. 15 for review). The reason for this is that direct recognition of allo-MHC molecules results in a 'strong' response, the number of T cells recognizing MHC molecules directly is 10–100 higher than those recognizing nominal antigen, resulting in a strong *in vitro* proliferative response.

In order to discover whether endothelial cells directly cause allostimulation of resting T cells, we and others have cultured stringently purified CD4 + T cells with pure passaged endothelial cells and looked for T cell proliferation (measured by uptake of 3H-thymidine) at day 6.[16,17] The endothelial cells are treated with mitomycin C to stop them proliferating; any proliferation which is detected is thus due to responding T cells (Fig. 4). The results in Fig. 5 show the response of CD4+ T cell to a human endothelial cell line (EAhy.926), porcine aortic endothelial cells (PAEC) and fetal lung fibroblasts. It can be seen that provided IFN-γ is used to upregulate MHC class II, there is a strong proliferative response to human endothelial cells, but not to fibroblasts. There is also a strong response to PAEC, which is independent of IFN-γ treatment. The reason for this is that PAEC class II expression persists in culture. That the response was direct and not indirect was proven by the findings that responder T cells were free of contaminating APC.[17]

It must be concluded therefore that donor endothelial cells can present alloantigen to recipient T cells. It is interesting to note that there is a species difference between rodents and humans, rodents do not constitutively express MHC class II antigens on their endothelial cells. This difference may explain why it is easier to suppress transplant rejection in rodents than it is in humans. It follows , that understanding the signals that allow human endothelial cells to stimulate T cells may lead to new

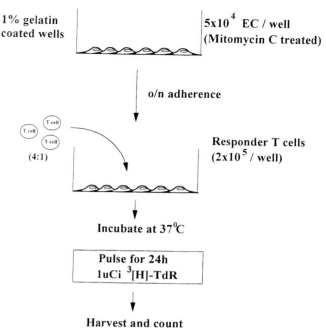

1% gelatin
coated wells

5×10^{4} EC / well
(Mitomycin C treated)

o/n adherence

(4:1)

Responder T cells
$(2 \times 10^{5} /$ well)

Incubate at 37^{0}C

Pulse for 24h
1uCi ^{3}[H]-TdR

Harvest and count

Fig. 4. Mixed endothelial-lymphocyte reaction. Method of measuring the proliferative response of purified CD4+ T cells to human endothelial cells. Addition of mitomycin-C (or irradiated) human endothelial cells to gelatin coated tissue culture wells results in a monolayer of endothelial cells to which can be added appropriate numbers of responder T cells. The endothelial cells and T cells are co-cultured for 6 days, in the presence of ^{3}[H]-thymidine (^{3}[H]-TdR) for the last 24 hours. The cultures are harvested and counted on a β-counter; the counts (cpm) represent the proliferative response of T cells. From ref. 29, with permission.

strategies of preventing rejection. One of the important concepts to emerge in recent years is the knowledge that T cells require two signals to become activated.[18] One signal occupancy of the T cell receptor and the second is activation of one of the many 'accessory molecules' present on T cells (Fig. 6). Much attention has focused on the B7 family of receptors, known to be essential as second signals on APC of bonemarrow origin (e.g., monocytes, B cells and dendritic cells) ; blockade of this pathway inhibits dendritic cell stimulated mixed lymphocyte responses *in vitro* and also inhibits allograft and indeed xenograft rejection in rodents.[19] We have questioned whether endothelial cells utilize the B7 pathway to stimulate T cells, and our results[20] and those of others[15] demonstrate that endothelial cells do not express B7 receptors and stimulate T cells via other accessory molecules.

Role of endothelial cells in chronic rejection

It is paradoxical that despite the heavy immunosuppression received by patients after solid organ transplantation, the majority make a vigorous antibody response against

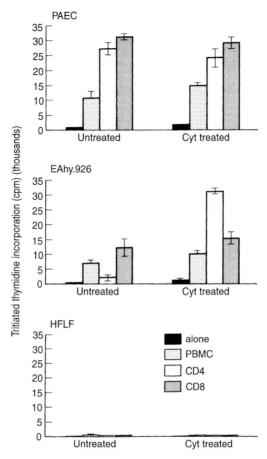

Fig 5. Response of purified peripheral blood mononuclear cells (PBMC) CD4+ and CD8+ T cells to untreated and IFN-γ treated PAEC, human endothelial cells (EAhy.926) and human fetal lung fibroblasts (HFLF). CD4+ and CD8+ T cells respond strongly to PAEC, regardless of cytokine (Cyt) treatment. CD4+ T cells respond well to human endothelial cells, providing they have been pre-treated with IFN-γ to upregulate MHC class II antigens. CD8+ T cells respond to human endothelial cells in the absence of cytokine treatment. There is no proliferative response of human lymphocytes to the fibroblasts. From ref. 29, with permission.

the allografted organ (reviewed in ref. 21). Many clinical studies have reported an association between antibody producers and development of chronic rejection.[21] Thus Suciu-Foca *et al*. reported a 90% 4-year actuarial survival in patients who had not made antibody following cardiac transplantation versus 38% 4-year survival in the antibody producers.[22] These authors looked for anti-HLA antibodies, but our own studies have shown a correlation between anti-endothelial antibodies and chronic rejection.[23] Using gel electrophoresis to separate endothelial peptides according to

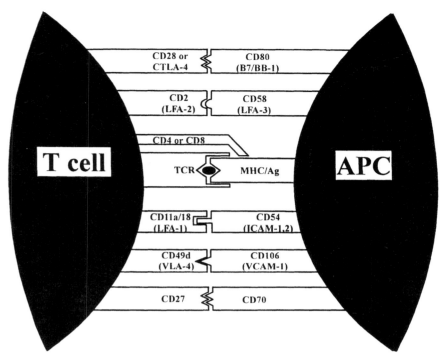

Fig. 6. Diagrammatic representation of possible interactions between receptors on T cells and their appropriate ligands on APC. From ref. 29, with permission.

molecular weight followed by probing blots with patients' sera, we found that the majority of patients with TxCAD had antibodies against endothelial peptides of 56/58kD. We have subsequently confirmed this association in a separate study of new patients using both Western blotting and flow cytometry.[24] A similar association between anti-endothelial antibodies, detected by flow cytometry and chronic rejection has been reported after renal transplantation.[25] Use of sodium dodecyl sulphate (SDS) gel electrophoresis and amino acid sequencing revealed that the most immunogenic endothelial protein (at 56/58kD) was the intermediate filament vimentin and other immunoreactive peptides were identified as triose phosphate isomerase and glucose regulating protein. In all, 40 different proteins were identified which reacted with patients immunoglobulin (IgM).[26] Vimentin is diffusely expressed in the intima and media of normal and diseased coronary arteries. Our working hypothesis is that antibodies to vimentin reflect disease activity in the coronary arteries – but the outstanding questions are how vimentin, a cytosolic protein is exposed to the immune system and whether and how the antibodies are damaging.

One of the major drawbacks to ascribing a role for antibodies in the pathogenesis of graft rejection is lack of understanding about the way antibodies interact with their cellular targets. The serum derived from our patients does not exhibit complement dependent cytotoxicity against endothelial cells derived from human umbilical vein or aorta, nor does it exhibit antibody dependent cellular cytotoxicity. Recent reports have demonstrated that antibodies from patients with autoimmune disease[27] or transplant patients[28] can upregulate adhesion molecules on endothelial cells. We believe the information that antibodies can activate endothelial cells is very promising and should be explored as a mechanism whereby antibodies could damage endothelial cells in both autoimmune disease and chronic rejection after solid organ transplantation.

REFERENCES

1. Rose ML: HLA antigens in tissues. In: Dyer P and Middleton D (Eds) *Methods in Clinical Histocompatibility Testing.* Oxford: IRL/Oxford University Press, 1992
2. Halloran PF, Wadgymar A, Autenreid P: The regulation of the expression of major histocompatibitly complex products. *Transplantation* **4**: 413–420, 1986
3. Briscoe DM, Schoen FJ, Rice GE *et al.:* Induced expression of endothelial-leukocyte adhesion molecules in human cardiac allografts. *Transplantation* **51**: 537–539, 1991
4. Taylor PM, Rose ML. Yacoub M H, Piggott R: Induction of vascular adhesion molecules during rejection of human cardiac allografts. *Transplantation* **54**: 451–457, 1992
5. Arbustini E, Grasso M, Diegoli M *et al.:* Expression of tumour necrosis factor in human acute cardiac rejection. An immunohistochemical and immunoblotting study. *Am J Pathol* **139**: 709–715, 1991
6. Cunningham DA, Dunn MJ, Yacoub MJ, Rose ML: Local production of cytokines in the human cardiac allograft. *Transplantation* **57**: 1333–1337, 1994
7. Gao SJ, Schroeder JS, Alderman EL, Hunt SA *et al.:* Prevalence of accelerated coronary artery disease in heart transplant survivors. Comparison of cyclosporine and azathioprine regimens. *Circulation* **8**: III100–105, 1989
8. Hosenpud JD, Shipley GD, Wagner CR: Cardiac allograft vasculopathy; current concepts, recent developments, and future directions. *J Heart Lung Transplant* **11**: 9–23, 1992
9. Ross R: The pathogeneis of atherosclerosis: a perspective for the 1990s. *Nature* **362**: 801–809, 1993
10. Tullius SG, Tilney NJ: Both alloantigen-dependent and independent factors influence chronic allograft rejection. *Transplantation* **59**: 313–318, 1995
11. Springer TA: Traffic signals for lymphocyte recirculation and leukocyte emigration; The mutistep paradigm. *Cell* **76**: 301–314, 1994
12. Page CS, Rose ML, Yacoub MH, Pigott R: Antigenic heterogeneity of vascular endothelium *Am J Path* **141**: 673–683, 1992
13. Pober JS, Cotran RS: The role of endothelial cells in inflammation. *Transplantation* **50**: 537–544, 1990
14. Shoskes DA, Wood KJ: Indirect presentation of MHC antigens in transplantation. *Immunology Today* **15**: 32–38, 1994
15. Pober JS, Orosz CG, Rose ML, Savage COS: Can graft endothelial cells initiate a host anti-graft immune response? *Transplantation* **61**: 343–349, 1996
16. Page CS, Holloway N, Smith H *et al.:* Alloproliferative responses of purified CD4+ and CD8+ T cell subsets to human vascular endothelial cells in the absence of contaminating accessory cells. *Transplantation* **57**: 1628–1636, 1994
17. Savage COS, Hughes CCW, McIntyre BW *et al.:* Human CD4+ T cells proliferate to HLA-DR + allogeneic vascular endothelium: identification of accessory interactions. *Transplantation* **56**: 128–138, 1993
18. Janeway CA, Bottomly K: Signals and signs for lymphocyte responses. *Cell* **76**: 275–285, 1994
19. Pearson TC, Alexander DZ, Winn KJ *et al.:* Transplantation tolerance induced by CTLA4-Ig. *Transplantation* **57**: 1701–1706, 1994
20. Page CS, Thompson C, Yacoub MH, Rose ML: Human endothelial cell stimulation of allogeneic T cells via a CTLA-4 independent pathway. *Transplant Immunol* **2**: 342–347, 1994

21. Rose ML: Antibody mediated rejection following cardiac transplantation. *Transplantation Rev* **7**: 140–152, 1993
22. Suciu-Foca N, Reed E, Marboe C *et al*.: The role of anti-HLA antibodies in heart transplantation. *Transplantation* **51**: 716–724, 1991
23. Dunn MJ, Crisp SJ, Rose ML *et al*.: Antiendothelial antibodies coronary artery disease after cardiac transplantation. *Lancet* **339**: 1566–70, 1992
24. Ferry BL, Welsh KI, Dunn MJ *et al*.: Anti-cell surface endothelial antiboides in sera from cardiac and kidney transplant recipients: association with chronic rejection. *Transplant Immunol* 1997 *(in press)*
25. Al Hussein KA, Talbot D, Proud G *et al*.: The clinical significance of post-transplantation non-HLA antibodies in renal transplantation. *Transplant Int* **8**: 214–220, 1995
26. Wheeler CH, Collins A, Dunn MJ *et al*.: Characterisation of endothelial antigens associated with transplant associated coronary artery disease. *J Heart Lung Transplantation* **14**: S188–97, 1995
27. Carvalho D, Savage COS, Black CM, Pearson JD: IgG antiendothelial cell autoantibodies from scleroderma patients induce leukocyte adhesion to human vascular endothelial cells *in vitro*. *J Clin Invest* **97**: 1–9, 1996
28. Pidwell DW, Heller MJ, Gabler D, Orosz C: *In vitro* stimulation of human endothelial cells by sera from a subpopulation of high percentage panel reactive antibody patients. *Transplantation* **60**: 563–569, 1995
29. Rose ML: Role of endothelial cells in transplant rejection. In: Poston L, Halliday A, Schachter M, Hunt B (Eds) *An Introduction to Vascular Biology*. Cambridge: Cambridge University Press, 1997 *(in press)*

Chronic Rejection – A Model for Atherosclerosis

P. R. F. Bell and N. Brindle

INTRODUCTION

Inflammation and thrombosis play a major role in a number of aspects of vascular surgery and also are an important part of the changes seen in the arteries following transplantation of organs. The results of transplantation are now excellent but long-term difficulties remain, in that organ function deteriorates gradually, and this decrease has been labelled 'chronic rejection'. Although there is no doubt that there is an element of ongoing inflammatory response due to antigenic differences between host and recipient, in the kidney and heart in particular, the eventual and progressive loss of function relates to changes very similar to those that occur in atherosclerosis with a narrowing of medium-sized blood vessels with their eventual thrombosis and infarction of the tissue they supply or its replacement by fibrosis.[1] This chapter is an attempt to look at the similarities and differences between these two processes, to perhaps gain some ideas on how research into one might help the other.

DEVELOPMENT OF ATHEROSCLEROSIS

This is summarized in Fig. 1. A number of factors cause damage, physical or functional, to the endothelial cell; these include hyperlipidaemia, smoking, hyperglycaemia, which is particularly important in diabetics, hypertension and abnormal shear stress. There are undoubtedly further factors yet to be determined. As with other tissue damage, this is associated with recruitment of inflammatory cells and elevation in local concentrations of inflammatory cytokines. Upregulation of adhesion molecules on the endothelial surface in response to tissue cytokines results in recruitment of mononuclear cells which migrate into the vessel wall and secrete a number of factors including interleukin 1 (IL-1), tumour necrosis factor (TNF), platelet-derived growth factor (PDGF) and insulin-like growth factor 1 (IGF1). The damaged endothelium also secretes basic fibroblast growth factor (bFGF), PDGF and IGF1.[2] All of these together have an effect on the smooth muscle cell and make it grow much more rapidly, producing intimal hyperplasia as the cells migrate towards the endothelium. In addition, the release of (IL-1) and TNF shifts the balance of tissue factor/thrombomodulin and plasminogen activator inhibitor/plasminogen activator production by endothelial cells to a prothrombotic antifibrinolytic phenotype.[3–6] Progression of this process is associated with lipid deposition and a matrix accumulation and the eventual formation of an atherosclerotic plaque.[2] This, as it gets

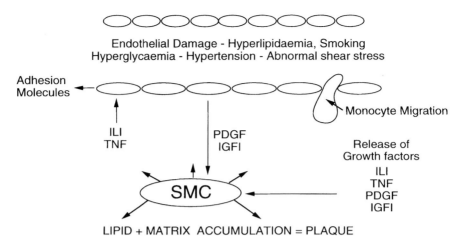

Fig. 1. The development of atherosclerosis.

bigger, ulcerates on the surface of the vessel leading to more thrombosis and eventual occlusion. Atherosclerotic lesions are essentially focal, many vessels are not affected at all and others affected badly. The reasons for this focal distribution of atherosclerosis remain to be determined. It may be that important elements such as abnormal shear stress in various localities lead to the exaggerated response of the endothelium or produce more damage leading to growth factor release and activation of smooth muscle cells. Recent studies have shown the presence of smooth muscle cell class 2 HLA antigens in the human atherosclerotic lesions of a typical variety.[7] Such lesions also contain a surprising number of T cells which suggests a degree of immune activation without an obvious stimulus. In the case of transplantation foreign class 2 antigens of course provide a trigger for the activation of these T cells and the release of a cascade of cytokines and growth factors leading to smooth muscle proliferation.

ARTERIOSCLEROSIS IN TRANSPLANTATION

The surface of most mammalian cells contain histocompatibility antigens, human leukocyte antigens (HLAI) which are normally expressed on the surface of endothelial cells and by peptides derived from foreign proteins allowing mobilization of the immune response in a defensive posture. Presentation of antigens to helper T cells requires another type of HLA, DR or class II, bearing a surface marker known as CD4. Class II antigens are responsible for recognition of class II molecules from another member of the species as foreign or antigenic. This interaction triggers off a sequence of events which leads to rejection of tissues transplanted across a major histocompatibility barrier. Although the expression of class II antigens was formerly thought to be restricted to bone marrow, it is now apparent that blood vessel wall cells can also express both classes of major HLA antigens.[7,8] Vascular endothelium normally expresses class I but exposure to a number of cytokines generated at the site of inflammation, for example interferon, increases the level of these antigens on the surface of the endothelial cells.[9,10] Class II expression is normally limited to venules but interferon is capable of inducing class II expression in arterial endothelial and smooth muscle cells. Another source of inflammatory cytokines is monocytes and other inflammatory cells. These cells adhere to the endothelium which has been activated by TNF or IL-1 and penetrate into the vessel wall. Once inside the vessel wall (Fig. 2) these cells produce a number of cytokines including TNF, IL-1, PDGF, bFGF and IGF. All of these factors in combination then cause stimulation of the smooth muscle cell. Again IL-1 and TNF activate vascular endothelial cells to express prothrombotic antifibrinolytic proteins. Thus locally produced IL-1 and TNF can dramatically alter a number of important functions in the vessel wall. This process is summarized in Fig. 2.

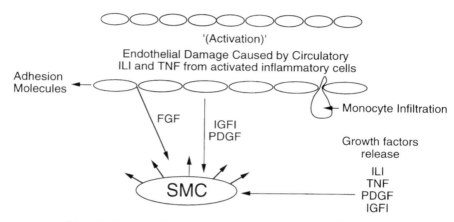

Fig. 2. The development of transplant arteriosclerosis.

In the accelerated atherosclerosis seen in allografts, leukocytes are often present and are a major source of cytokine and growth factors. These cells are also able to secrete, transforming growth factors (TGF) which appear to promote the growth of smooth muscle cells and are likely to enhance extracellular matrix deposition in the newly forming neointima.[11] The continuing presence of a low grade inflammatory response with activated white cells entering the arteries at all levels in an allograft means that the ongoing process shown occurs with the continuous production of cytokines and growth factors, the stimulation of smooth muscle cells leading to a widespread proliferation of these cells with intimal hyperplasia and eventual thrombosis of the vessels concerned as the narrowing becomes critical. An example of the proliferative response in human kidneys is seen in Fig. 3. An excellent model for chronic rejection is the Fischer to Lewis renal transplant model where rejection is mild and chronic changes appear.[12] These changes in the vessel walls, which mirror those seen in human transplants, are shown in Fig. 4. Similarities and differences are seen in atherosclerosis and transplant arterial sclerosis. The big difference between the arterial lesions seen in chronic rejection and those seen in atherosclerosis relates to the extent of the inflammation and the degree of atherosclerosis generated. The

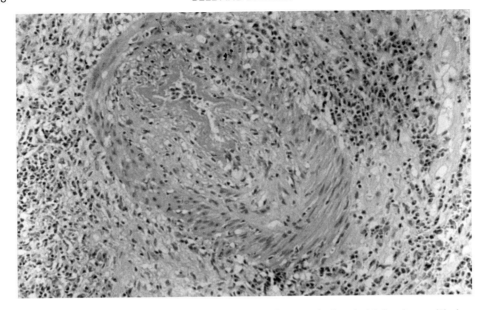

Fig. 3. Chronic rejection in a human kidney. Severe intimal thickening with lumen reduction is present.

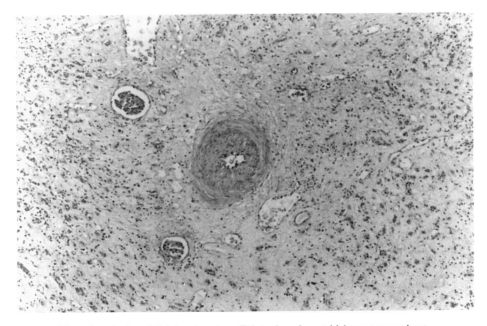

Fig. 4. Intimal thickening in a DA to Lewis rat kidney transplant.

transplant-associated form of arterial damage tends to be concentric and diffuse whereas the disease seen with atherosclerosis tends to be focal.[1] As far as the heart is concerned, the other interesting feature about transplant arterosclerosis is that it appears to be independent of other atherosclerotic risk factors such as smoking, dislipoproteinaemia of family predisposition.[13] Another important feature of transplant-associated arteriosclerosis or chronic rejection is that although the grafted organs are affected the host's own native vessels are usually spared.[1] These lesions are therefore not caused by immunosuppression but result from a continuing injury or immune activation. This could either be the ischaemia produced during harvest and implantation or an immune mechanism could be implicated. Although the latter seems likely the involvement of the immune system in this form of atherosclerosis remains obscure and difficult to be sure of. However, participation of a number of the intrinsic cells of the blood vessel wall, in particular the endothelium and smooth muscle cells undoubtedly involve an inflammatory reaction.

Excessive proliferation of vascular smooth muscle cells appears to contribute decisively to the genesis of transplantation arteriosclerosis. The difference between the two forms of the disease, i.e. transplant-generated and true atherosclerosis, is perhaps not surprising in that the former is more widespread and the latter focal. In addition, the progression of transplant atherosclerosis is far more rapid. It has been speculated that development of transplant-associated atherosclerosis may represent a sustained antigeneic reaction localized to the vessel wall. This process resembles a chronic hypersensitivity reaction.

Research into transplantation, particularly in animal models, suggests that allograft arteriosclerosis is a very similar phenomenon to that seen in the early stages of atherosclerosis whatever its cause. The use of models such as the Fischer to Lewis rat renal transplant model could provide an opportunity to study the effects of inhibition of growth factors in particular and cytokines on smooth muscle proliferation which could in turn lead to rational therapies for the prevention and progression of atherosclerosis. Vascular smooth muscle cell proliferation and intimal hyperplasia with vessel occlusion seen in chronic rejection is undoubtedly an inflammatory response triggered by an ongoing endothelial damage and monocyte activation. The release of growth factors in response to this damage is initially non-specific and activates the final common pathway to vessel thickening and occlusion.

REFERENCES

1. Hayry P, Isoniemi H, Yilmaz S *et al.*: Chronic allograft rejection. *Immunol Rev.* **134**: 33–81, 1993
2. Ross R. The pathogenesis of atherosclerosis: a perspective for the 1990s. *Nature* **362**: 801–809, 1993
3. Bevilacqua MP, Pober JS, Majeau GR: Interleukin-1 [IL-1] induces biosynthesis and cell surface expression of procoagulant activity in human vascular endothelial cells. *J Exp Med* **160**: 618–623, 1984
4. Nawroth PP, Stern DM: Modulation of endothelial cell hemostatic properties by tumour necrosis factor. *J Exp Med* **163**: 740–745, 1986
5. Moore KL, Esmon CT, Esmon NL: Tumour necrosis factor leads to internalisation and

degradation of thrombomodulin from the surfaces of bovine aoric endothelial cells in culture. *Blood* **73**: 159–165, 1989

6. Bevilacqua MP, Schleef RR, Grimbone MAJ, Loskutoff DJ: Regulation of the fibrinolytic system of cultured human vascular endothelium by interleukin-1. *J Clin Invest* **78**: 587–591, 1986

7. Libby P, Hansson GK: Involvement of the immune system in human atherogensis: Current knowledge and unanswered questions. *Lab Invest* **64**: 5, 1991

8. Hayry P, von Willebrand E, Parthenais E *et al.*: The inflammatory mechanisms of allograft rejection. *Immunol Rev* **77**: 85–142, 1984

9. Lapierre LA, Fiers W, Pober JS: Three distinct classes of regulatory cytokines control endothelial cell MHC antigen expression. *J Exp Med* **167**: 794–804, 1988

10. Turner RR, Beckstead JH, Warnke RA, Wood GS: Endothelial cell phenotypic diversity: *in-situ* demonstration of immunologic and specific morphologic subtypes, *Am J Clin Pathol* **87**: 569–575, 1987

11. McCaffrey TA, Consigli S, Du B *et al.*: Decreased type II/type I TGF-beta receptor ratio in cells derived from human atherosclerotic lesions. Conversion from an antiproliferative to profibrotic response to TGF-beta 1. *J Clin Invest* **96**: 2667–2675, 1995

12. White E, Hildemann WH, Mullen Y: Chronic kidney allograft reactions in rats. *Transplantation* **8**: 602–617, 1969

13. Libby P, Solomon RN, Payne DD *et al.*: Functions of vascular wall cells related to development of transplantation associated coronary atherosclerosis. *Trans Proc* **21**: 3677–3684, 1989

Imaging Endothelial Activation

Dorian O. Haskard and A. Michael Peters

INTRODUCTION

Over the last decade there has been a considerable increase in understanding of the role of endothelium in inflammation. Endothelium is no longer seen as a passive inner lining to blood vessels but as an active participant in the control of vascular tone and permeability and in the recruitment of leukocytes into the tissues. The capacity of endothelial cells (EC) to contribute to an inflammatory response is mediated by a number of separate but overlapping programmes of cellular activation involving the redistribution of presynthesized proteins and the activation of genes encoding factors for surface expression or secretion. Perhaps the best characterized of the EC activation programmes in inflammation is the cellular response to stimulation with the interleukin-1 (IL-1) or tumour necrosis factor (TNF).[1]

The importance of changes in EC function in inflammation has fostered the need for new techniques to assess the state of EC activation, both in experimental studies and in the clinic. To this end we have explored the possible use of targeting radiolabelled monoclonal antibodies (mAb) to antigens expressed by the EC lumenal surface, focusing in the first instance on E-selectin. In this chapter we will briefly introduce the biology of E-selectin and describe our experience using an anti-E-selectin mAb to quantify and localize activated endothelium *in vivo*.

E-SELECTIN

E-Selectin is a cytokine-inducible adhesion molecule for leukocytes on the surface of activated EC. It was first identified by Bevilacqua *et al.* as a result of functional studies which showed that stimulating EC with IL-1 rendered them more adhesive for neutrophils.[2] Monoclonal antibodies were subsequently generated against IL-1 stimulated EC, one of which (mAb H4/18) reacted specifically with stimulated and not unstimulated EC.[3] Whilst this antibody had little inhibitory effect on leukocyte adhesion, a further antibody (mAb 18/7) against the same molecule significantly reduced the adhesion of neutrophils and monocytic cell lines to cytokine-activated EC. On these grounds the antigen was initially designated endothelial leukocyte adhesion molecule-1 (ELAM-1).[4] The subsequent cloning of ELAM-1 cDNA led to the appreciation that the molecule was structurally similar to the platelet antigen GMP-140/(PADGEM) and the leukocyte MEL-14 antigen. On these grounds the three molecules were respectively redesignated E-, P- and L-selectin.[5]

Each of the three selectins is a single chain transmembrane glycoprotein, the extracellular component of which consists of an N-terminal outer lectin domain, an epidermal-growth factor-like domain and a series of short consensus repeats (SCR) with homology to those found in complement regulatory proteins. The three molecules differ in the number of SCRs, with human E-selectin having six. As might be expected from the presence of the lectin domain, the selectins primarily bind carbohydrate ligands, although these need to be presented by the opposing cell on specific glyoproteins or glycolipids. The best characterized carbohydrate to which E-selectin binds is the fucosylated tetrasaccharide sialyl-Lewis X which is expressed by most granulocytes.[6] E-Selectin can also bind a related carbohydrate known as the cutaneous lymphocyte antigen (CLA) on memory T lymphocytes found in skin.[7]

Experiments examining the adhesion of leukocytes to endothelium under conditions of flow have established that the primary role of selectins is to initiate leukocyte-EC interactions rather than to promote leukocyte arrest.[8] The binding of selectins to their ligands generally has a high affinity but fast on–off kinetics and selectins are insufficient by themselves to immobilize the circulating leukocyte. However, since the bonds have a high tensile strength, selectin-mediated leukocyte adhesion tends to result in the rolling of leukocytes on the vessel wall.[9] The subsequent activation of leukocyte integrin function then leads to firm adhesion which is followed by the transmigration of leukocytes through endothelium into the tissues. In addition to mediating leukocyte rolling, it is possible that E-selectin may have a signalling role[10] and may also be involved in angiogenesis.[11]

Our choice of E-selectin as a target for imaging was very much influenced by the fact that most resting EC express the molecule at a barely detectable level. Stimulation of cultured EC with IL-1 or TNF leads to peak expression of E-selectin in 4–6 hours, after which expression may decline to near basal levels by 24 hours in the continuous presence of stimulant.[3] However, the degree to which E-selectin declines after peak expression is somewhat dependent on the type of cultured EC, being most marked with human umbilical vein EC (HUVEC) and less pronounced with cutaneous microvascular EC. As is the case for several proteins, the induction of E-selectin expression is mediated by the nuclear translocation of NFκB and the activation of gene transcription and *de novo* protein synthesis.[12] The transient nature of expression seen in HUVEC is thought to be related to the capacity of NFκB to induce its own inhibitor IκBα.[13] A number of other factors apart from IL-1 and TNF have been reported to be capable of inducing E-selectin expression, including bacterial lipopolysaccharide,[3] thrombin,[14] IL-3[15] and cross-linking CD40.[16]

PORCINE E-SELECTIN

The anti-E-selectin mAb 1.2B6 was generated against cytokine-activated EC,[17] but was found to react also with porcine aortic EC and with COS-7 cells transfected with porcine E-selectin cDNA (Fig. 1).[18] We therefore used mAb 1.2B6 to screen porcine tissues immunohistochemically for basal and inducible expression of E-selectin. In most tissues E-selectin was not detectable in the resting state but could be induced by the intravenous infusion of IL-1. An exception to this rule was endothelium in porcine skin which was found to stain positively for E-selectin in the absence of

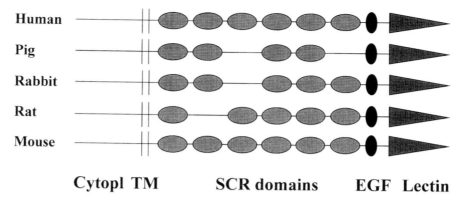

Fig. 1. Cartoon of the structure of E-selectin in different species. The molecule consists of a cytoplasmic domain (Cytopl), a transmembrane domain (TM), a series of short consensus repeats (SCR), an epidermal growth factor-like domain (EGF), and an N-terminal lectin domain.

obvious inflammation. This constituitive expression of E-selectin in pig skin seems to be different to human skin, in which there tends to be a very low level of constitutive E-selectin expression.[19]

SIMPLE MODELS OF INFLAMMATION IN THE PIG

Systemic activation

In order to establish that mAb 1.2B6 could specifically bind E-selectin when injected *in vivo*, we performed some experiments examining the clearance of radiolabelled mAb 1.2B6 compared with the clearance of a differentially radiolabelled control IgG$_1$.[20] These experiments showed that the clearance of mAb 1.2B6 but not that of the control antibody was dramatically accelerated 35–40 minutes after the intravenous injection of IL-1, presumably through binding of the antibody to E-selectin as soon as it was expressed on the EC luminal surface. Besides establishing the specificity of mAb 1.2B6 binding *in vivo*, this experiment therefore also told us the latency with which E-selectin is expressed following IL-1 stimulation *in vivo*.

Cutaneous activation

The large surface area of pig abdominal skin allows the simultaneous investigation of inflammatory responses in separate skin lesions established at different times and with different concentrations of mediators. In collaboration with Dr Richard Binns (The Babraham Institute) and Dr Martyn Robinson (Celltech Ltd), we used a model system already established for studying lymphocyte trafficking into inflamed tissue[21] to analyse the relationship between uptake of mAb 1.2B6 (reflecting E-selectin expression) and the capacity of neutrophils and lymphocytes to localize in inflammatory lesions. Although blocking studies with saturating concentrations of anti-E-selectin mAb demonstrated that E-selectin is necessary for optimal accumulation of both neutrophils or lymphocytes into IL-1- or TNF-stimulated lesions (Fig. 2) or into delayed-type hypersensitivity reactions, we found that the kinetics of E-selectin expression during inflammatory responses *in vivo* stretched

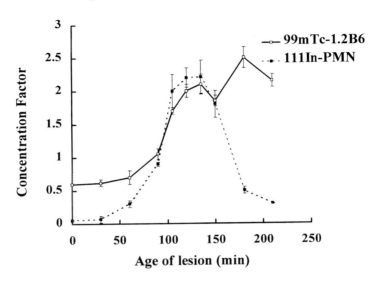

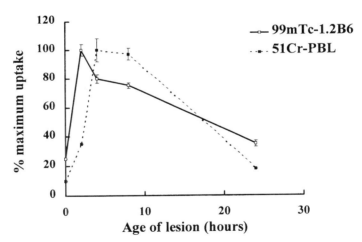

Fig. 2. The time-course of expression of E-selectin was studied by measuring the uptake of intravenously injected ^{99m}Tc-labelled mAb 1.2B6 (anti-E-selectin) into porcine skin lesions stimulated for different lengths of time with TNF. Uptake of anti-E-selectin was compared with the capacity of the lesions to recruit ^{111}In-labelled neutrophils (PMN) (upper) or ^{51}Cr-labelled lymphocytes (PBL) (lower). The early phase of E-selectin expression (up to 150 min) is characterized by neutrophil uptake, whilst lymphocyte accumulation occurs with E-selectin expression at later time-points. (Data from ref. 22, with permission.)

across those of early neutrophil accumulation and those of later lymphocyte accumulation, and therefore could not account for the time-course of traffic of either type of leukocyte.[22,23] The additional mechanisms controlling the timing of leukocyte entry into these skin lesions remain to be determined but obviously could include the regulated expression of other adhesion molecules and also of chemoattractants. From an imaging perspective, the importance of these observations is that uptake of anti-E-selectin mAb during inflammatory responses may take place across a broader time-frame than the accumulation of labelled neutrophils, and radiolabelled anti-E-selectin imaging may therefore have a wider range of applications, including that of imaging chronic inflammation.

Imaging porcine monoarthritis

Having established that mAb 1.2B6 is taken up specifically by inflamed tissues, we were in a position to test whether the antibody could be used for imaging. Initially we approached this question using models of porcine monoarthritis in which one of the knees is injected either with phytohaemagglutinin[24] or monosodium urate crystals.[25] In both these models ^{111}In-labelled mAb 1.2B6 was shown to accumulate in the inflamed knee over 24 hours, giving readily detectable images of inflamed synovium that were not observed with ^{111}In-labelled control IgG_1. Furthermore, the specificity of mAb 1.2B6 uptake was validated post mortem by showing that there was thirteen-fold accumulation of radioactivity in the inflamed knee compared with the uninflamed knee, in comparison with less than three-fold increase in control antibody. Interestingly, we were also able to image accumulation of E-selectin in uninflamed skin (reflecting the low grade constitutive expression of E-selectin seen by immunohistochemistry) and in the activated regional lymph node draining the inflamed synovium. Since the binding of a whole IgG_1 antibody to the EC surface could lead to endothelial injury through the Fc-mediated binding of neutrophils,[26] we repeated these studies with a F(ab')$_2$ fragment of mAb 1.2B6. The fragment gave superior images of monoarthritis compared with those obtained with the whole molecule. The images were also superior to those obtained with ^{99m}Tc-labelled neutrophils, partly because the antibody, unlike neutrophils, is not taken up by local bone marrow.[27]

CLINICAL IMAGING WITH ANTI-E-SELECTIN

Our experience with imaging E-selectin expression in the pig was sufficiently encouraging to warrant development of the technique for clinical imaging. Accordingly, we have tested the capacity of ^{111}In-labelled mAb 1.2B6 F(ab')$_2$ fragments to image inflamed tissues in patients with inflammatory diseases, focusing in the first instance on rheumatoid arthritis (RA). We have observed focal uptake of mAb 1.2B6 in inflamed joints in all of the 14 patients with active RA that we have scanned.[28] Since it is undesirable to give patients irrelevant mouse antibodies and not possible to count radioactivity in tissues at the end of the clinical imaging, validating the specificity of antibody uptake is obviously more difficult in humans than in the pig. However, we have scanned six patients with stable arthritis with both ^{111}In-labelled mAb 1.2B6 and ^{111}In-labelled human immunoglobulin (HIG) and found that ^{111}In-labelled mAb 1.2B6 imaging gives significantly more focal imaging of inflamed tissues (Fig. 3) and is also more sensitive than ^{111}In-labelled HIG. In particular, mAb 1.2B6 but not HIG could identify joints which were not clinically inflamed. Preliminary imaging in patients with inflammatory bowel disease has also indicated ^{111}In-labelled anti-E-selectin in segments of inflamed bowel that were positive on contemporaneous ^{99m}Tc-leukocyte scanning.[29]

PROSPECTS FOR FUTURE IMAGING OF ENDOTHELIAL ACTIVATION

Now that we have established that it is possible to target and image an endothelial activation antigen, the work could follow a number of directions. First, it will be interesting to determine the capacity of anti-E-selectin to identify endothelial activation in other inflammatory conditions with a view both to the localization of inflamed tissues and to the monitoring of the response to treatment. In the light of the detection by immunohistology of E-selectin expression at the base of atherosclerotic plaques and in inflamed adventitial tissue,[30] a particular goal is to image endothelial

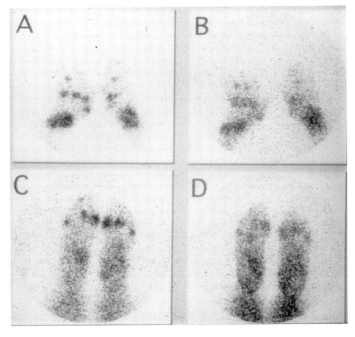

Fig. 3. Imaging of the small joints of the hands (A, B) and feet (C, D) in a patient with rheumatoid arthritis. Scans were performed 2 weeks apart with ^{111}In-labelled mAb 1.2B6 (anti-E-selectin) (A, C) and ^{111}In-labelled human immunoglobulin (B, D). It can be seen that the imaging of the inflamed joints is more intense and focal with anti-E-selectin compared with control immunoglobulin. (Reproduced from ref. 28, with permission.)

activation in arterial disease, although this presents an obvious technical challenge in terms of image resolution.

A second direction for further development is the application of the same approach to targeting and imaging other EC activation antigens which are regulated differentially to E-selectin, thereby increasing our repertoire of molecular 'reporters' of different programmes of EC response. It is possible, however, that not all EC activation antigens will be suitable as targets for imaging. We believe that the capacity to image E-selectin expression is related not only to endothelial expression of the antigen and the affinity of the antibody, but also to the mechanism of removal of the antigen from the cell surface. The majority of cell surface E-selectin molecules are removed from the EC surface by internalization, and it is likely that antibody that has bound E-selectin is taken along with the radiolabel into the cell.[31] This is especially evident in inflammatory bowel disease in which positive imaging with anti-E-selectin remains localized to the segment of inflamed bowel. In contrast, ^{99m}Tc-leukocytes that have gained access to the inflamed segment then migrate into the bowel lumen and move distally with the bowel contents.[29] It is possible that antigens that are predominantly shed from the cell surface rather than internalized may not allow the localization of labelled antibody for long enough to successfully obtain images.

ACKNOWLEDGEMENTS

The authors gratefully acknowledge the contributions that many colleagues have made to the work described in this chapter. These include Drs Mansoor Bhatti, Ted Keelan, Andrew Harrison, Humphrey Hodgson, Peter Chapman and Francois Jamar (RPMS), Martyn Robinson and Yvonne Tsang (Celltech Ltd) and Richard Binns, Steve Licence and Tony Whyte (The Babraham Institute).

REFERENCES

1. Pober JS, Cotran RS: Cytokines and endothelial cell biology. *Physiol Rev* 70; 427–51: 1990
2. Bevilacqua MP, Pober JS, Wheeler ME *et al.*: Interleukin-1 acts on cultured human vascular endothelium to increase the adhesion of polymorphonuclear leukocytes, monocytes, and related cell lines. *J Clin Invest* **76**: 2003–2011, 1985
3. Pober JS, Bevilacqua MP, Mendrick DL *et al.*: Two distinct monokines, interleukin-1 and tumor necrosis factor, each independently induce the biosynthesis and transient expression of the same antigen on the surface of cultured human vascular endothelial cells. *J Immunol* **136**: 1680–1687, 1986
4. Bevilacqua MP, Pober JS, Mendrick DL *et al.*: Identification of an inducible endothelial-leukocyte adhesion molecule. *Proc Natl Acad Sci USA* **84**: 9238–9242, 1987
5. Bevilacqua M, Butcher E, Furie B *et al.*: Selectins: A family of adhesion receptors. *Cell* **67**: 233, 1991
6. Brandley BK, Swiedler SJ, Robbins PW: Carbohydrate ligands of the LEC cell adhesion molecules. *Cell* **63**: 861–863, 1990
7. Berg EL, Yoshino T, Rott LS *et al.*: The cutaneous lymphocyte antigen is a skin lymphocyte homing receptor for the vascular lectin endothelial cell-leukocyte adhesion molecule 1. *J Exp Med*, **174**: 1461–1466, 1991

8. Lawrence MB, Springer TA: Neutrophils roll on E-selectin. *J Immunol* **151:** 6338–6346, 1993

9. Alon R, Hammer DA, Springer TA: Lifetime of the P-selectin-carbohydrate bond and its response to tensile force in hydrodymanic flow. *Nature* **374:** 539–542, 1995

10. Kaplanski G, Farnarier C, Benoliel A-M *et al.*: A novel role for E- and P-selectins: shape control of endothelial cell monolayers. *J Cell Sci* **107:** 2449–2457, 1994

11. Kralin BM, Razon MJ, Boon LM *et al.*: E-selectin is present in proliferating endoithelial cells in human hemangiomas. *Am J Pathol* **148:** 1181–1191, 1996

12. Collins T, Read MA, Neish AS *et al.*: Transcriptional regulation of endothelial cell adhesion molecules: NF-κB and cytokine-inducible enhancers. *FASEB J* **9:** 899–909, 1995

13. De Martin R, Vanhove B, Cheng Q *et al.*: Cytokine-inducible expression in endothelial cells of an IκBκ-like gene is regulated by NFκB. *EMBO J* **12:** 2773–2779, 1993

14. Shankar R, de la Motte CA, DiCorleto PE: 3-Deazaadenosine inhibits thrombin-stimulated platelet-derived growth factor production and endothelial-leukocyte adhesion molecule-1-mediated monocytic cell adhesion in human aortic endothelial cells. *J Biol Chem* **267:** 9376–9382, 1992

15. Brizzi MF, Garbarino G, Rossi PR *et al.*: Interleukin 3 stimulates proliferation and triggers endothelial-leukocyte adhesion molecule 1 gene activation of human endothelial cells. *J Clin Invest* **91:** 2887–2892, 1993

16. Karmann K, Hughes CCW, Schechner J *et al.*: CD40 on human endothelial cells: inducibility by cytokines and functional regulation of adhesion molecule expression. *Proc Natl Acad Sci USA* **92:** 4342–4346, 1995

17. Wellicome SM, Thornhill MH, Pitzalis C *et al.*: A monoclonal antibody that detects a novel antigen on endothelial cells that is induced by tumor necrosis factor, IL-1 or lipopolysaccharide. *J Immunol* **144:** 2558–2565, 1990

18. Tsang Y, Stevens PE, Licence ST *et al.*: Porcine E-selectin: cloning and functional characterization. *Immunology* **85:** 140–145, 1995

19. Norris P, Poston RN, Thomas DS *et al.*: The expression of endothelial leukocyte adhesion molecule-1 (ELAM-1), Intercellular adhesion molecule-1 (ICAM-1) and vascular cell adhesion molecule-1 (VCAM-1) in experimental cutaneous inflammation: a comparison of ultraviolet- B erythema and delayed hypersensitivity. *J Invest Dermatol* **96:** 763–770, 1991

20. Keelan ETM, Licence ST, Peters AM *et al.*: Characterization of E-selectin expression *in vivo* using a radiolabelled monoclonal antibody. *Am J Physiol* **266:** H279–290, 1994

21. Binns RM, Licence ST, Wooding FBP, Duffus WPH: Active lymphocyte traffic induced in the periphery by cytokines and phytohemagglutinin: three different mechanisms? *Eur J Immunol* **22,** 2195–2203, 1992

22. Binns RM, Licence ST, Harrison AA *et al.*: In vivo E-selectin upregulation correlates with early infiltration of PMN, later with PBL-entry: mAbs block both. *Am J Physiol* **270:** H183–193, 1996

23. Binns RM, Whyte A, Licence ST *et al.*: The role of E-selectin in lymphocyte and polymorphonuclear cell recruitment into cutaneous delayed hypersensitivity reactions in sensitised pigs. *J Immunol* **157:** 4094–4099, 1996

24. Keelan ETM, Harrison AA, Chapman PT *et al.*: Imaging vascular endothelial activation: an approach using radiolabelled monoclonal antibody against the endothelial cell adhesion molecule E-selectin. *J Nucl Med* **35:** 276–281, 1994

25. Chapman PT, Jamar F, Harrison AA *et al.*: Non-invasive imaging of E-selectin expression by activated endothelium in urate crystal-induced arthritis. *Arthritis Rheum* **37:** 1752–1756, 1994

26. Leeuwenberg JF, Jeunhomme GM, Buurman WA: Adhesion of polymorphonuclear cells to human endothelial cells. Adhesion-molecule-dependent, and Fc receptor-mediated adhesion-molecule-independent mechanisms. *Clin Exp Immunol* **81:** 496–500, 1990

27. Jamar F, Chapman PT, Harrison AA *et al.*: Inflammatory arthritis: imaging of endothelial activation with an indium-111-labeled F(ab')2 fragment of anti-E-selectin monoclonal antibody. *Radiology* **194:** 843–850, 1995

28. Chapman PT, Jamar F, Keelan ETM *et al.*: Use of a radiolabeled monoclonal antibody

against E-selectin for imaging endothelial activation in rheumatoid arthritis. *Arthritis Rheum* **39:** 1371–1375, 1996

29. Bhatti MA, Chapman PT, Jamar F *et al.*: Immunolocalization of active inflammatory bowel disease using a monoclonal antibody against E-selectin. *J Nucl Med* **37:** 114P, 1996
30. Parums DV: The distribution of adhesion molecules in normal and atherosclerotic arteries and aortas. In: Gallo LL (Ed) *Cardiovascular Disease* Vol 2, pp. 159–171. New York: Plenum Press, 1995
31. von Asmuth EJU, Smeets EF, Ginsel LA *et al.*: Buurman WA, Evidence for endocytosis of E-selectin in human endothelial cells. *Eur J Immunol* **22:** 2519–2526, 1992

AORTIC ANEURYSMS

Imaging of Inflammation in Inflammatory Abdominal Aortic Aneurysms

William G. Tennant and Roger N. Baird

INCIDENCE

Current estimates of the incidence of inflammatory change in aortic aneurysms are about 7%, and vary from 2% to 23%[1,2] of all abdominal aortic aneurysms (AAA). Higher figures are probably biased by the clustering of cases in specialist centres, and the true incidence is towards the lower end of this range.

SYMPTOMS AND SIGNS

Most unruptured inflammatory aneurysms are symptomatic, unlike their non-inflammatory counterparts. There is remarkable consistency in the clinical features of inflammatory aneurysms. Pain in the abdomen or back is a frequent finding,[1,3–6] usually caused by vertebral erosion or by visceral obstruction by the inflammatory

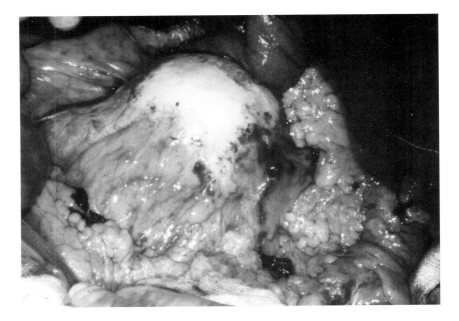

Fig. 1. Inflammatory abdominal aortic aneurysm seen at operation.

mass.[3,5,7] The pain may be severe, mimicking a contained rupture, and the patient is treated by urgent operation.[1,8,9] Weight loss is a common complaint,[1,5,7] and there may be other signs of systemic illness, such as pyrexia.[7] On examination, the aneurysm is often tender in the absence of free or contained rupture.[1] Patients may also present with symptoms of obstruction of adjacent structures secondary to fibrous invasion of the retroperitoneum. The effects include swelling of the lower limbs from venous obstruction arising from inferior vena caval stenosis or aortocaval fistula; vomiting because of duodenal stenosis, and loin pain from hydronephrosis caused by ureteric obstruction. These symptoms and signs can be misleading and result in referrals to physicians and urological surgeons.

The most common finding on haematological examination is of a raised erythrocyte sedimentation rate (ESR) and plasma viscosity, but anaemia has been noted in some series.[3,6,7,10] The white blood count is usually normal.[6] Obstruction of the ureters may lead to a raised blood urea and creatinine.[1] A number of non-specific inflammatory markers such as C-reactive peptide (CRP) may be raised in patients with inflammatory aneurysms, but there is no specific immunological test for the presence of inflammatory change.[11]

PATHOLOGY

The aetiology and pathogenesis of inflammatory change are unknown. The most plausible theory is that some material, probably oxidized lipid, is extruded through the damaged medial coat of some aortic aneurysms, so initiating an inflammatory

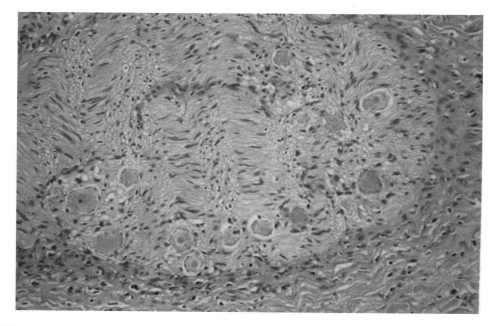

Fig. 2. A sympathetic ganglion trapped in the fibrosis surrounding an inflammatory aneurysm.

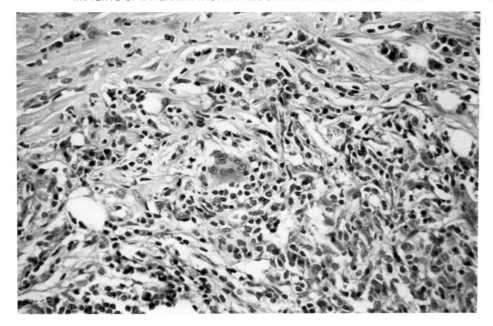

Fig. 3.   Giant cells in the wall of an inflammatory aneurysm.

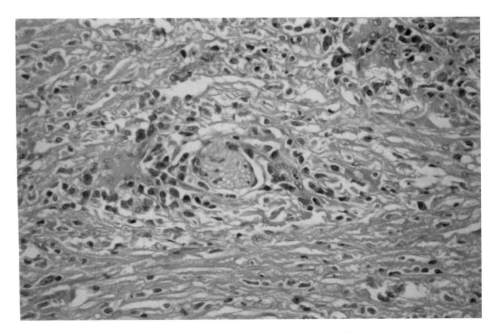

Fig. 4.   A peripheral nerve trapped in the wall of an inflammatory aneurysm.

response.[12-15] This would explain the findings in 'early' inflammatory change of discrete plaques of inflammatory tissue on the surface of the aneurysm rather than an overall covering.

Inflammatory change may be simply a slightly thickened aneurysm wall with the duodenum adherent to the right and anterior surface. In more florid cases, the aneurysm is encased in a thick white coating giving rise to the epithet 'sugar icing aneurysm'.

Histologically, the thickened wall of inflammatory aneurysms is composed of fibrous tissue infiltrated with lymphocytes and displaying early germinal centre formation. There is frequently a perivascular and perineural infiltrate of plasma cells and both haemosiderin laden macrophages and giant cells may be present. Engulfed sympathetic ganglia may be seen in tissue sections of the outer fibrous layers of inflammatory tissue (Figs 2–4).

WHY SHOULD WE IMAGE INFLAMMATION IN THIS DISEASE?

Extensive inflammatory change can represent a considerable technical challenge to the vascular surgeon. Within the mass of inflammatory tissue may lie the ureters, duodenum, left renal vein and inferior vena cava. The small bowel or sigmoid mesentery may be shortened by fibrosis. All of these features make for a dissection of the neck of the aneurysm that can be difficult or even dangerous. In particular, if the duodenum is entered, the hole should be sutured and the aneurysm operation abandoned for the time being, as the Dacron prosthesis is likely to be contaminated by intestinal organisms. If florid inflammatory tissue is present up to the level of the diaphragm open operative repair may be impossible. Because of these potential difficulties, safe open surgery on inflammatory aneurysms is time consuming and the services of an experienced operating team are required. Operative blood loss is increased, and a red cell scavenging system is useful.

The need to demonstrate a thickened aneurysm wall may become less important with the advent of endovascular techniques. As it becomes possible to replace aneurysms with stent prostheses, the presence of extralumenal inflammatory change will become less relevant. Imaging will still be required to demonstrate inflammatory change in cases where visceral obstruction is symptomatic, where steroid treatment is contemplated, and where the anatomy of the aneurysm renders it unsuitable for endovascular repair.

WHAT INFORMATION IS REQUIRED?

In order to assess the patient's suitability for open aortic replacement, it is necessary to know three things about inflammatory change in aortic aneurysm disease:

1. its presence or absence (i.e. false negative and false positive detection);
2. its extent in relation to the renal and other visceral arteries;
3. its effect on adjacent organs.

The first two items go hand in hand, in that those investigations most reliable at detecting inflammatory change are able to determine its extent most accurately. While these examinations *may* define the degree of involvement of adjacent organs, this is by no means guaranteed. Supplementary investigations may be required depending on the organ system thought to be involved.

KEY FEATURES FOR DETECTION

The basis of radiological detection of inflammatory change is the demonstration of an abnormal soft tissue mass lying anterior to an aortic aneurysm. The posterior aspect of the aorta is usually spared. The retroperitoneal thickening may spread laterally to encase other structures, most notably the duodenum, ureters and inferior vena cava. Other features which may be detected radiologically include all the consequences of visceral obstruction from florid inflammatory change. Thus each of hydronephrosis (Fig. 6), inferior vena caval obstruction and deep venous thrombosis, duodenal obstruction, small bowel and sigmoid obstruction can be demonstrated preoperatively.

IMAGING MODALITIES

Plain and contrast radiography, ultrasound, computerized tomography (CT) and magnetic resonance imaging (MRI) can all be used to demonstrate aneurysm formation in the abdominal aorta. Each will be considered in turn and its sensitivity in detecting the presence and extent of inflammatory change discussed.

Plain radiography (Fig. 5)

'Eggshell' calcification can be seen in a few aneurysms on plain abdominal radiography because of calcification of the dilated arterial wall. This is usually most easily seen in the lateral projection because of reduced interference anteriorly from overlying bowel gas and posteriorly from the lumbar vertebrae. The absence of calcification does not rule out an aneurysm. Inflammatory change cannot be seen on a plain radiograph.

Contrast radiography

Aortography does not reliably serve to demonstrate the full extent of aneurysmal change in the aorta because of the presence of intralumenal thrombus.[16,17] Angiography is helpful if there is arterial occlusive disease affecting the renal or iliofemoral arteries, or if there is unusual renal anatomy as in horseshoe kidney and multiple renal arteries. The role of intravenous urography, upper and lower gastrointestinal barium studies and venography is limited to the demonstration of the effects of inflammatory change on adjacent organs.

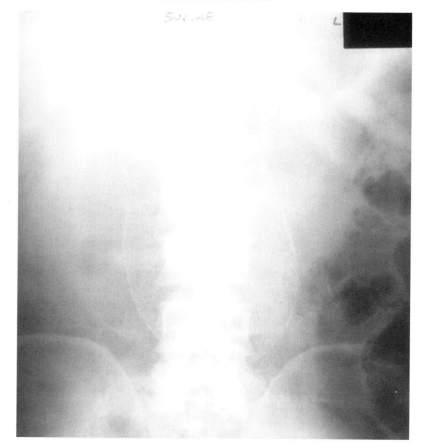

Fig. 5.   'Eggshell' calcification seen in the wall of an aortic aneurysm.

Ultrasound (Fig. 7)

While ultrasound is highly sensitive in detecting aneurysm formation in the abdominal aorta,[18] inflammatory change in the aortic wall is seldom seen. The renal artery origins may be obscured by overlying bowel gas, and the relationship of the aneurysm neck to the renal arteries is usually inferred from the level of the closely adjacent superior mesenteric artery. Dilation of the renal pelvis can be demonstrated using ultrasound, as can gastric, small and large bowel dilatation. Urinary and biliary calculi may also be seen.

Contrast enhanced computerized tomography (Figs 8 and 10)

Computerized tomography is moderately good at demonstrating both the presence and extent of inflammatory change with a sensitivity of 50–70%.[19] Higher figures usually come from retrospective studies where the features of inflammatory change

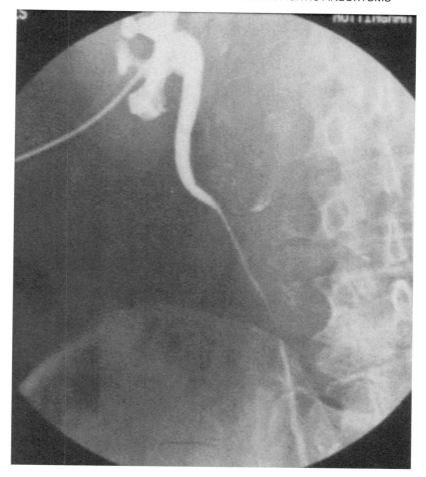

Fig. 6. Ureteric deviation and stenosis in inflammatory aortic aneurysm. A neprostomy tube has been inserted in the hydronephrotic kidney.

have been specifically sought. The renal vessels enhance with contrast and are often visible on one or more slices. Using systems only capable of transverse imaging, the plane of the scan slices cannot be adjusted to provide an optimal view, particularly when the aneurysm overhangs the renal arteries proximally. Further scans may be required, increasing the patient's radiation dose. A recent prospective series shows a sensitivity of 82% in the preoperative diagnosis of inflammatory aneurysm using contrast enhanced CT.[20] At present there are no studies on the use of helical CT scanning in inflammatory aneurysm disease, but preliminary studies of this modality in assessing aneurysms for endovascular repair shows that the relationship of the renal and visceral arteries to the aneurysm neck can be accurately defined.[21]

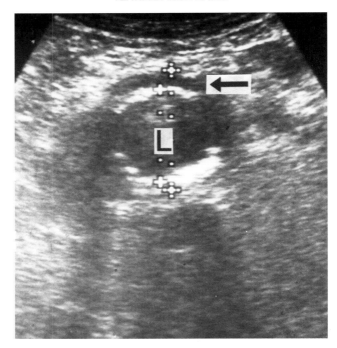

Fig. 7.   Ultrasound of inflammatory change. The thickened wall is visible (arrow). The lumen of the aorta is marked (L).

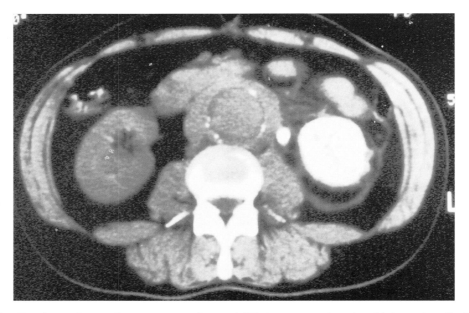

Fig. 8.   Late phase of a contrast-enhanced CT demonstrating the thickened wall of an inflammatory aneurysm with a left hydronephrosis. The dilated left ureter can be seen adherent to the wall of the aneurysm.

Magnetic resonance imaging (Fig. 9)

Magnetic resonance imaging is the newest imaging modality. It is highly sensitive and specific in the detection of aneurysmal dilatation, and does not require intravenous contrast agents. Studies of MRI in detecting inflammatory tissue have demonstrated characteristic appearances in short tau inversion recovery sequences. These show that inflammatory tissue has a complex layered appearance.[19] Histologically there is layering of inflammatory aortic wall caused by alternating bands of fibrosis and cellular infiltrate, but this finding has not been linked to the MR appearance.[22] The use of gadolinium DTPA contrast has been reported in one case,[23] but it is not yet known whether the use of contrast enhances the sensitivity of MRI.

SELECTING PATIENTS FOR DETAILED IMAGING OF INFLAMMATORY CHANGE – WHEN SHOULD WE BE SUSPICIOUS?

No specific haematological or immunological test exists for inflammatory change. In consequence, clinical features and simple blood tests are used to aid selection. The diagnostic features of malaise, weight loss, and a 'flu-like' illness coupled with tenderness of the aneurysm, back pain and pyrexia are typically associated with a raised ESR and plasma viscosity and (more rarely) a raised neutrophil count. The clinical sequelae of visceral obstruction may also be present.

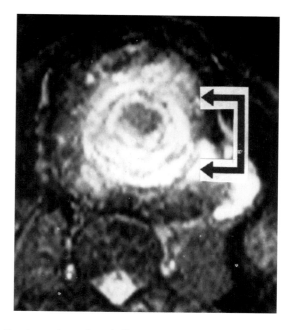

Fig. 9. Layering of an inflammatory aortic aneurysm seen on short-tau inversion recovery sequence magnetic resonance scan.

Most patients reach the vascular surgeon having had an ultrasound scan to confirm the diagnosis. In thin patients where a non-tender aneurysm can be felt well below the costal margin, and where there are no clinical or haematological features of inflammatory change, no further imaging may be required. In practice, it is usual to evaluate patients prior to elective surgery with contrast enhanced CT scans of the abdomen. This will unexpectedly demonstrate inflammatory change in a few asymptomatic patients, and will confirm its presence where there is a high degree of clinical suspicion. In patients where clinical suspicion is high, but CT scanning does not show an inflammatory aneurysm, magnetic resonance scanning is the next step as it is currently the most sensitive method.

ENDOVASCULAR REPAIR OF INFLAMMATORY ANEURYSMS

A few highly selected inflammatory aneurysms may be suitable for endovascular treatment which offers a less invasive and possibly less risky alternative to open operation in patients who are unfit or unsuitable for open surgery. Imaging

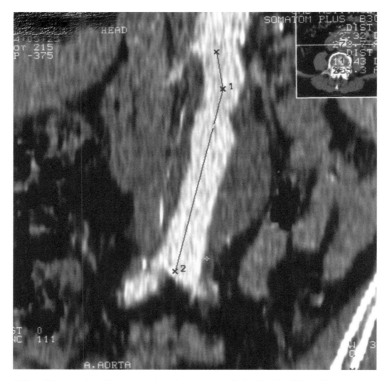

Fig. 10. Reconstructed contrast-enhanced helical CT of an aneurysm demonstrating the right renal artery and calipers to measure the neck length and length of the aneurysm lumen

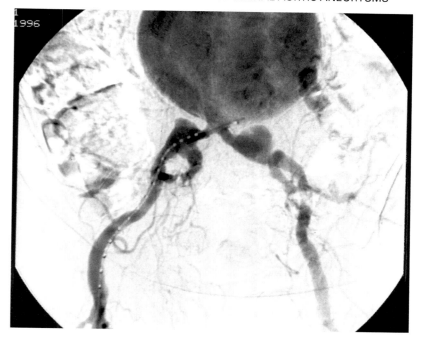

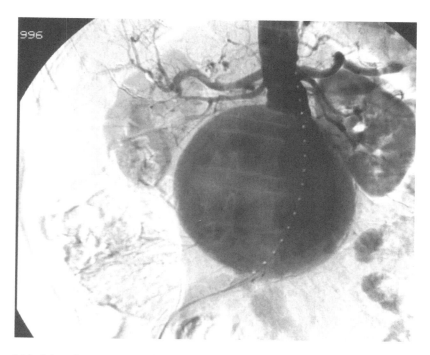

Fig. 11(a,b). Assessment of the length of the lumen and the iliac arteries of an aneurysm intended for endovascular treatment. An angiographic catheter is used which carries radio-opaque markers at 1 cm intervals.

requirements for this are different. No information need be sought for the proximal or lateral extent of the inflammatory change. Similarly, accurate information about the position of the ureters, inferior vena cava and duodenum are unnecessary. Lumenal measurements are essential and accurate measurements of the length and diameter of the neck of the aneurysm, diameter and tortuosity of the iliac systems and the total length of the aneurysm are needed. Helical CT images may be manipulated to give accurate positional information on the iliac systems and measurement of the length of the aneurysm neck (Fig. 10) and an angiographic catheter carrying radio-opaque 1 cm markers gives accurate measurement of the longitudinal length of aneurysms when angiography is carried out in several planes (Figs 11a, b).

SUMMARY

Inflammatory aortic aneurysms are encountered moderately frequently in clinical practice. Because of the technical difficulties which may accompany open operation, a preoperative diagnosis of the presence and extent of inflammatory change is desirable. History, examination and non-specific inflammatory markers are useful in alerting the clinician to the possibility of an inflammatory aneurysm. The mainstay of diagnosis is radiological, and ultrasound, contrast enhanced CT and MRI are all helpful. Involvement of other organ systems in the inflammatory process may require the use of other radiological techniques.

Despite clinical awareness and advances in imaging technology, inflammatory aneurysms are occasionally encountered unexpectedly, and all surgeons should be prepared to handle inflammatory aneurysms by the transperitoneal route.

ACKNOWLEDGMENTS

The authors would like to thank Professor B.R. Hopkinson and Professor M. Horrocks, Consultant Surgeons, for permission to include patients under their care, and Dr Simon Whitaker and Dr Roger Gregson, Consultant Radiologists, for their permission to use the images displayed in Figs 6, 8, 10 and 11.

REFERENCES

1. Crawford JL, Stowe CL, Safi HJ et al.: Inflammatory aneurysms of the aorta. J Vasc Surg 2: 113–124, 1985
2. Darke SG, Glass RE, Eadie DGA: Abdominal aortic aneurysm: Perianeurysmal fibrosis and ureteric obstruction and deviation. Br J Surg 64: 649–652, 1977
3. Walker DI, Bloor K, Williams G, Gillie I: Inflammatory aneurysms of the abdominal aorta. Br J Surg 59: 609–614, 1972
4. Goldstone J, Malone JM, Moore WS: Inflammatory aneurysms of the abdominal aorta. Surgery 83: 425–430, 1978
5. Pennell RC, Hollier LH, Lie JT et al.: Inflammatory abdominal aortic aneurysms: A thirty year review. J Vasc Surg 2: 859–869, 1985

6. Plate G, Forsby N, Stigsson L *et al.*: Management of inflammatory abdominal aortic aneurysm. *Acta Chir Scand* **154:** 19–24, 1988
7. Sethia B, Darke SG: Abdominal aortic aneurysm with retroperitoneal fibrosis and ureteric entrapment. *Br J Surg* **70:** 434–436, 1983
8. Stringer MD, Bentley PG: Inflammatory aortic aneurysms. *Br J Hosp Med* June: 512–515, 1987
9. Koep L, Zuidema GD. The clinical significance of retroperitoneal fibrosis. *Surgery* **81:** 250–257, 1977
10. Baskerville PA, Blakeney CG, Young AE, Browse NL: The diagnosis and treatment of peri-aortic fibrosis ('Inflammatory' aneurysms). *Br J Surg* **70:** 381–385, 1983
11. Tennant WG, Baird RN, Horrocks M: Metabolic activity in inflammatory and non-inflammatory aneurysms of the abdominal aorta. *Eur J Vasc Surg* **6:** 199–203, 1992
12. Mitchinson MJ: Chronic periaortitis and periarteritis. *Histopathology* **8:** 589–600, 1984
13. Parums D. Mitchinson MJ: Demonstration of immunoglobulins in the neighbourhood of advanced atherosclerotic plaques. *Atherosclerosis* **38:** 217–228, 1981
14. Mitchinson MJ: Insoluble lipids in human atherosclerotic plaques. *Atherosclerosis* **45:** 11–15, 1982
15. Munro JM, Van der Walt JD, Cox EL: A comparison of cytoplasm immunoglobulins in retroperitoneal fibrosis and abdominal aortic aneurysms. *Histopathology* **10:** 1163–1169, 1986
16. Andersen PE, Lorentzen JE: Comparison of computed tomography and aortography in abdominal aortic aneurysm. *J Comput Assist Tomog* **7:** 670–673, 1983
17. Eriksson I, Forsberg JO, Hemmingsson A, Lindgren PG: Pre-operative evaluation of abdominal aortic aneurysms: Is there a need for aortography? *Acta Chir Scand* **147:** 533–537, 1981
18. Leopold GR, Goldberger LE, Bernstein EF: Ultrasonic detection and evaluation of abdominal aortic aneurysms. *Surgery* **72:** 939–945, 1972
19. Tennant WG, Hartnell GG, Baird RN, Horrocks M: Radiological investigation of aneurysm disease: Comparison of three modalities in staging and the detection of inflammatory change. *J Vasc Surg* **17:** 703–709, 1993
20. Arroyo A, Rodriguez C, Rodriguez J *et al.*: Inflammatory aneurysms: A diagnostic and therapeutic challenge to the vascular surgeon. *Eur J Vasc Surg* (1997) (in press)
21. Balm R, van Leeuwen MS, Noordzij J, Eikelboom BC: Spiral CT for aortic aneurysms. In: Greenhalgh RM (Ed) *Vascular Imaging for Surgeons* pp 191–202. London: WB Saunders, 1995
22. Tennant WG, Hartnell GG, Baird RN, Horrocks M: Inflammatory aortic aneurysms: Characteristic appearance on magnetic resonance imaging. *Eur J Vasc Surg* **6:** 399–402, 1992
23. Hyashi H, Kumazaki T: Case Report: Inflammatory abdominal aortic aneurysm. Dynamic Gd-DTPA enhanced magnetic resonance imaging features. *Br J Radiol* **68:** 321–323, 1995

Medical Management of Inflammatory Abdominal Aortic Aneurysms

Massimo D'Addato, Andrea Stella and Mauro Gargiulo

INTRODUCTION

In 1935 James first described a periaortic inflammatory process in a patient with abdominal aortic aneurysm (AAA).[1] The inflammatory reaction led to entrapment and occlusion of both ureters resulting in kidney failure and death.[1] Since then a number of reports have described cases of AAA with periaortic inflammation.[2–8] In 1972 Walker et al. defined this feature as 'inflammatory aneurysm'.[9]

Inflammatory abdominal aortic aneurysm (IAAA) is a well-defined clinical entity[9–15] with an incidence ranging from 2%[16] to 18.1%[17] of all cases of AAA. Macroscopically, the lesion presents a whitish, thickened aortic wall (> 0.5 cm thick) adhering to adjacent tissues and organs (duodenum, sigmoid colon, ureters, inferior vena cava, left renal vein, left gonadal vein, loops of small bowel, pancreas). Thickening of the vessel wall is caused by centrifugal development of a parietal fibroinflammatory process whose aetiology and mechanisms of onset remain unsettled.[9–11,13,16–27]

Thickening of the wall of the aorta does not seem to reduce the risk of aneurysm rupture[9,28–31] so that surgery remains the treatment of choice. In addition a graft appears to arrest the centrifugal expansion of the parietal inflammatory process, leading to inflammatory mantle regression in a high percentage of cases.[15,24,28,32–38]

Surgical management of IAAA is technically difficult due to the presence of the parietal inflammatory process. The relations between the aorta and proximal structures are impaired, hampering isolation of the aneurysm and increasing the risk of iatrogenic damage to periaortic structures with a consequent rise in morbidity and mortality associated with aneurysmal resection.[14–17,32] These technical drawbacks and the high morbidity-mortality rate spurred the search for an alternative therapeutic approach that would resolve the periaortic inflammatory process and release the periaortic structures entrapped in the fibroinflammatory tissue.[9,14,17,34,39–46] In 1977 Clyne and Abercrombie were the first to recommend the use of steroids in the treatment of 'perianeurysmal retroperitoneal fibrosis'.[39] They administered prednisolone to two patients with symptomatic IAAA, elevated erythrocyte sedimentation rate (ESR) and bilateral ureteral obstruction. Steroid therapy led to a remission of symptoms, release of the ureters and normalization of ESR in both cases (Table 1).

Following their success, many authors advocated the use of steroids to treat the parietal inflammatory process in AAA.[17,28,29,34,36,41–46] The literature reports 23 cases of medical management, of perianeurysmal fibrosis of which 22 received

Table 1. Medical treatment and outcome in patients with IAAA

Authors/year	Age/sex	Symptoms/preop. IVU	Preop. serum creatinine (μmol/l)	Preop. ESR (mm/h)
Clyne and Abercrombie 1977[39]	51 M	Right loin pain IVU: Non-functioning left kidney	160	70
	64 M	Upper abdominal pain, backache, weight loss IVU: Obstruction of both ureters	?	?
Baskerville *et al.* 1983[34]	58 M	Abdominal pain IVU: Medial ureteric deviation	?	30
	73 M	Loin pain IVU: Bilateral hydronephrosis	?	76
	53 M	Abdominal and right loin pain IVU: Non-functioning right kidney	?	41
	49 M	Abdominal and back pain IVU: Normal	?	91
	48 M	None IVU: ?	?	46
Sethia and Darke 1983[41]	74 M	Backache IVU: Bilateral medial ureteric deviation and hydronephrosis	?	120
Feldberg and Hene 1983[42]	56 M	Loin pain IVU: Obstruction of both ureters	200	?
Hedges and Bentley 1986[43]	56 M	Left loin and lower back pain IVU: Normal	?	65
Higgins *et al.* 1988[46]	71 M	Loin pain, anorexia, weight loss IVU: ?	798	141
	61 M	Anemia, renal failure IVU: ?	666	68
	64 M	Renal failure IVU: ?	1276	79
Gaylis and Isaacson 1989[17]	51 M	Asympyomatic IVU: ?	?	1
	50 M	Backache IVU: ?	?	?
Stella *et al.* 1996[44]	67 M	Fever, abdominal and loin pain, renal failure IVU = left hydronephrosis	?	?
	52 M	Bilateral hydrocele, left loin pain IVU: Normal	Normal	?

IVU = intravenous urography

Table 1 *continued*

IAAA diameter (cm)	Treatment	Follow-up
?	Prednisolone 5 mg three times per day	6 weeks: alive and well, creatinine: 110 mmol/l, IVU: normal 8 months: alive and well, ESR: 10 mm/h
?	Prednisolone 5 mg three times per day	2 months: alive and well, IVU: dilatation upper calyces on the right only 30 months: alive and well
5.7	Prednisone 5 mg three times per day	4 months: alive and well, ESR <20 mm/h, CT: partial regression fibrosis 16 months: alive and well, ESR <20mm/h, IVU: normal
3.1	Prednisone 5 mg three times per day	7 and 16 months: alive and well, ESR <20 mm/h, IVU: normal, CT: partial regression fibrosis
4.3	Prednisone 5 mg three times per day	7 and 26 months: alive and well, ESR <20 mm/h, CT: partial regression fibrosis
3.3	Prednisone 5 mg three times per day	7 months: alive and well, ESR <20 mm/h, CT: partial regression fibrosis
4.6	Prednisone 5 mg three times per day	3 and 12 months: alive and well, ESR <20 mm/h, CT: partial regression fibrosis
?	?	6 months: alive and well, ESR: 35 mm/h, IVU: improved
?	Methylprednisolone 1 g x 4 + prednisone 100 mg / day	3 weeks: alive and well, ESR: ?, IVU: improved, CT: partial regression fibrosis 7 months: alive and well, aneurysm resected
6	Prednisolone 15 mg/day	2 months: alive and well, ESR: 8 mm/h, 6 months: back pain, aneurysm diameter: 7 cm, aneurysm resected
?	Prednisolone 30–60 mg/day	24 months: alive and well, ESR: 45 mm/h, creatinine: 136 μmol/l, CT: improved
?	Prednisolone 30–60 mg/day	48 months: alive and well, ESR: 45 mm/h, creatinine: 296 μmol/l, CT: improved
?	Prednisolone 30–60 mg/day	24 months: alive and well, ESR: 14 mm/h, creatinine: 274 μmol/l, CT: improved
8	Prednisone 5 mg/day	8 months: alive and well 24 months: IAAA rupture (died)
6	Prednisone 5 mg/day	13 months: backache 31 months: minimal backache
3.9	Prednisolone 8 mg/day	6 weeks: alive and well, ESR <20 mm/h 3 months: alive and well 6 months: abdominal and loin pain, CT: unchanged 52 months: alive and well
3.5	Tamoxifen 10 mg/day	3 months: hydrocele improved, CT: unchanged 6 months: complete regression of hydrocele, CT: unchanged 12 months: bilateral hydrocele, ESR > 20 mm/h, CT: progression of fibrosis, IAAA diameter 3.8 cm., right hydronephrosis, aneurysm resected

steroids.[17,28,29,34,36,39,41–46] These studies offer different indications for steroid therapy at varying dosage. In some cases steroids are administered as an alternative to surgery (high surgical risk patients with small symptomatic IAAA; patients refusing surgery),[34,39,44,46] in others they serve as a preoperative treatment (patients with extensive retroperitoneal involvement[28,42,43]); in yet others, steroids are given postoperatively (patients with postoperative progression of the fibroinflammatory process; patients in whom aneurysm resection was abandoned due to extensive retroperitoneal involvement).[17,34,36,39,41–43,45] Some authors have advocated high doses of steroids,[46] while others recommend low doses.[17,34] These discrepancies account for the variance of clinical and radiological outcome in IAAA patients receiving steroid therapy.

Stella *et al.* recently introduced tamoxifen in the treatment of IAAA with severe interstitial collagen deposition.[44] Their proposal was based on the histological similarities between IAAA with a cell/fibrosis ratio <1[38] and other diseases characterized by fibrosis responding to tamoxifen treatment (desmoid tumours, retroperitoneal fibrosis).[47,48]

This chapter summarizes the rationale and clinical and radiological outcome of medical management of IAAA and its indications.

RATIONALE

The rationale of medical treatment of the parietal fibroinflammatory process of IAAA is based on the three hallmarks of these lesions: 1) composition of the parietal inflammatory process, 2) parietal thickening, 3) operative mortality and morbidity.

Inflammation in AAA

Non-specific AAA are characterized by severe disruption of the aortic wall which presents macroscopic thinning. This is largely due to an impairment of the extracellular matrix, especially quantitative changes in its two major components (elastin and collagen). Histological and biochemical studies of the AAA wall have disclosed both elastin depletion and a significant increase in insoluble collagen.[10,49–55] These changes may result from a genetic abnormality of the ratio between proteases and their inhibitors.[56,57]

Parietal inflammatory processes are among the factors which may determine or exacerbate changes in the extracellular matrix of the aortic wall. Collagen synthesis and deposition as well as elastin degradation are particularly enhanced in aortic lesions presenting histological features of a parietal inflammatory infiltrate.[54,56] The infiltrate is frequently found in histological analysis of aortic aneurysms,[10,11,56,58–60] encountered in 83.3% of aneurysms examined by Rijbroek *et al.*[60]

Inflammation in the wall of an AAA resembles a chronic inflammatory infiltrate. It is composed of a cell population in the active phase mainly comprising lymphocytes and macrophages[61] while large immunoglobilin deposits are found in the insterstitial space.[56] Since the extent of inflammatory infiltrate varies histologically, in 1981 Rose and Dent[10] classified the inflammation in relation to the severity of the infiltrate. This classification, recently updated by Rijbroek *et al.*,[60] divides the chronic parietal inflammation into different degrees according to which grade three (severe chronic inflammation) corresponds to histological evidence of the aneurysmatic lesions that Walker *et al.* defined as IAAA.[9] Histological findings in IAAA include a large inflammatory infiltrate which appeared to consist of lymphocytes, plasma cells and monocytes in the active phase, involving vasa and nerva vasorum.[9,13,30] These lesions also reveal immunoglobulin (IgG, IgM) deposition in the interstitial space.[13] The similarity in composition and distribution of the inflammatory infiltrate in the wall of AAA and IAAA led Rose and Dent[10] to define IAAA as an inflammatory 'variant' of 'atherosclerotic' aneurysms. This definition is based solely on the histological features of the aneurysm, especially its cell component. It readily applies to IAAA with histological features of a large inflammatory infiltrate (Fig. 1), but is less applicable to aneurysms which are macroscopically 'inflammatory'[9] and histologically characterized by severe fibrosis and mild inflammatory infiltrate[38] (Fig. 2). Although the inflammatory infiltrate is an important histological aspect and often the morphological and clinical hallmark of IAAA,[10,13,60] the walls of these lesions usually present a marked modification of the extracellular matrix resulting in massive collagen deposition.[54]

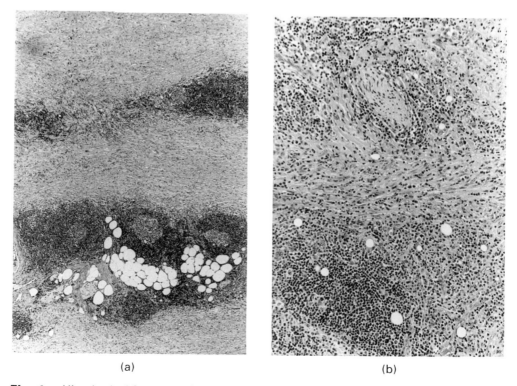

(a)   (b)

Fig. 1. Histological features of the media and adventitia of an IAAA with a cell/fibrosis ratio >1 (haematoxylin-eosin; a x 50, b x 136).

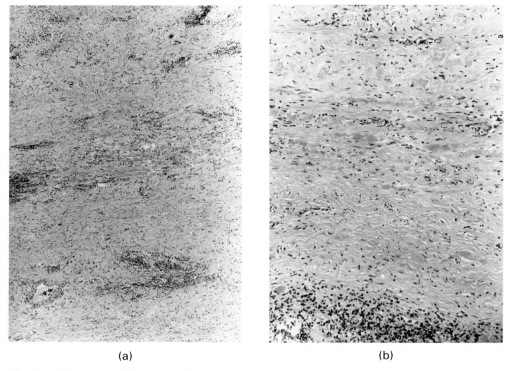

(a)   (b)

Fig. 2.   Histological features of the media and adventitia of an IAAA with a cell/fibrosis
ratio <1 (haematoxylin-eosin; a x 50, b x 136).

The parietal inflammatory process in IAAA is thus characterized by cellular and interstitial (collagen) components. The ratio between these two components (cells/fibrosis ratio) fluctuates with the cell component predominating in some IAAA and the interstitital component in others.[38] IAAA with a cell/fibrosis ratio >1 usually have a good clinical and radiological response to anti-inflammatory steroid treatment. When the ratio is <1, the predicted response is partial or absent. This may account for the negative clinical and radiological results obtained in the medical management of some IAAA.[17,28,29] In view of this, it is important to establish the cell/fibrosis ratio before drug therapy. Our approach envisages ^{99m}Tc hexamethylpropylene amioneoxime (HM-PAO)-labelled leukocyte scan[62] which determines leukocyte uptake by the aortic wall in the 4 hours following their administration (Fig. 3). No uptake signifies a large collagen deposition with a cell/fibrosis ratio < 1; patients with these findings cannot expect to benefit from steroid therapy[44] and should receive drugs which ensure a remission of parietal fibrosis. The successful treatment of desmoid tumours[47] and retroperitoneal fibrosis[48] with tamoxifen is encouraging for the use of this drug therapy for IAAA with mild chronic inflammatory infiltrate.[44]

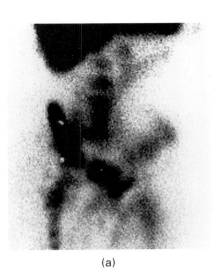 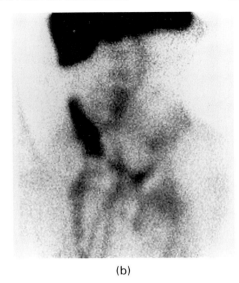

(a)   (b)

Fig. 3. [99m]Tc HM-PAO leukocyte-labelled scan of an IAAA. One hour after the administration of leukocytes, intense leukocyte uptake is visible anteriorly to the spine (a) persisting up to the fourth hour (b) (fibroinflammatory infiltrate with a cell/fibrosis ratio >1).

Parietal thickening and risk of IAAA rupture

The natural history of IAAA is characterized by the centrifugal development of the parietal fibroinflammatory process with involvement and entrapment of the periaortic structures (Fig. 4) and thickening of the wall which exceeds 0.5 cm (Fig.4).

Some investigators claim that this thickening of the aortic wall protects the aneurysm against rupture.[30,35] Indeed, Savarese et al.[35] noted a marked difference in the incidence of this complication between IAAA and AAA (7.7% vs 22%), a difference which proved statistically significant in a comparative study by Sterpetti et al. (3% vs 17%).[30]

Since the risk of IAAA rupture is low, some authors have advocated the medical management of small symptomatic IAAA (<4 cm).[39,44]

Mortality and morbidity in surgery for IAAA

Nitecki et al. recently published a case control study to define the postoperative outcome of IAAA and AAA approached by median transperitoneal laparotomy.[15] Their results show that the surgical morbidity and mortality of IAAA are significantly higher than the rates encountered in surgery for NSA, mortality being 6.8% and 0% and morbidity 45% and 26% for IAAA and AAA respectively.[15] Similar results were reported by Gaylis and Isaacson in 1989,[17] Fiorani et al. in 1990[32] and Lindblad et al. in 1991.[16] The higher incidence of mortality and morbidity in surgery for IAAA is mainly due to the high risk of iatrogenic injury entailed in surgical

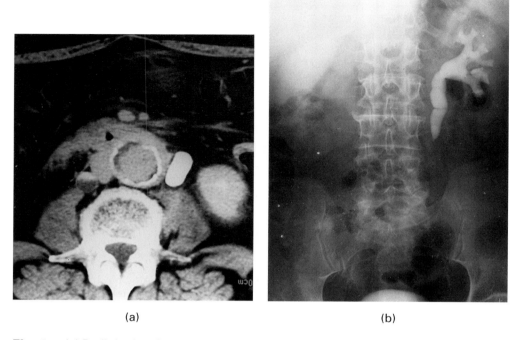

(a)   (b)

Fig. 4. (a) Radiological features of an IAAA. The abdominal aorta is dilated with a perianeurysmatic sheath extending over the anterior and both lateral surfaces of the aortic
wall. The inflammatory process involves the duodenum and inferior vena cava; both
ureters are dilated. (b) Intravenous urography in the same patient shows left
hydroureteronephrosis and functional exclusion of the right kidney.

dissection of IAAA.[14] In 1985 Pennel *et al.*[14] described damage to the duodenum in
4.7% of IAAA treated surgically, injury to the left renal vein in 3.2%, spleen in 2.4%,
ureters in 1.6%, inferior vena cava and small intestine in 0.8%.

Since the incidence of these complications is directly proportional to the extension
of the parietal fibroinflammatory process, some authors have recommended medical
treatment in patients with extensive retroperitoneal involvement either as the
treatment of choice (small symptomatic IAAA)[44] or prior to resection (IAAA >4cm in
diameter).[42,43]

CLINICAL AND RADIOLOGICAL RESULTS

The results of medical treatment of perianeurysmatic fibrosis of IAAA are assessed in
terms of remission of symptoms, inflammatory indices (ESR, C-reactive protein),
kidney function and the radiological features of the perianeurysmatic inflammatory
rind and the periaortic structures it envelops.

In the following section we summarize the results of medical therapy in the management of IAAA divided into groups on the basis of therapeutic indications.

Medical therapy as an alternative to surgery

Medical therapy was deemed an alternative to surgery in two groups of patients: a) patients refusing surgery,[34] b) patients at high surgical risk with small symptomatic IAAA.[39,44] The overall results of this approach were positive irrespective of the drug chosen or the administered dose. Steroid therapy in these patients led to a remission of symptoms with normalization of ESR, kidney function and release of the ureters. Benefit from drug therapy appeared within 7–10 days in patients treated at high doses (prednisolone 30–60 mg daily)[46] and in a few weeks in those who received low doses of steroids (prednisone 10 mg daily, prednisolone 8-10 mg daily).[34,39,44] These results contrast with those of Suy et al.[28] and Hill and Charlesworth[29] who reported unsuccessful steroid treatment in three IAAA. However, these reports did not include clinical and radiological data on the aneurysms or the type of drug treatment used which precludes any comparison with the findings of studies by Baskerville et al.,[34] Clyne and Abercrombie,[39] Stella et al.[44] and Higgins et al.[46]

According to Higgins et al.[46] steroid treatment should be prolonged at low doses (prednisolone 5–10 mg/day) for about 2 years since suspension of therapy within this period could result in a recurrence of symptoms leading to kidney failure.[46] Such a long treatment, however, must be monitored to exclude the possible side-effects of chronic steroid administration.[63,64]

Medical therapy prior to aneurysm resection

This indication is only recommended in patients presenting an inflammatory process with extensive retroperitoneal involvement in whom surgery for IAAA is indicated. Medical management reduced the parietal thickening and the extension of the inflammatory process, making the periaortic inflammatory tissue less fibrotic.[42] In this pathologic condition, dissection of the aneurysm and its replacement with a graft are facilitated. Hedges and Bentley[43] advocated the surgical treatment of IAAA after 6 months of steroid therapy with prednisolone (15 mg daily for 8 weeks; 5 mg daily thereafter).[42] Feldberg and Hene resected an aneurysm after high doses of methylprednisolone and prednisone (methylprednisolone 1g i.v. four times with prednisone 100 mg daily).[43] In both instances steroid therapy was instituted after failure to resect an aneurysm due to extensive perianeurysmal fibrosis. Laparotomy performed after steroid treatment disclosed a marked improvement in the pathological features of the retroperitoneum which proved surgically accessible allowing aortic reconstruction.

Contrasting results have been reported by other investigators. Sethia and Darke[41] performed laparotomy for aneurysm resection after 3 months of steroid therapy. Despite medical treatment (drug and dosage not reported), their attempt to reconstruct the aorta was abandoned due to the fibrosis of periaortic inflammatory tissue and the high risk of damage to venous structures adjacent to the aorta.[41] Gaylis and Issacson[17] were also forced to abandon aortic reconstruction despite preoperative administration of 5 mg/day prednisone and access to the IAAA via the left extraperitoneal approach.

Medical therapy after surgery

Medical treatment has also been recommended as a postoperative treatment for IAAA in two clinical presentations: a) patients in whom aortic reconstruction was abandoned intraoperatively due to retroperitoneal fibrosis and b) patients who present postoperative clinical and radiological progression of perianeurysmal fibrosis.

The first indication applies to IAAA electively operated, but where there is a high risk of serious complications to periaortic structures. While some authors do not administer any treatment in this situation,[9,14,40] others prefer to give steroids to accelerate clinical and radiological regression of the inflammatory infiltrate.[17,34,39,41] Accordingly, Baskerville et al.[34] administered prednisone 5mg/twice a day in four patients (Table 1). Within a few weeks, all patients had a full remission of preoperative symptoms, a normalization of ESR and release of the ureters. Computed tomography (CT) findings also disclosed major changes with a gradual regression of the fibroinflammatory tissue in follow-up scans over subsequent months. Although this finding reflects drug efficacy, it enhances the risk of aneurysm rupture, a complication encountered in 20% of IAAA treated with steroids.[34]

In about 2% of IAAA which are repaired, there is evidence of postoperative progression of the parietal fibroinflammatory tissue.[38] This evolution gives rise to clinical postoperative symptoms directly correlated to the extension of the inflammatory process and the involvement of periaortic structures (bowel, ureters).[36,45] Only two literature reports describe postoperative clinical and radiological progression of the periaortic inflammatory infiltrate. In the first patient, reported by Stotter et al.,[36] symptoms appeared 22 days after aneurysm resection; in the second, reported, by Baskerville and Prowse,[45] symptoms appeared 4 months after surgery. Steroid therapy led to a full remission of symptoms with release of the ureters in both patients. Stotter's patient also showed a marked improvement in radiological findings after 4 weeks of steroid treatment.[36]

Personal experience

In the last decade (January 1986 to August 1996) 1598 AAAs were treated at the Vascular Surgery Unit of the Department of Surgical and Anaethesiological Sciences at the University of Bologna. Of these, 82 (5.1%) had radiological and/or macroscopic features diagnostic for IAAA. Two lesions were small (<4cm) symptomatic IAAA at high surgical risk and these were treated by medical management (Table 1).[44]

Case 1

A 67-year-old male, smoker, under dialysis since 1985 for chronic kidney failure was hospitalized in 1989 for hyperpyrexia and abdominal-lumbar pain. An abdominal ultrasound scan and a CT scan revealed an infrarenal aortic aneurysm (diameter 3.9 cm) and a left hydroureteronephrosis (Figs. 5, 6). A soft-tissue rind (inflammatory tissue) surrounded the aneurysm extending as far as the origin of the common iliac arteries and involved their first segment (Fig. 6); the left ureter appeared to be entrapped by the left periiliac inflammatory tissue (Fig. 6). In 1990 the patient underwent a left nephrectomy. In 1991 the patient presented with abdominal-lumbar

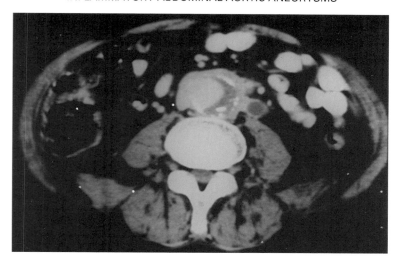

Fig. 5. Case 1. CT scan of the infrarenal abdominal aorta. The abdominal aorta is dilated and its wall shows the typical four-layer aspect of IAAA (lumen, thrombus, parietal calcifications, perianeurysmatic inflammatory sheath). The left ureter is entrapped within the perianeurysmal fibroinflammatory process and shows hydroureteronephrosis (from ref 44, with permission).

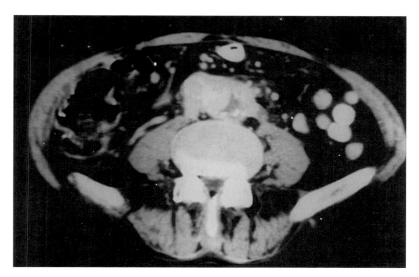

Fig. 6. Case 1. CT scan of the aortic bifurcation. An aneurysm can be seen in the left common iliac artery together with a large bilateral periiliac fibroinflammatory process. The left ureter is entrapped within the left periiliac inflammatory mantle (from ref. 44, with permission).

pain with increased ESR and C-reactive protein; an abdominal CT scan revealed no changes of the aortic diameter and periaortic inflammation. The patient was referred to our department.

Cardiological examination revealed left ventricular hypertrophy, while a chest X-ray and respiratory function tests identified signs of obstructive lung disease and a 22% restrictive ventilatory deficit. A ^{99m}Tc HM-PAO leukocyte scan[62] revealed persistent leukocyte deposition on the distal third of the aorta (cell/fibrosis ratio > 1) (Fig. 7). In view of CT appearance of the aortic lesion (diameter < 4 cm, no blister) and renal failure, non-operative management was instituted and prednisolone 8 mg daily was given. After 45 days there was a complete remission of pain and normalization of ESR; the leukocyte scan revealed absence of the aortic uptake. The patient was evaluated by ultrasound scan at 3-month intervals during the first year and at 6-month intervals thereafter, with CT scans every 6 months. At 3 months the patient was pain-free and the aneurysm showed no morphological alterations. At 6 months the patient presented with abdominal-lumbar pain but no radiological alteration of the aneurysm and inflammation The patient was treated with prednisolone which produced a total remission of symptoms. At 40 months the clinicoradiological picture was unchanged.

Case 2

A 52-year-old male, smoker, was referred to us in November 1992 with a small inflammatory aneurysm of the abdominal aorta.

The aortic lesion had been identified during abdominal ultrasound and CT scans performed, elsewhere, to identify the aetiopathogenesis of bilateral hydrocele

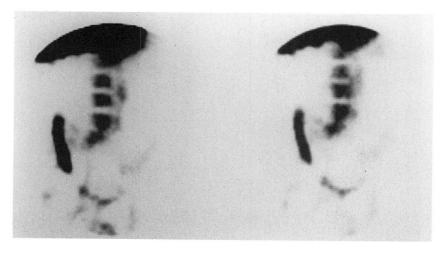

Fig. 7. Case 1. [99m]Tc HM-PAO leukocyte-labelled scan of the abdominal aorta. Anteriorly to the spine there is strong uptake of labelled leukocyte at the second and fourth hour (fibroinflammatory infiltrate with a cell/fibrosis ratio > 1) (from ref. 44, with permission).

associated with left abdominal and lumbar pain. The radiologic investigation revealed a 3.5 cm aneurysm on the abdominal aorta (Fig. 8), dilatation of both common iliac arteries, periaortic (Fig. 8) and periiliac inflammatory mantle. The non-operative management was instituted (prednisolone 8 mg daily); after 5 months there was still no improvement in the clinical and radiological features.

In our department the patient was subjected to cardiological examination which revealed concentric hypertrophy of the left ventricle and a 25% ejection fraction together with slight aortic and pulmonary insufficiency. Blood tests revealed that ESR, C-reactive protein, kidney and liver function parameters were all within normal limits. A chest X-ray and respiratory function tests revealed obstructive lung disease and an 18% restrictive ventilatory deficit. A 99mTc HM-PAO leukocyte scan[62] revealed an absence of aortic and iliac uptake in the fourth hour (cell/fibrosis ratio < 1) (Fig. 9).

The small size of the aneurysm as well as the patient's heart disease suggested a non-operative management; the results of the leukocyte scan led us to replace the steroid treatment with tamoxifen (20 mg daily).

The patient was evaluated by ultrasound scan at 3-month intervals during the first year and at 6-month intervals thereafter, with CT scans every 6 months. At 3 months we found partial regression of the hydrocele but no change in the radiological features. At 6 months the hydrocele was completely cured but the radiological picture had still not changed. We therefore reduced the tamoxifen dose (10 mg daily).

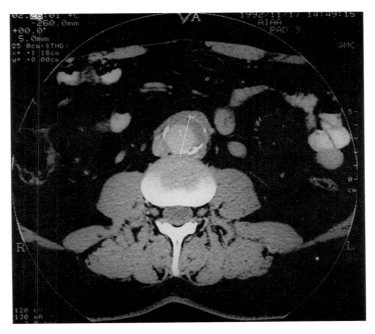

Fig. 8. Case 2. CT of the infrarenal abdominal aorta. The abdominal aorta is dilated and its wall presents the typical four-layer feature of IAAA (from ref. 44, with permission).

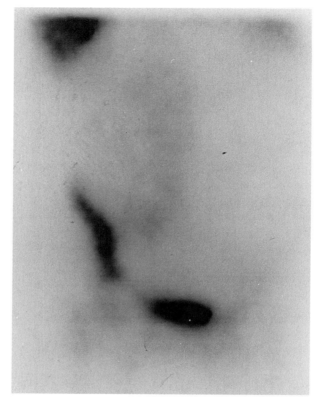

Fig. 9. Case 2. ^{99m}Tc HM-PAO leucocyte-labelled scan. At the fourth hour no leukocyte uptake is visible anteriorly to the spine (fibroinflammatory infiltrate with a cell/fibrosis ratio <1) (from ref. 44, with permission).

At 12 months we found a new bilateral hydrocele together with increased ESR and C-reactive protein and a further reduction in kidney function (blood creatinine 1.9 mg/dl, blood nitrogen 0.89 g/l). Meanwhile the CT scan of the abdomen revealed an increase in the diameter of the aorta (diameter 3.8 cm) and a pronounced centrifugal development of the periarterial inflammatory process at aortic and right iliac artery levels (Fig. 10); entrapment of the right ureter with hydroureteronephrosis, functional exclusion of the kidney and reduced cortical thickness were evident (Fig. 11). The leukocyte scan revealed significant leukocyte uptake on the aorta, the right common iliac artery and on terminal ileum (Fig. 12). We therefore inserted a right ureteral stent that to restore kidney function. The ventricular ejection fraction had improved to 40%. Therefore we elected to implant an aortic prosthesis. Given the morphology of the right kidney and the appendix we performed a right nephrectomy and an appendectomy simultaneously. After 30 days we observed partial regression of the bilateral hydrocele, normal ESR and C-reactive protein levels and improved kidney function (blood creatinine 1.4 mg/dl, blood nitrogen 0.45 g/l).

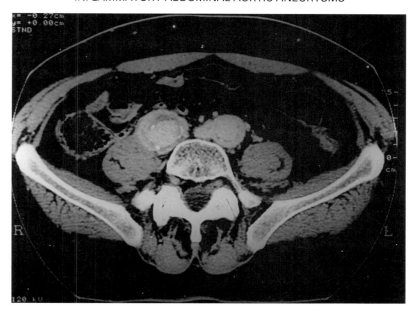

Fig. 10.   Case 2. CT scan of the common iliac arteries. Both common iliac arteries are dilated with a thick periiliac inflammatory sheath. On the right the ureter appears entrapped within the periiliac fibroinflammatory infiltrate (from ref. 44, with permission).

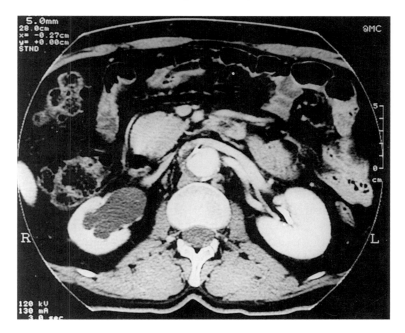

Fig. 11.   Case 2. CT scan of juxtarenal abdominal aorta. The aorta does not appear aneurysmal. There is hydroureteronephrosis with functional exclusion of the right kidney and cortical kidney thinning (from ref. 44, with permission).

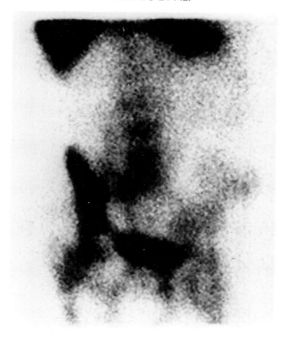

Fig. 12.   Case 2. 99mTc HM-PAO leukocyte-labelled scan.
At the fourth hour there is strong leukocyte uptake in the
terminal aorta, right common iliac artery and an ileal loop
in the right iliac fossa (fibroinflammatory infiltrate with
cell/fibrosis ratio >1) (from ref. 44, with permission).

At 3 months the hydrocele had completely disappeared while ESR, Creactive protein
and kidney function had not changed. The patient died of a myocardial infarct 6
months after surgery.

CURRENT INDICATIONS

Although some investigators claim that surgery is the only treatment for
inflammatory aneurysms,[24,29] medical treatment for IAAA may have a place in
certain clinical situations as an adjunct or alternative to a graft.

Medical treatment may provide an alternative to surgery for symptomatic IAAA in
patients refusing surgery or for small (<4 cm) symptomatic IAAA at low risk of
rupture[65] in patients at high surgical risk because of associated cardiopulmonary or
renal disease.[66] As medical therapy does not reduce the risk of aneurysm rupture or
the risk of increase in aneurysm diameter and the evolution of the inflammatory
process is unpredictable (case 2), clinical and radiological monitoring is mandatory
in these patients frequent intervals (not exceeding 6 months). The onset of signs of
parietal rupture or a reduced surgical risk in patients with an increased diameter of

the aneurysm and/or periaortic inflammatory mantle warrants prompt surgical resection.

For patients presenting extensive perianeurysmal fibrosis with retroperitoneal involvment without contraindications to surgery, short-term (2–3 months) preoperative medical therapy can be instituted. Lastly, medical therapy can also be given postoperatively following surgical resection of the aneurysm when there is clinical and/or radiological evidence of progression of the fibroinflammatory infiltrate.

REFERENCES

1. James TGI: Uremia due to aneurysm of the abdominal aorta. *Br J Urol* **7:** 157, 1935
2. DeWeerd JH, Ringer MG Jr, Pool TL, Gambill EE: Aortic aneurysm causing bilateral ureteral obstruction: report of case. *J Urol* **74:** 78–81, 1955
3. Shumacker HB Jr, Garrett R: Obstructive uropathy from abdominal aortic aneurysm. *Surg Gynecol Obstet* **100:** 758–761, 1955
4. Abercrombie GF, Hendry WF: Ureteric obstruction due to perianeurysmal fibrosis. *Br J Urol* **43:** 170–173, 1971
5. Albers DD, Bettaglio A: Ureteral obstruction from an unsuspected aortic aneurysm: case report. *J Urol* **85:** 249–250, 1961
6. Boontje AH, Groenwold H, Hekking JH: Ureteral obstruction secondary to abdominal aortic aneurysm. *J Cardiovasc Surg* **15:** 606–610, 1974
7. Branch WT, Turley K, Crowell BH et al.: Aortic aneurysm with a retroperitoneal fibrosis and ureteral obstruction. *Urology* **9:** 299–302, 1977
8. Darke SG, Glass RE, Eadie DGA: Abdominal aortic aneurysm: perianeurysmal fibrosis and ureteric obstruction and deviation. *Br J Surg* **64:** 649–652, 1977
9. Walker DJ, Bloor K, Williams G et al.: Inflammatory aneurysms of the abdominal aorta. *Br J Surg* **59:** 609–614, 1972
10. Rose AG, Dent DM: Inflammatory variant of abdominal atherosclerotic aneurysm. *Arch Pathol Lab Med* **105:** 409–413, 1981
11. Mitchinson MJ: Chronic periaortitis and periarteritis. *Histopathology* **8:** 589–600, 1984
12. McMahon JN, Davies JD, Scott DJA et al.: The microscopic features of inflammatory abdominal aortic aneurysms: Discriminant analysis. *Histopathology* **16:** 557–564, 1990
13. Stella A, Gargiulo M, Pasquinelli G et al.: The cellular component in the parietal infiltrate of inflammatory abdominal aortic aneurysms (IAAA). *Eur J Vasc Surg* **5:** 65–70, 1991
14. Pennell RC, Hollier LH, Lie JT et al.: Inflammatory abdominal aortic aneurysms: a thirty-year review. *J Vasc Surg* **2:** 859-69, 1985
15. Nitecki SS, Hallett JW, Stanson AW et al.: Inflammatory abdominal aortic aneurysms: a case-control study. *J Vasc Surg* **23:** 860–869, 1996.
16. Lindblad B, Almgren B, Bergqvist D et al.: Abdominal aortic aneurysm with perianeurysmal fibrosis: experience from 11 Swedish vascular centers. *J Vasc Surg* **13:** 231–239, 1991
17. Gaylis H, Isaacson C: Abdominal aortic inflammatory aneurysms. In: Bergan JJ, Yao JST (Eds) *Aortic Surgery* pp. 267–292. Philadelphia: WB Saunders, 1989
18. Leu HJ: Inflammatory abdominal aortic aneurysms: a disease entity? Histological analysis of 60 cases of inflammatory aortic aneurysms of unknown aetiology. *Virchows Arch A Pathol Anat Histopathol* **417:** 427–433, 1990
19. West AB, Patch MRC, Ryan PC et al.: Inflammatory aortic aneurysm: report of a case suggesting athero-ischemic aetiology. *J Cardiovasc Surg* **29:** 213–215, 1988
20. Duckett G, Laperriere J, Fontaine S et al.: Anevrisme inflammatoire de l'aorta. Utilité de la tomodensitometrie et de l'echographie dans le diagnostic d'un cas et revue de la litterature. *J Radiol* **67:** 911–915, 1986

21. Tanaka S, Komori K, Okadome K *et al.*: Detection of active cytomegalovirus infection in inflammatory aortic aneurysms with RNA polymerase chain reaction. *J Vasc Surg* **20:** 235–243, 1994

22. Pasquinelli G, Preda P, Gargiulo M *et al.*: An immunohistochemical study of inflammatory abdominal aortic aneurysms. *J Submicrosc Cytol Pathol* **25:** 103–112, 1993

23. Newman KM, Jean-Claude J, Li H *et al.*: Cytokines that activate proteolysis are increased in abdominal aortic aneurysms. *Circulation* **90:** II224–II227, 1994

24. Crawford JL, Stowe CL, Safi HJ *et al.*: Inflammatory aneurysms of the aorta. *J Vasc Surg* **2:** 113–124, 1985

25. Kittredge RD, Gordon R: Inflammatory aneurysm of aorta: development documented by computed tomography. *J Comput Tomogr* **11:** 128–131, 1987

26. Latifi HR, Heihen JP: CT of inflammatory abdominal aortic aneurysm: development from an uncomplicated atherosclerotic aneurysm. *J Comput Assist Tomogr* **16:** 484–486, 1992

27. Pistolese GR, Ippoliti A, PienaBarca A *et al.* Può un aneurisma infiammatorio dell'aorta addominale rappresentare l'evoluzione di un aneurisma aterosclerotico? Caso clinico. *G Ital Chir Vasc* **2:** 129–135, 1995

28. Suy R, Vanvambeke K, De Gheldere C *et al.*: Anevrismes inflammatoires de l'aorte abdominale sous-renale. In: Kieffer E (Ed) *Les anevrismes de l'aorte abdominale sous-renale* pp. 357–365. Paris: AERCV, 1990

29. Hill J, Charlesworth D: Inflammatory abdominal aortic aneurysms: a report of thirty-seven cases. *Ann Vasc Surg* **2:** 352–357, 1988

30. Sterpetti AV, Hunter WJ, Feldhaus RJ *et al.*: Inflammatory aneurysms of the abdominal aorta: incidence, pathologic, and etiologic consideration. *J Vasc Surg* **9:** 643–650, 1989

31. Boontje AH, van den Dungen J, Blanksma C: Inflammatory abdominal aortic aneurysms. *J Cardiovasc Surg* **31:** 611–616, 1990

32. Fiorani P, Lauri D, Faraglia V *et al.*: The recognition and management of the non-specific European inflammatory aortic aneurysm. In: Greenhalgh RM, Mannick JA (Eds) T*he Cause and Management of Aneurysms* pp. 189–202. Philadelphia: WB Saunders, 1990

33. Vint VC, Usselman JA, Warmath MA, Dilley RB: Aortic perianeurysmal fibrosis: CT density enhancement and ureteral obstruction. *Am J Roentgenol* **134:** 577–580, 1980

34. Baskerville PA, Blakeney CG, Young AE *et al.*: The diagnosis and treatment of peri-aortic fibrosis. (inflammatory aneurysms). *Br J Surg* **70:** 381–385, 1983

35. Savarese RP, Rosenfeld JC, DeLaurentis DA: Inflammatory abdominal aortic aneurysm. *Surg Gynec Obstet* **162:** 405–410, 1986

36. Stotter AT, Grigg MJ, Mansfield AO: The response of peri-aneurysmal fibrosis – the "inflammatory" aneurysm – to surgery and steroid therapy. *Eur J Vasc* **4:** 201–205, 1990

37. Nachbur B, Marincek B, Jacob R *et al.*: The impact of computed tomography in the diagnosis and postoperative follow-up of ureteric obstruction in aorto-iliac aneurysmal disease. *Eur J Vasc Surg* **3:** 475–492, 1989

38. Stella A, Gargiulo M, Faggioli GL *et al.*: Postoperative course of inflammatory abdominal aortic aneurysms. *Ann Vasc Surg* **7:** 229–238, 1993

39. Clyne CAC, Abercrombie GF: Perianeurysmal retroperitoneal fibrosis: two cases responding to steroids. *Br J Urol* **49:** 463–467, 1977

40. Goldstone J, Malone JM: Inflammatory aneurysms of the abdominal aorta. *Surgery* **83:** 425–430, 1978

41. Sethia B, Darke SG: Abdominal aortic aneurysm with retroperitoneal fibrosis and ureteric entrapment. *Br J Surg* **70:** 434–436, 1983

42. Feldberg MAM, Hene RJ: Perianeurysmal fibrosis and its response to corticosteroid treatment: a computed tomography follow up in one case. *J Urol* **130:** 1163–1164, 1983

43. Hedges AR, Bentley PG: Resection of inflammatory aneurysm after steroid therapy. *Br J Surg* **73:** 374, 1986

44. Stella A, Gargiulo M, Faggioli GL *et al.*: Antiinfiammatori ed antiestrogeni nel trattamento di due aneurismi infiammatori dell'aorta addominale. *G Ital Chir Vasc* **3:** 45–55, 1996

45. Baskerville PA, Browse NL: Peri-aortic fibrosis: progression and regression. *J Cardiovasc Surg* **28:** 30–31, 1987

46. Higgins PM, Bennett-Jones DN, Naish PF, Aber GM: Non-operative management of retroperitoneal fibrosis. *Br J Surg* **75:** 573–577, 1988
47. Kinzbrunner B, Ritter S, Domingo J, Rosenthal CJ: Remission of rapidly growing desmoid tumors after tamoxifen therapy. *Cancer* **52:** 2201–2204, 1983
48. Clark CP, Vanderpool D Preskitt JT: The response of retroperitoneal fibrosis to tamoxifen. *Surgery* **109:** 502–506, 1991
49. Bussuttil RW, Rinderbriecht H, Flescher A, Carmack C: Elastase activity: the role of elastase in aortic aneurysm formation. *J Surg Res* **32:** 214–217, 1982
50. Campa JS, Greenhalgh RM, Powell JT: Elastin degradation in abdominal aortic aneurysms. *Atherosclerosis* **65:** 13–21, 1987
51. Menashi S, Campa JS, Greenhalgh RM, Powell JT: Collagen in abdominal aortic aneurysm: typing, content and degradation. *J Vasc Surg* **6:** 578–582, 1987
52. Rizzo RJ, McCarthy WJ, Dixit SN *et al.*: Collagen types and matrix protein content in human abdominal aortic aneurysms. *J Vasc Surg* **10:** 365–373, 1989
53. Powell JT, Greenhalgh RM: Cellular, enzymatic and genetic factors in the pathogenesis of abdominal aortic aneurysms. *J Vasc Surg* **9:** 297–304, 1989
54. Gargiulo M, Stella A, Spina M *et al.*: Content and turnover of extracellular matrix protein in human 'non-specific' and 'inflammatory' abdominal aortic aneurysms. *Eur J Vasc Surg* **7:** 546–553, 1993
55. Cenacchi G, Guiducci G, Pasquinelli G *et al.*: The morphology of elastin in non-specific and inflammatory abdominal aortic aneurysms. A comparative transmission, scanning and immunoelectronmicroscopy study. *J Submicrosc Cytol Pathol* **27:** 75–81, 1995
56. Brophy CM, Reilly JM, Smith GJW, Tilson MD: The role of inflammation in nonspecific abdominal aortic aneurysm disease. *Ann Vasc Surg* **5:** 229–233, 1991
57. Powell JT, Greenhalgh RM: Genetic variation chromosome 16 and the growth of abdominal aortic aneurysms. In: Yao JST, Pearce WH (Eds) *Technologies in Vascular Surgery* pp. 40–46. Philadelphia: WB Saunders, 1992
58. Beckman EN: Plasma cell infiltrates in atherosclerotic abdominal aortic aneurysms. *Am J Clin Pathol* **85:** 21–24, 1986
59. Imakita M, Yutani C, Ishibashi-Ueda H, Nakajima N: Atherosclerotic abdominal aortic aneurysms: a comparative data of different types based on the degree of inflammatory reaction. *Cardiovasc Pathol* **1:** 65–73, 1992
60. Rijbroek A, Moll FL, Dijk HAV *et al.*: Inflammation of the abdominal aortic aneurysm wall. *Eur J Vasc Surg* **8:** 41–46.
61. Ramshaw AL, Parums DV: Immunohistochemical characterization of inflammatory cells associated with advanced atherosclerosis. *Histopathology* **17:** 543–552, 1990
62. Gargiulo M, Levorato M, Faggioli GL *et al.*: Aneurismi infiammatori dell'aorta addominale: ruolo diagnostico della scintigrafia con leucociti marcati. *Atti XVII Congresso Nazionale SIRC* pp. 127–131. Trieste: OCT Editore, 1992
63. Tiptaft RC, Costello AJ, Paris AMI, Blandy JP: The long-term follow-up of retroperitoneal fibrosis. *Br J Urol* **54:** 620–634, 1982
64. Mitchinson MJ, Withycombe JFR, Arden Jones R: The response of idiopathic retroperitoneal fibrosis to corticosteroids. *Br J Urol* **43:** 444–449, 1971
65. Faggioli GL, Stella A, Gargiulo M *et al.*: Morphology of small aneurysms: definition and impact on risk of rupture. *Am J Surg* **168:** 131–135, 1994
66. Johnston KW: Multicenter prospective study of nonruptured abdominal aortic aneurysm. Part II. Variables predicting morbidity and mortality. *J Vasc Surg* **9:** 437–447, 1989

Inflammation and the Aetiology of Abdominal Aortic Aneurysms

J. T. Powell

INTRODUCTION

Two opposing theories concerning the pathogenesis of abdominal aortic aneurysms (AAA) have been developed. For many years it has been assumed that environmental insults, particularly smoking, lead to aortic atherosclerosis and aneurysms are just one of the complications of atherosclerosis.[1-3] During the past decade the strong familial clustering of aneurysms has been recognized, leading to the hypothesis that AAA is a late onset genetic disorder.[4-8] It has proved difficult to identify the genes involved and although most of the evidence relates to mutations in type III collagen, such mutations are the cause of but few aortic aneurysms.[9-11] Few have considered that inflammation is an important factor in the pathogenesis of aortic aneurysms. In the light of recent evidence it is timely to redress this situation and consider how inflammation contributes to the development of AAA.[12-14]

Over 200 years ago Lancisi proposed that all aneurysms had a syphilitic aetiology and even at the beginning of this century, if a patient presented with an aortic aneurysm, usually in the thoracic aorta, syphilis was suspected.[15] Some 20 years ago when DeBakey reviewed a series of 100 consecutive patients with ascending aortic aneurysm only 10% had a syphilitic aetiology.[16] Today syphilis almost is forgotten. In 1955 the American Society for the Study of Arteriosclerosis provided the following definition for syphilitic arteriopathy: 'Widespread vascular abnormalities characterized principally by adventitial cellular infiltration, especially by plasma cells. . . . In the aorta, the gross changes follow on obliteration of vasa vasorum and consist in destruction of the elastica with a tendency to aneurysm formation'.[17] Aneurysm formation was attributed to an immunoinflammatory response to the spirochete, localized in the adventitia. Contemporary studies of coronary arteries, published a year later, provided evidence for the hypothesis that focal adventitial infiltrations in the coronary arteries were caused by a state of anoxia.[18] Spasm or occlusion of a coronary artery was suggested to cause local anoxia in the adventitia, with subsequent lymphocytic infiltration of the adventitia. This hypothesis is consistent with the observation that cellular infiltration of the human arterial adventitia is associated with atheromatous plaques.[19] These observations have been neglected, perhaps because the striking atherosclerotic changes in the diseased intima have diverted attention away from the medial and outer layers of the vessel wall. The adventitia of the abdominal aorta, with its sparse vasa vasorum,[20] may be particularly susceptible to anoxic injury and hence aneurysmal dilatation.

Adventitial inflammation is a feature of almost all AAA although the amount of inflammation is very variable.[21] There is the possibility that active inflammation is associated with active disease and dilatation and that little inflammation represents early, static or 'burnt out' end-stage disease. Many vascular surgeons consider that the inflammatory aortic aneurysm is a separate entity from the common atherosclerotic AAA. Certainly surgical repair is technically more difficult when ureters and other retroperitoneal structures have become adherent to the dense adventitial fibrotic inflammatory tissue and the disease process has been considered a variant of retroperitoneal fibrosis.[22] The intensity of the inflammatory response in retroperitoneal fibrosis, with foci of lymphocytes and plasma cells, has caused pathologists to consider whether this was a response to specific antigens, including oxidized lipoproteins, which had breached the intima and media of the aortic wall.[23] Many of these patients have high titres of antibodies to oxidized low density lipoproteins (LDL) but high titres of these antibodies are common in patients with other manifestations of atherosclerosis, including carotid atherosclerosis.[23,24]

Several studies have shown that the extent of inflammation is a factor which discriminates AAA from occlusive aortic atherosclerosis. Serum markers of inflammation, including C-reactive protein and soluble intercellular adhesion molecule 1 (ICAM-1) are present at higher concentrations in patients with AAA than in patients with occlusive aortic atherosclerosis.[25,26] Histopathological investigations also have shown that inflammatory infiltration of the media and adventitia is much more prominent in the aneurysmal wall than in atherosclerotic aorta.[12] The detailed description of the inflammatory infiltrate in the media and adventitia varies in different patient series, although macrophages always are prominent. Koch *et al.* provide a detailed description of the T cells present in the outer aneurysmal wall: the presence of CD3 positive T cells was a feature which distinguished aneurysms from normal and occluded atherosclerotic aorta.[12] The CD4 positive : CD8 positive ratio was greater in aneurysmal tissue and CD19 positive lymphocytes (B cells) were present in all pathological tissues. The B cells were most prominent in atherosclerotic aneurysms rather than frank inflammatory aneurysms.[12] In contrast, Ramshaw and Parums have described the chronic inflammatory response in the vessel wall, with macrophages and B cells being the dominant cell types, together with the presence of B cell follicles in the adventitia of some aneurysmal aortas.[27] This is concordant with our own findings of a chronic inflammatory infiltrate in the outer aneurysmal wall,[14] with macrophage and B cells being common, together with the presence of scarcer plasma cells (Fig. 1).

The evidence to associate inflammation in the outer layers of the aortic wall with the presence of aortic aneurysm is strong. Two important questions need to be answered. First, is the chronic inflammatory response causative or consequential to the aneurysm dilatation? Second, is the inflammation a non-specific response or a response to specific antigens generated by disease in the aortic wall?

INFLAMMATION AND THE GROWTH OF ABDOMINAL AORTIC ANEURYSMS

For many studies the accepted definition of an AAA is a maximum infrarenal aortic diameter of >3cm. It has been difficult to obtain any evidence about the

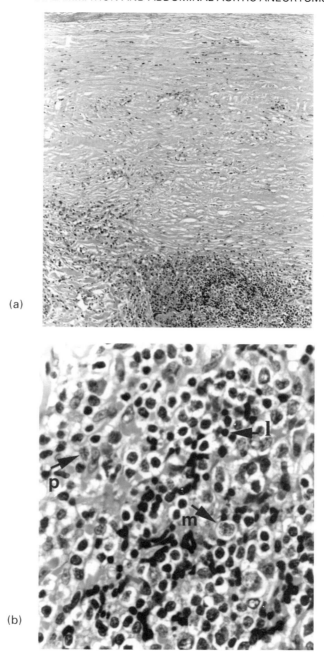

Fig. 1. The cellular infiltrate in an aneurysm wall. At lower power (a) the atheromatous intima is at the top, the fibrotic media contains scattered inflammatory cells and in the adventitia a lymphoid follicle is developing. At higher power (b) the lymphoid follicle is seen to contain macrophages (m), lymphocytes (l) and plasma cells (p).

pathophysiology of these early aneurysms, since they are too small for surgeons to consider surgical repair. Many surgeons will not consider surgical repair until the aneurysm diameter is >5.5cm in diameter. In these large aneurysms the disease process is well advanced and the separation of underlying cause and the response to the cause and consequent connective tissue remodelling becomes impossible. There has been a considerable debate concerning the benefits of operating on smaller aneurysms, between 4.0 and 5.5 cm in diameter, where the disease process may not be as advanced. The UK Small Aneurysm Trial was established to determine whether early elective surgery or a period of ultrasound surveillance provided the better management for these smaller aneurysms.[28] This has provided the opportunity to investigate what histological, and other features, might discriminate between smaller and large aneurysms.

INFLAMMATION AND OTHER HISTOLOGICAL CHARACTERISTICS IN ANEURYSM BIOPSIES

Aortic biopsies were obtained from 64 patients undergoing elective repair of an AAA, where the maximum anterior–posterior aneurysm diameters, measured by ultrasonography ranged from 4 to 10cm (median 6.2cm). The biopsy (~1 x 2cm) was obtained from the anterior abdominal wall, opposite the origin of the inferior mesenteric artery, close to the point of maximum dilatation. The biopsy was subdivided for histology and biochemical studies. The histology was reported by a single pathologist, who described the specimens on a standard reporting form which included, degree of atherosclerosis (graded 0–3), wall thickness (in mm), plaque cholesterol, plaque and vessel calcification, haemosiderin, degree of medial and adventitial inflammation, (both graded from 0–3), fibrosis (graded from 0–3), vascularity of media and adventitia (both grade 0–3) and presence of bacteria. To obtain reassurance about the objectivity of the pathological grading, 6 biopsies were divided and sent for duplicate pathological descriptions.

Immunohistochemistry was used to determine the lineage of lymphocytes using formal saline fixed biopsies embedded in paraffin, using monoclonal antibodies to CD3 or CD22, to discriminate T and B lymphocytes respectively. Some sections were incubated with monoclonal antibodies to TNF-α to localize this proinflammatory cytokine.

Multivariate regression analysis was used to discern which histological features of the aneurysm wall were associated with wall thickness and maximum anterior–posterior aneurysm diameter. Associations between graded characteristics and aneurysm diameter or thickness also were assessed using the χ^2 test.

The aneurysm biopsies showed evidence of extensive atherosclerosis, graded either 2 or 3 in all biopsies. The blind reporting of thickness and other pathological characteristics, in the six biopsies sent in duplicate, was closely similar in the duplicates. The infiltration of both the media and the adventitia by inflammatory cells was very variable and the full extent of the grading range, 0–3, was used. The infiltrate was usually non-specific, with a mixture of macrophages and B cells: polymorphonuclear and other inflammatory cells were not prominent. Immunohistochemistry showed that the majority of the lymphocytes were of B cell lineage (CD22 positive). A dense network of capillaries was observed in the adventitia. In the most inflamed biopsies the endothelium of these capillaries showed positive staining for TNF-α, often with a perivascular cuff of TNF-α positive T-lymphocytes (Fig. 2).

Aneurysm diameter was associated significantly with the extent of adventitial inflammation (ANOVA, p=0.011), the largest aneurysms having the most inflammatory infiltrate. The distribution of grading for adventitial inflammation according to tertile of aneurysm diameter is shown in Table 1: diameter was associated with the extent of adventitial inflammation, χ^2 trend 8.61, p=0.018. After adjustment for the degree of atherosclerosis, medial inflammation, vascularity and adventitial fibrosis, adventitial inflammation remained as the only histological variable associated with aneurysm diameter, p=0.022. There was no evidence of bacteria, or other remarkable findings, in any of the biopsies.

The thickness of the aortic wall ranged from 0.2 to 0.8mm. The tendency for the larger aneurysms to have thicker walls did not achieve statistical significance (univariate analysis, p=0.089). The thickness of the aneurysmal wall was most closely associated with the amount of adventitial fibrosis (univariate analysis p=0.086, multivariate analysis p=0.005, Table 2).

In summary, this biopsy study clearly showed that smaller aneurysms had a lower density of inflammatory cells in the aortic wall than larger aneurysms. The inflammation was characteristic of a chronic response and there was a very significant association between aneurysm diameter and the extent of adventitial inflammation.

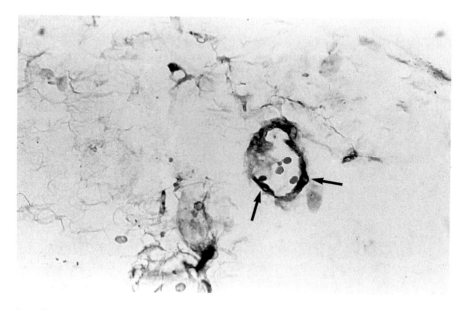

Fig. 2. Activated neovasculature in the adventitia. The endothelium of a new vessel in the adventitia shows positive staining for TNF-α (arrows).

Table 1.   Aneurysm diameter and adventital inflammation in 64 biopsies

Aneurysm diameter	Grading of adventitial inflammation			
(cm) tertile	0	1	2	3
4.0–5.5 (n=21)	7	9	4	1
5.6–6.5 (n=22)	2	10	10	0
6.6–10 (n=21)	0	10	9	2

$\chi^2 = 13.52$, p=0.035, χ^2 trend = 8.61, p=0.018.

Table 2.   Multivariate regression analysis for determinants of aneurysm wall thickness in 64 biopsies

Variable	Partial regression coefficient	p
Diameter	0.030	0.025
Atherosclerosis	0.034	0.419
Medial inflammation	0.012	0.648
Adventitial inflammation	−0.062	0.024
Vascularity	0.038	0.179
Adventitial fibrosis	0.065	0.005
Constant=0.127	F ratio=4.13	Probability level=0.003

CHRONIC INFLAMMATION – CAUSE OR CONSEQUENCE?

Inspection of any biopsy from an AAA reveals the extent of degeneration and vascular remodelling that has accompanied the dilatation of the aorta from 2 to 6 times the normal aortic diameter. This pathological picture is just one snapshot in time and may not always provide insight into the mechanism of disease. Comparison of the changes that have occurred when the aorta has dilated from its normal diameter (range 1.5–2.2cm) to 2–6 times this diameter is an alternative approach that we have exploited here. We have benefitted from access to biopsies of small aneurysms (4.0–5.5cm in diameter) from patients randomized to elective surgery in the UK Small Aneurysm Trial, which provided one-third of the biopsies in this series. In many centres only patients with larger aneurysms proceed to elective surgery.

As the aorta enlarges, and the risk of rupture increases, it might be assumed that, like a balloon, the aortic wall would become thinner. Our studies show that this premise is untrue. The larger aneurysms have thicker, but probably weaker, walls than the smaller aneurysms. These observations, even in the absence of detailed histology, underscore the extent of vascular remodelling that has taken place as the aorta dilates. More particularly, as the aorta dilates the media is attenuated and the increased thickness of aneurysmal walls results from compensatory adventitial remodelling and fibrosis. At a fixed arterial pressure load, this thickening of the aortic wall will act to reduce wall tension (Laplace's law). The fibrotic thickening of the adventitia appears to arise principally from vascular remodelling with which the deposition of new collagen fibres, which are not organized in concentric lamellae. Inflammation, through activation of cytokine cascades, could provide the stimulus for this remodelling. Inflammation also may be a response to atherosclerosis. In our study the extent of atherosclerosis and associated intimal inflammation was similar in biopsies from small and large aneurysms. The striking differences in inflammatory characteristics were observed in the adventitia and to a lesser extent in the media.

Our findings of the strong association between the density of inflammatory cells provide circumstantial evidence that the presence of these inflammatory cells contributes to aneurysmal dilatation. Since the growth rate of aneurysms may be exponential,[29] as the aneurysm dilates the density of inflammatory cells and the pace of vascular remodelling is likely to increase. Our study indicates that the growth of aneurysms is associated with an increased concentration of inflammatory cells in the adventitia, principally macrophages and B cells. These inflammatory cells are likely to be the source of both the increased amount of enzymes involved in vascular remodelling and a cascade of cytokines involved in the vascular remodelling.[30,31]

EXPERIMENTAL STUDIES OF INFLAMMATION AND ANEURYSM GROWTH

Our results showing a very significant association between aneurysm diameter and the extent of adventitial inflammation in aortic biopsies are mirrored by animal experiments, where non-specific activation of the immune system potentiates the growth of elastase-induced aneurysms in rats.[32] In these elastase-induced aneurysms the inflammatory response was observed in the media, where the cells were characterized as principally T cells and macrophages. The period of dilation of these experimental aneurysms covers the period of the first 2 weeks after the intraluminal instillation of elastase.[32] The inflammatory cells were observed during the period of active dilatation, but after the aortic diameter stabilized the inflammatory infiltrate regressed. Newer evidence also indicates that the infusion of a monoclonal antibody to the leucocyte adhesion molecule CD18 slows the expansion of these experimental aneurysms, without altering circulating neutrophil count.[33] These associations between inflammation and dilatation in experimental aneurysms provide stronger evidence that the inflammatory cells participate in the connective tissue destruction and remodelling which characterizes aneurysmal enlargement.

Other evidence on the important role of the macrophage in aneurysmal dilatation comes from a different animal model of aortic aneurysm, where aneurysms were induced in rabbits by periarterial application of calcium chloride.[34] The development of aneurysmal dilatation was associated with an influx of foamy, lipid laden macrophages into the adventitia and a reduction in collagen concentration.[34] In the absence of stimuli to activate macrophages there was thickening of the aortic wall without dilatation, whereas in the presence of thioglycollate and hypercholesterolaemic aneurysmal dilatation occurred. Activated macrophages appear to have a crucial role in experimentally induced aneurysms.

IS THE INFLAMMATORY RESPONSE SPECIFIC OR NON-SPECIFIC?

The inflammation which characterizes AAA is similar to that observed in chronic periaortitis, which is a local adventitial response associated with advanced atherosclerosis.[23] The first detailed description of the difference of inflammatory cells found in stenosing aortic atherosclerosis and aortic aneurysm was by Koch et al.[12] Aneurysmal tissue contained more inflammatory cells, both CD3 positive T cells and CD19 positive B cells were prominent in the adventitia of aneurysmal aorta but rare in stenosed aorta. The adventitia of aneurysmal aorta also was characterized by the presence of many CD11c positive macrophages, which were often surrounded by lymphoid aggregates. Koch et al.[12] suggested that this was the result of an immune-mediated response, with components of the elastic fibres of modified lipoproteins as potential antigens. Oxidized lipoproteins are known to be very antigenic and elastin peptides are chemotactic for inflammatory cells. In chronic periaortitis, antibodies to oxidized LDL are found in serum and it has been suggested that the adventitial response arises in response to oxidized lipids which have breached the media and stimulated an immune response in the outer layers of the vessel wall.[23] If the inflammation in the aneurysmal wall was a response to specific antigens, one would expect to find plasma cells in the infiltrate. Plasma cells are present in the inflammatory infiltrate (Fig. 1). If these plasma cells were secreting immunoglobulins in response to stimulation with a specific antigen(s), DNA analysis should reveal monoclonal or oligoclonal immunoglobulin genes. This can be investigated by a method known as 'immunoglobulin gene fingerprinting'.[35]

Methods have been described for the analysis of immunoglobulin genes using the polymerase chain reaction to amplify the VDJ region of the heavy chain.[35,36] We selected 20 aortic biopsies which had shown a heavy B lymphocyte infiltrate and purified genomic DNA from these samples, using a protocol with an extended proteinase K digestion; B cells and plasma cells are not a feature of the atherosclerotic plaque, so that contamination from this part of the biopsy does not provide a problem in analysis of B or plasma cell DNA. The purity of the DNA was assessed by agarose gel electrophoresis prior to amplification of the VDJ region using framework 3 primers.[36] A polyclonal control was provided by DNA prepared from tonsil and DNA from Raji cells (and other lymphoma cell lines) provided monoclonal controls. The PCR amplified products were analysed by polyacrylamide gel electrophoresis.

Analysis of 20 samples of aneurysm wall DNA has been performed (Fig. 3). The results clearly show that the immunoglobulin heavy chain genes are polyclonal in all samples, even those where distinct B cell follicles were present in the adventitia. This provides initial evidence that the inflammatory infiltrate is not in response to a limited number of tissue antigens (e.g. lastin fragments) or neoantigens (e.g. oxidized LDL). However, even in the well characterized autoimmune diseases only a proportion of the tissues analysed show evidence of monoclonal immunoglobulin heavy chain genes and use of the framework 2 primers, which we have used, may give a false negative result in up to 20% of samples. For these reasons we need to continue to analyse the variable region of the immunoglobulin heavy chain gene using framework 3 primers.[36] If this new analysis also demonstrates that all samples have polyclonal immunoglobulin genes, we shall have provided convincing evidence that the inflammatory response in the adventitia of aortic aneurysms is not

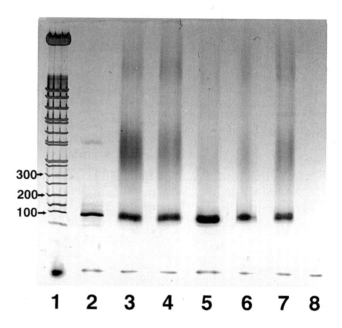

Fig. 3. Immunoglobulin gene fingerprinting. Amplification of DNA purified from four separate AAA biopsies are shown, together with DNA purified from Raji cells and tonsil and a negative control with no added DNA: lane 1: molecular weight markers (size in bp); lane 4: AAA DNA polyclonal smear; lane 5: AAA DNA polyclonal smear; lane 6: AAA DNA polyclonal smear; lane 7: AAA DNA polyclonal smear; lane 3: tonsil polyclonal control; lane 2: Raji cell monoclonal control; lane 8: negative control, no DNA.

a response to specific antigens such as oxidized LDL or elastin fragments. Such results would contradict the findings of Gregory *et al.*, who have suggested that, since antibodies to components of normal wall have been identified in aneurysm extracts, aortic aneurysm is an autoimmune disorder.[37] The DNA evidence will be more powerful.

INFLAMMATION AS A RESPONSE TO AORTIC WALL HYPOXIA

If we can exclude the possibility that the inflammation which characterizes the aneurysmal aortic wall is a response to specific antigens, we might consider whether the inflammation is a response to hypoxia. Cytokines coordinate the immune response. There is enhanced production of interleukins 1β and 8, monocyte chemoattractant protein-1 (MCP-1), and TNF-α in the aneurysmal wall.[36,37] The TNF-α plays an important role in the regulation of endothelial function, lymphocyte adhesion and trafficking. In aneurysmal tissue we have demonstrated the presence of TNF-α in and around mononuclear cells close to vasa vasorum in the adventitia and in the endothelial cells of new vessels (Fig. 2). The most potent chemoattractant for monocytes, MCP-1, can by synthesized by endothelium, smooth muscle cells and lymphocytes. Activated macrophages recruited into the adventitia also may synthesize and secrete TNF-α, so perpetuating the inflammatory response. There is evidence of extensive neovascularization in both the aortic media and the adventitia. This neovascularization may be stimulated by hypoxia. The cells of the normal aorta receive most of their oxygen and nutrients by diffusion from the lumen and there are only a limited number of vasa vasorum in the adventitia.[20] As the aneurysm enlarges, the lumen fills with dense laminated thrombus leaving a main flow channel of normal aortic calibre. This laminated thrombus may restrict the supply of oxygen and nutrients to the aortic wall, resulting in hypoxia: there are no reports concerning the oxygen tension in the aneurysmal aortic wall, although studies are underway in both the UK and the USA. Hypoxia is a potent stimulus to neovascularization.[38] Activation of this neovasculature would stimulate the recruitment of inflammatory cells into the adventitia. Amongst the growth factors which stimulate angiogenesis, vascular endothelial growth factor (VEGF) is probably the only one that acts exclusively by directly stimulating the endothelium. Hypoxia selectively upregulates the production of VEGF from vascular smooth muscle cells and enhances endothelial cell permeability, consequently allowing the migration of monocytes and other inflammatory cells into the vessel wall.

Currently, hypoxic stimulation of an activated neovasculature provides an attractive hypothesis for the origin of the inflammatory infiltrate in the adventitia of the aneurysmal aortic wall. Alternatively, recent evidence has suggested that cytomegalovirus infection might stimulate an intense inflammatory response in the vessel wall.[39]

CONCLUSIONS

The possibility that the recruitment of inflammatory cells into the aortic media is the critical pathology underlying aneurysmal dilatation has been raised in experimental studies of elastase-induced aneurysms.[31] The association between the extent of inflammatory infiltrate and aneurysm diameter has been confirmed in a human biopsy study, although the strongest association was between adventitial, rather than medial, inflammation and aortic diameter.[14] The inflammatory cells have the potential to synthesize and secrete both cytokines, which perpetuate the inflammatory response, and enzymes which participate in the continuing enlargement and remodelling of the vessel wall. Perhaps those aneurysms which have little evidence of inflammation through the aortic wall are 'burnt out', stable and not enlarging, which would account for the variable spectrum of the inflammatory infiltrate. The evidence to date suggests that the inflammation is chronic, although there is some dispute as to whether T cells or B cells are the most prominent lymphocyte, and that the macrophages are a source of potent enzymes which participate in connective tissue remodelling.[12,23,30]

Having established the crucial role of inflammation in aneurysm expansion some important clinical questions can be asked. First, do anti-inflammatory drugs limit aneurysm growth rates? Second, would imaging of aortic inflammation permit identification of rapidly growing aneurysms at high risk of rupture? Third, should a course of anti-inflammatory drugs precede the resection of any inflammatory aortic aneurysms? Fourth, does treatment with tetracycline analogues to inhibit the matrix metalloproteinases secreted by adventitial macrophages limit aneurysm growth? Some information on the first of these questions will be available when the aneurysm growth rates of patients in the observational arm of the UK Small Aneurysm Trial are analysed. Given the apparent increase in the incidence of AAA and the increasing longevity of the population these questions need urgent investigation.

ACKNOWLEDGEMENTS

Original research was supported by the British Heart Foundation. The immunoglobulin gene fingerprinting was performed by Lesley Walton, and Dinah Parums was the pathology consultant.

REFERENCES

1. Hammond EC, Garfinkel L: Coronary heart disease, stroke and aortic aneurysm. Factors in the etiology. *Arch Environ Hlth* **19:** 167–182, 1967
2. Davies MJ, Woolf N: Atherosclerosis: what is it and how does it occur? *Br Heart J* **69:** S3–11, 1993
3. Reed D, Reed C, Stemmermann G, Hayashi T: Are aortic aneurysms caused by atherosclerosis? *Circulation* **85:** 205–211, 1992
4. Johansen K, Keopsell T: Familial tendency for abdominal aortic aneurysms. *J Am Med Assoc* **256:** 1934, 1986
5. Bengtsson H, Norrgard O, Angqvist K *et al.*: Ultrasonographic screening of the abdominal aorta among siblings of patients with abdominal aortic aneurysms. *Br J Surg* **76:** 589–591, 1989
6. Adamson J, Powell JT, Greenhalgh RM: Selection for screening for familial aortic aneurysm. *Br J Surg* **79:** 897, 1992
7. Majumder PP, St Jean PL, Ferrell RE *et al.*: The inheritance of abdominal aortic aneurysm. *Am J Hum Genet* **48:** 164, 1991
8. Kuivaniemi H, Tromp G, Prockop DJ: Genetic causes of aortic aneurysms. *J Clin Invest* **88:** 1141–1444, 1991
9. Kontusaari S, Tromp G, Kuivaniemi H *et al.*: A mutation in the gene for type III procollagen (COL3A1) in a family with aortic aneurysms *J Clin Invest* **86:** 1465, 1990
10. Powell JT, Adamson J, MacSweeney STR *et al.*: Influence of type III collagen genotype on aortic diameter and disease. *Br J Surg* **80:** 1246, 1993
11. Tromp G, Wu Y, Prockop DJ *et al.*: Sequencing of cDNA from 50 unrelated patients reveals that mutations in the triple-helical domain of type III procollagen are an infrequent cause of aortic aneurysms. *J Clin Invest* **91:** 2539, 1993
12. Koch AE, Haines GK, Rizzo RJ *et al.*: Human abdominal aortic aneurysms. Immunophenotypic analysis suggesting an immune-mediated response. *Am J Pathol* **137:** 1199–1213, 1990
13. Parums DV: The spectrum of chronic periaortitis. *Histopathology* **16:** 423–431, 1990

14. Freestone T, Turner RJ, Coady A *et al.*: Inflammation and matrix metalloproteinases in the enlarging abdominal aortic aneurysm. *Arterioscler Thromb Vasc Biol* **15**: 1145–1151, 1995
15. Lancisi GM: *De aneurysmatibus, Opus Posthumum.* (Translation of 1745 version by WC Wright) New York: Macmillan, 1952
16. Liddicoat JE, Bekassy SM, Rubio PA: Ascending aortic aneurysms – review of 100 consecutive cases. *Circulation* **51/52:** I202–209, 1975
17. Report of Committee on Nomenclature of the American Society for the Study of Arteriosclerosis. Tentative classification of arteriopathies. *Circulation* **12**: 1065–1067, 1955
18. Gerlis LM: The significance of adventitial infiltrations in coronary atherosclerosis. *Br Heart J* **18**: 166–172, 1955
19. Schwartz CJ, Mitchell JRA: Cellular infiltration of the human arterial adventitia associated with atheromatous plaques. *Circulation* **26**: 73–78, 1962
20. Wolinsky H, Glagov S: Nature of the species difference in the medial distribution of vasa vasorum in mammals. *Cirulat Res* **25**: 677–686, 1969
21. Rose AG, Dent DM: Inflammatory variant of abdominal atherosclerotic aneurysm. *Arch Pathol Lab Med* **105**: 409–413, 1981
22. Mitchinson MJ: Retroperitoneal fibrosis revisited. *Arch Pathol* **110**: 784–786, 1986
23. Parums DV, Brown DL, Mitchinson DJ: Serum antibodies to oxidised LDL and ceroid in chronic periaortitis. *Arch Pathol* **114**: 383–387, 1990
24. Salonen JT, Yla-Herttuala S, Yamamoto R *et al.*: Autoantibody against oxidised LDL and progression of carotid atherosclerosis. *Lancet* **339**: 883–887, 1992
25. Powell JT, Muller BR, Greenhalgh RM: Acute phase proteins in patients with abdominal aortic aneurysms. *J Cardiovasc Surg* **28**: 528–530, 1987
26. Szekanecz Z, Shah MR, Pearce WH, Koch AE: Intercellular adhesion molecule-1 (ICAM-1) expression and soluble ICAM-1 (sICAM-1) production by cytokine-activated human aortic endothelial cells: a possible role for ICAM-1 and sICAM-1 in atherosclerotic aortic aneurysms. *Clin Exp Immunol* **98**: 337–343, 1994
27. Ramshaw AL, Parums DV: Immunohistochemical characterization of inflammatory cells associated with advanced atherosclerosis. *Histopathology* **17**: 543–552, 1990
28. UK Small Aneurysm Trial Participants: The UK Small Aneurysm Trial : methods and progress. *Eur J Vasc Surg* **9**: 42–48, 1995
29. Powell JT, MacSweeney STR, Greenhalgh RM: The spontaneous course of small aortic aneurysm. In: Yao JST, Pearce WH (Ed) *Aneurysms: New Findings and Treatments* pp. 71–77. Norwalk, Connecticut: Appleton and Lange, 1994
30. Newman KM, Jean-Claude J, Li H *et al.*: Cellular localization of matrix metalloproteinases in the abdominal aortic aneurysm wall. *J Vasc Surg* **20**: 814–820, 1994
31. Thompson RW, Holmes DR, Mertens RA *et al.*: Production and localization of 92-kilodalton gelatinase in abdominal aortic aneurysms. *J Clin Invest* **96**: 318–326, 1995
32. Anidjar S, Dobrin PB, Eichorst M *et al.*: Correlation of inflammatory infiltrate with the enlargement of experimental aortic aneurysms. *J Vasc Surg* **16**: 139–147, 1992
33. Ricci MA, Strindberg F, Slaiby JM *et al.*: Anti-CD 18 monoclonal antibody slows experimental aortic aneurysm expansion. *J Vasc Surg* **23**: 301–307, 1996
34. Freestone T, Turner RJ, Higman DJ *et al.*: The influence of hypercholesterolaemia and adventitial inflammation on the development of aortic aneurysm in rabbits. *Arterioscler Thromb Vasc Biol* **17**: 10–17, 1997
35. Deane M, Norton JD: Immunoglobulin gene 'fingerprinting': an approach to analysis of B lymphoid clonality in lymphoproliferative disorders. *Br J Haematol* **77**: 274–281, 1991
36. Diss TC, Peng H, Wotherspoon AC *et al.*: Detection of monoclonality in low-grade B cell lymphomas using the PCR is dependent on primer selection and lymphoma type. *J Pathol* **169**: 291–295, 1993
37. Gregory AK, Yin NX, Capella J *et al.*: Features of autoimmunity in the abdominal aortic aneurysm. *Arch Surg* **131**: 85–88, 1996
38. Koch AE, Kunkel SL, Pearce WH *et al.*: Enhanced production of the chemotactic cytokines IL-8 and MCP-1 in human abdominal aortic aneurysms. *Am J Pathol* **142**: 1423–1431, 1993
39. Newman KM, Jean-Claude J, Ramey WG, Tilson MD: Cytokines that activate proteolysis are increased in abdominal aortic aneurysms. *Circulation* **90**: 224–227, 1994

Neutrophil Activation During Aortic Surgery

N. J. Cheshire, M. Mireskandari, J. H. N. Wolfe and A. O. Mansfield

INTRODUCTION

Acute renal failure (ARF), adult respiratory distress (ARDS) and multiple organ failure (MOF) are important postoperative complications associated with high mortality rates,[1-3] prolonged intensive care unit and in-hospital stay and increased management costs.[2-5] The incidence of these problems following aortic surgery is not known but it has been estimated that MOF is the primary cause of over 50% of deaths following elective abdominal aneurysm repair and over 90% of deaths after initially succesful repair of ruptured infrarenal aneurysms.[5-8] Incidence rates are higher after extensive operations such as thoracoabdominal aneurysm repair[4,9-11] in which recognized aetiological factors, such as visceral ischaemia, large volume blood transfusion and pulmonary trauma may act synergistically. However, it is only during the last 5–10 years that a satisfactory explanation for the development of single or multiple organ impairment after seemingly uncomplicated aortic surgery has been suggested.

Recent work on the aetiology of ARF, ARDS and MOF suggests that these complications develop secondary to an abnormal systemic inflammatory response,[1,2,12] which may be triggered by a variety of stimuli with or without bacterial infection.[2,3] It is believed that the effects of the initial stimulus are amplified by production of humoral inflammatory mediators and consequent activation of endothelial cells, circulating polymorphonuclear neutrophils (PMN), monocytes and other immunocompetent cell species. This results in an extensive endothelial injury by both the direct effect of the mediating agents and neutrophil/endothelial interaction,[1,13] producing generalized endothelial cell swelling, capillary leak, oedema and organ dysfunction.[14-17] These effects may compromise the function of all major systems, but the kidney and lung (followed closely by the liver[3]) usually develop clinical manifestations first. This results in the common situation of a ventilator-dependent patient with deteriorating renal function who develops abnormal liver function and jaundice, cardiovascular instability and coagulation abnormalities prior to death. The mortality rate associated with MOF is directly related to the number of systems or organs clinically affected by the process[2,3] and ranges from 5–20% in single system failure to over 90% when four systems are involved.[3] The average mortality for all patients in reported series is approximately 50%.

The most common underlying causes of MOF are major trauma and serious bacterial infections but studies of the pathophysiology of the systemic inflammatory response and MOF in these groups of patients are complicated by the wide variability in the nature of their injuries, uncertainty about the time of onset of sepsis and the relatively small number of patients seen in any individual centre. Aortic surgery on the other hand provides a readily available, well defined, non-infective insult at a specified time and has been used by a number of authors to study the pathophysiology of the sytemic inflammatory response and organ impairment, with varying degrees of success; one evident problem is that almost all studies have looked at infrarenal aneurysms and the incidence of MOF in this group is sufficiently low that very large numbers of patients are required in order to produce meaningful results.

At St Mary's Hospital we have been studying the inflammatory and immunological changes occurring during thoracoabdominal aortic aneurysm repair and have correlated our observations with postoperative organ dysfunction, multiple organ failure and outcome. This chapter reviews the data available from other centres on white cell function after aortic surgery and presents our results to date.

For the sake of clarity no attempt has been made to review the exhaustive animal literature on neutrophil function in ischaemia and reperfusion except where essential. Similarly, experimental data regarding potential mediators of PMN activation are not referenced except where evidence relating to man is presented.

WHITE CELL ACTIVATION DURING INFRARENAL AORTIC SURGERY

The local effects of reperfusion of ischaemic tissues on the polymorphonuclear neutrophil are well recognized: experimental work in animals has clearly shown that reintroduction of oxygenated blood into non-infected ischaemic tissues results in local activation of PMN (and endothelium) and recruitment of these inflammatory cells into the reperfused tissue by mechanisms possibly involving the generation of oxygen-free radical species and peroxidation of cell surface lipids.[13,18]

Furthermore, depletion or inhibition of PMN in animal models prior to revascularization of previously ischaemic organs has been shown to reduce endothelial and tissue injury.[15,19] For obvious reasons little of this work has been undertaken in man although in one notable study, Formigli *et al.*, by obtaining repeated postoperative quadriceps muscle biopsies demonstrated granulocyte accumulation in skeletal muscle after aortic cross-clamping for abdominal aortic aneurysm (AAA) repair,[20] confirming the ability of sterile human tissues to activate and recruit PMN on reperfusion.

The possibility that reperfusion of large volumes of tissue, such as the lower limbs, may result in escape of inflammatory mediators or activated neutrophils into the systemic circulation provoking a systemic inflammatory response and remote organ injury has encouraged a number of authors to investigate white cell function and outcome after infrarenal aortic aneurysm repair. Fosse and colleagues[21] in 1987 demonstrated increased numbers of PMN in bronchial lavage fluid from a small series of patients undergoing abdominal aneurysm repair but were unable to correlate these findings with the development of respiratory compromise leading them to conclude that the white cells were not responsible pulmonary injury. In contrast, Paterson *et al.* demonstrated an acute reduction in circulating neutrophil levels early after aortic declamping following infrarenal aneurysm repair which was associated with acute increases in mean pulmonary artery pressures and pulmonary vascular resistance, and transient non-cardiac pulmonary oedema on chest X-ray.[22] These findings were interpreted as evidence of white cell trapping within the lung after lower limb and pelvic ischaemia. The same author subsequently showed that patient plasma taken from the inferior vena cava during reperfusion after aneurysm repair could recruit rabbit neutrophils into an elaborate skin chamber model, suggesting the plasma contained agents capable of PMN activation.[23]

Less direct evidence was provided by Soong et al. in Belfast who showed a fall in sigmoid colon mucosal pH following aortic aneurysm repair, indicating relative sigmoid ischaemia and thus neutrophil activation (although this was not directly measured), was associated with impaired postoperative pulmonary function (measured as FiO2/PaO$_2$ ratio) compared with patients who maintained a normal sigmoid pH.[24]

Recently, Barry et al. in Dublin[25] have demonstrated direct evidence of neutrophil activation (measured as cell surface expression of the adhesion molecule CD11b – see section on thoracoabdominal aneurysm repair below) in venous and arterial blood samples taken within 30 minutes of aortic cross-clamp removal from eight patients undergoing AAA repair. We studied PMN surface CD11b expression during AAA repair in a similar fashion but were unable to demonstrate significant adhesion molecule upregulation intra- or postoperatively (Fig. 1). Our findings are supported

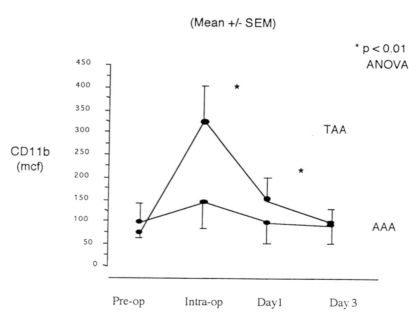

Fig. 1. Neutrophil surface CD11b expression (expressed as mean channel flourescence) in patients undergoing thoracoabdominal aortic aneurysm repair (TAA, n=8) compared with patients undergoing infrarenal aortic aneurysm repair (AAA, n=6). Intraoperative and early postoperative neutrophil activation was significantly greater in TAA patients. There was no significant elevation from baseline in patients undergoing AAA repair.

by Hill *et al.* who were also unable to show significant increase from baseline in PMN activation markers following infrarenal aortic cross-clamping.[26]

The mechanisms by which neutrophils may become activated during infrarenal aneurysm surgery are complex and have not been been clearly documented. Paterson and colleagues[22] have shown that plasma thromboxane B2 levels rise significantly in association with pulmonary white cell trapping, increased pulmonary resistance and oedema. As thromboxane B2 is known to stimulate neutrophils *in vitro* and in animal models, this finding suggests that it may be causally linked to neutrophil activation after aneurysm repair. Raised plasma levels of a number of other arachidonic acid metabolites have been demonstrated after lower limb reperfusion in animal models,[27,28] and thus may be important following infrarenal aortic cross-clamp removal but to date no clear data exists.

In patients who developed subclinical ischaemia of the sigmoid colon and pulmonary impairment, Soong *et al.*[29] were able to demonstrate increased circulating levels of endotoxin and tumour necrosis factor compared with controls but this study did not directly examine neutrophil activation and no further assumptions can be made.

An interesting study by Corson[30] in rats suggested that reperfusion following lower limb ischaemia can alter gut permeability to endotoxin. Endotoxaemia is a powerful potential trigger for systemic inflammatory response (see below) as well as an indicator of bacterial absorption from the gut, and some evidence exists that similar gut permeability changes may occur after infrarenal cross-clamp removal in man.[31] Although this interesting finding may explain some of the observations seen after aortic surgery, the clinical importance of gut permeability changes after infrarenal aortic cross-clamping remains to be established.

THORACOABDOMINAL AORTIC ANEURYSM REPAIR

Thoracoabdominal aortic aneurysms involve the infrarenal aorta and a variable portion of the descending thoracic and proximal abdominal aortic segments such that thoracotomy and laparotomy are required for exposure. The Crawford classification is shown in Fig. 2. Although there is great variation in the extent of the disease, aortic reconstruction in all patterns requires supracoeliac cross-clamping and temporary interuption of visceral arterial flow. This feature of thoracoabdominal aortic aneurysm repair is responsible for many of intraoperative challenges to both the surgeon and anaesthetist and also for many of the postoperative problems.

Renal and respiratory impairment are common postoperative complications.[4,9,11] In Crawford's large series of over 1500 procedures, postoperative renal failure occurred in 18% of patients and was statistically associated with death.[9] Respiratory complications developed in 8%, carrying a 40% mortality.[10] In our own series, acute renal failure requiring haemofiltration or dialysis occurred in 15% of patients and both renal failure and prolonged ventilation were associated with postoperative mortality.[11]

Published perioperative mortality rates for thoracoabdominal aortic aneurysms series vary between 0% and 66%.[9–11,32–36,37] Despite these apparently wide discrepancies, it has been suggested by some authors that most results are relatively similar when confounding factors are taken into account.

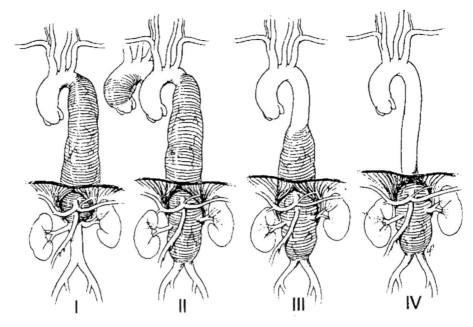

Fig. 2. Classification of thoracoabdominal aortic aneurysms according to Crawford.

WHITE CELL ACTIVATION DURING THORACOABDOMINAL AORTIC ANEURYSM REPAIR

Neutrophil adhesion molecule expression

We have studied neutrophil and plasma changes in a series of 20 consecutive patients undergoing thoracoabdominal aortic aneurysm repair.

In all patients venous blood samples were taken preoperatively and at regular intervals during visceral and lower limb reperfusion. Further samples were then obtained on the first 3 postoperative days. Polymorphonuclear neutrophil activation was measured as cell surface expression of the adhesion molecule CD11b by flow cytometry; CD11b is an important component of the CD18/CD11 adhesion molecule complex by which activated neutrophils bind to receptors expressed by the endothelial cell (including intercellular adhesion molecule I :ICAM-1). Cell–cell adhesion in this manner is an essential requirement for neutrophil-mediated endothelial injury as postulated in the current theories of MOF pathophysiology.[13]

During follow-up 11 patients developed acute renal failure (defined in this study as renal impairment requiring temporary or permanent renal replacement therapy) or pulmonary failure (ventilatory support for 5 days or more). Most patients (nine of the eleven) developed both complications indicating multiple organ dysfunction. Postoperative plasma creatinine and the duration of ventilatory support are compared between complicated and uncomplicated patients in Fig. 3. Overall

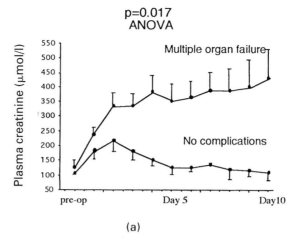

(a)

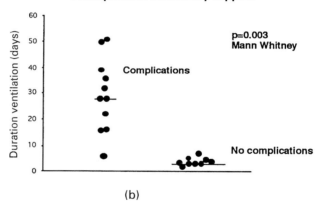

(b)

Fig. 3. Plasma creatinine levels (a) and duration of ventilatory support (b) in patients who developed multiple organ failure following thoracoabdominal aortic aneurysm repair compared with those who made an uneventful recovery.

survival at 30 days was 70% with all deaths occurring in the complicated group. This results in a mortality for MOF in this group of patients of 54% – similar to reported figures from other centres.

Figure 4 shows perioperative neutrophil CD11b expression in patients undergoing thoracoabdominal aortic aneurysm repair separated into those who developed complications and those who made an uneventful recovery. It can be seen that neutrophil CD11b expression rises serially for the first hour following thoracic aortic cross-clamp removal and that intraoperative neutrophil activation is significantly greater in the eleven patients who subsequently went on to develop MOF, indicating that neutrophil surface CD11b expression is a marker for postoperative organ

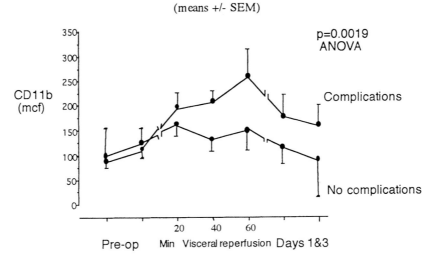

Fig. 4. Neutrophil surface CD11b expression (mean channel flourescence) in 20 patients who developed postoperative multiple-organ impairment (renal and respiratory failure, n=11) after thoracoabdominal aortic aneurysm repair compared with patients who made an uneventful recovery (n=9). Intraoperative neutrophil activation was significantly greater in those patients who went on to develop postoperative complications.

dysfunction and death following thoracoabdominal aortic aneurysm repair. These findings were independent of the extent of the aneurysm repair, the duration of aortic cross-clamping and the volumes of blood transfused during the operation.

Furthermore, we were able to demonstrate a positive correlation between peak intraoperative neutrophil CD11b expression and postoperative peak creatinine levels suggesting that the observed neutrophil changes may be causally related to the development of renal failure.

Significant increases in neutrophil adhesion receptor expression after supracoeliac aortic cross-clamping have been described by Hill et al., in the USA[26] but these findings were not correlated with organ dysfunction.

Mechanisms of neutrophil activation

There are a large number of mechanisms by which the neutrophil may be activated during thoracoabdominal aortic aneurysm repair in addition to those which may act during infrarenal surgery. We have studied plasma levels of endotoxin (potentially absorbed from the lumen of the ischaemic gut during thoracic aortic cross-clamping) and the acute phase cytokines – tumour necrosis factor-α (TNF), interleukin-1 and interleukin-6 (IL-1, IL-6).

Endotoxin, derived from the cell wall of Gram-negative bacteria has potent effects on the mediators of the acute inflammatory response in man and is believed to be important in the development of septic shock and organ dysfunction in gut-origin sepsis.[38–41] The acute-phase cytokines are thought to be the primary immunological mediators of sepsis, particularly after exposure to endotoxin, and increased plasma levels have been shown experimentally and clinically during sepsis.[42–46]

Endotoxin

Perioperative changes in endotoxin were measured directly by chromogenic limulus assay and indirectly by ELISA estimation of circulating IgG class anti-endotoxin-core antibodies (EndoCab assay – IgG to the endotoxin core is present constitutively and plasma levels fall during acute endotoxaemia due to binding).[47] Results are shown in in Figs 5 and 6.

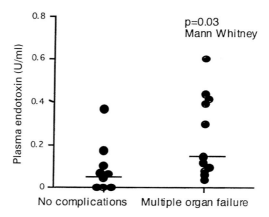

Fig. 5. Plasma endotoxin levels (measured by chromogenic limulus assay) were significantly higher in 11 patients who developed multiple organ failure after thoracoabdominal aortic aneurysm repair compared with those who made an uneventful recovery (medians shown).

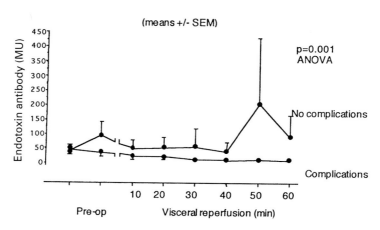

Fig. 6. Plasma anti-endotoxin antibody levels (EndoCab) in nine patients who made an uneventful recovery after thoracoabdominal aortic aneurysm repair compared with 11 patients who developed multiple organ failure. The significantly lower intraoperative levels seen in the complicated group suggest acute exposure to endotoxin.

It can be seen that thoracic aortic cross-clamping during thoracoabdominal aortic aneurysm repair is associated with endotoxin exposure and that intraoperative levels of endotoxin are significantly higher in patients who subsequently develop neutrophil activation and postoperative organ dysfunction compared with those who make an uncomplicated recovery.

We were also able to demonstrate close correlation between peak intraoperative endotoxin and PMN CD11b expression suggesting that endotoxaemia may be important in PMN activation.

Cytokines

In contrast to the differences in endotoxin exposure seen between patients who developed complications and those who made an uneventful recovery, the results of the cytokine assays demonstrated no significant differences in plasma acute phase cytokine levels between the two groups. This finding was suprising and as yet has not been satisfactorily answered; however, there are a number of alternative mechanisms by which endotoxin can influence the neutrophil and we are now turning our attention to these. We are currently interested in the role of the transcription factor NFkB which may be central in neutrophil activation in response to a variety of stimuli in addition to endotoxin and thus may prove to be a suitable target to prevent neutrophil activation in a complex system such as thoracoabdominal aneurysm repair.

SUMMARY

The systemic inflammatory response syndrome and MOF are believed to represent an inappropriate inflammatory reaction in which the neutrophil plays an important role. A systemic inflammatory response with or without organ impairment can develop after any form of aortic surgery but is particularly common after thoracoabdominal aneurysm repair.

There is indirect evidence that neutrophils may be activated and sequestered in both local (reperfused) and remote sites following infrarenal aortic surgery in humans but the results of direct studies are contradictory. The mechanisms of neutrophil activation in this group are unclear but arachidonic acid derivatives (from reperfused skeletal muscle) and subclinical colonic ischaemia may play a role.

There is direct evidence that neutrophils are activated during visceral reperfusion in thoracoabdominal aortic aneurysm repair and we suggest that this is causally related to postoperative organ injury. At the present time the mechanisms of PMN activation are not clear but gut and visceral ischaemia is one of the unique features of thoracoabdominal aortic aneurysm repair and we have some evidence that absorption of endotoxin occurs during cross-clamping. The mechanisms of endotoxin-PMN interaction following thoracoabdominal aortic aneurysm repair are complex but do not seem to involve the acute phase cytokines and further studies are required to clarify this.

Intervention to prevent PMN-endotoxin interaction, PMN activation or PMN-endothelial interaction may reduce the incidence of the systemic inflammatory response and MOF following all types of aortic surgery, improve outcome and reduce costs.

REFERENCES

1. Goris RJA: MODS/SIRS: Result of an overwhelming inflammatory response. *World J Surg*, **20**: 418–421, 1996
2. Rangel-Frausto MS *et al.*: The natural history of the sytemic inflammatory response syndrome (SIRS). *JAMA* **273**: 117–123, 1995
3. Regel G *et al.*: Pattern of organ failure following severe trauma. *World J Surg* **20**: 422–429, 1996
4. Harward TRS *et al.*: Visceral ischaemia and organ dysfunction after thoracoabdominal aortic aneurysm repair. *Ann Surg* **223**: 729–736, 1996
5. Meesters, RC *et al.*: Ruptured aortic aneurysm: early postoperative prediction of mortality using an organ system failure score. *Br J Surg* **81**: 512–516, 1994
6. Huber TS *et al.*: Operative mortality rates after elective infrarenal aortic reconstructions. *J Vasc Surg* **22**: 287–293, 1995
7. Henderson A, Effeney D: Morbidity and mortality after abdominal aortic surgery in a population of patients with high cardiovascular risk. *Aust N Z J Surg* **65**: 417–420, 1995
8. Kurihara H. *et al.*: [A review of post-operative multiple organ failure in peripheral arterial diseases]. *Nippon Geka Gakkai Zasshi* **89**: 1908–1913, 1988
9. Svensson LG *et al.*: Experience with 1509 patients undergoing thoracoabdominal aortic operations. *J Vasc Surg* **17**: 357–368, 1993
10. Svensson LG *et al.*: A prospective study of respiratory failure after high-risk surgery on the thoracoabdominal aorta. *J Vasc Surg* **14**: 271–282, 1991
11. Gilling-Smith G *et al.*: Surgical repair of thoracoabdominal aortic aneurysm: 10 years' experience. *Br J Surg* **82**: 624–629, 1995
12. Klausner JM *et al.*: Lower torso ischemia-induced lung injury is leukocyte dependent. *Ann Surg* **208**: 761–767, 1988
13. Grace PA: Ischaemia-reperfusion injury. *Br J Surg* **81**: 637–647, 1994
14. Craig I *et al.*: Pulmonary permeability edema in a large animal model of nonpulmonary sepsis. A morphologic study. *Am J Pathol* **128**: 241–251, 1987
15. Duran WN Dillon PK: Effects of ischemia-reperfusion injury on microvascular permeability in skeletal muscle. *Microcirc Endothelium Lymph* **5**: 223–239, 1989
16. Nuytinck JK *et al.*: Acute generalized microvascular injury by activated complement and hypoxia: the basis of the adult respiratory distress syndrome and multiple organ failure? *Br J Exp Pathol* **67**: 537–548, 1986
17. Pretorius JP *et al.*: The 'lung in shock' as a result of hypovolemic-traumatic shock in baboons. *J Trauma* **27**: 1344–1353, 1987
18. Belkin M *et al.*: The role of leukocytes in the pathophysiology of skeletal muscle ischemic injury. *J Vasc Surg* **10**: 14–18, 1989
19. Eiermann GJ, Dickey BF, Thrall RS: Polymorphonuclear leukocyte participation in acute oleic-acid-induced lung injury. *Am Rev Resp Dis* **128**: 845–850, 1983
20. Formigli L *et al.*: Neutrophils as mediators of human skeletal muscle ischemia-reperfusion syndrome. *Hum Pathol* **23**: 627–634, 1992
21. Fosse E *et al.*: Granulocytes in bronchial lavage fluid after major vascular surgery. *Acta Anaesthesiol Scand* **31**: 33–37, 1987
22. Paterson IS *et al.*: Noncardiogenic pulmonary edema after abdominal aortic aneurysm surgery. *Ann Surg* **209**: 231–236, 1989
23. Paterson IS *et al.*: Reperfusion plasma contains a neutrophil activator. *Ann Vasc Surg* **7**: 68–75, 1993
24. Soong CV *et al.*: Bowel ischaemia and organ impairment in elective abdominal aortic aneurysm repair [see comments]. *Br J Surg* **81**: 965–968, 1994
25. Barry MC *et al.*: Limb revascularisation increases neutrophil adhesion receptor

expression. Presented at the 80th meeting of the Surgical Research Society Glasgow: 1994

26. Hill GE *et al.*: Supraceliac, but not infrarenal, aortic cross-clamping upregulates neutrophil integrin CD11b. *J Cardiothorac Vasc Anesth* **9**: 515–518, 1995

27. Welbourn R *et al.* Role of neutrophil adherence receptors (CD 18) in lung permeability following lower torso ischemia. *Circ Res* **71**: 82–86, 1992

28. Klausner JM, *et al.*: Thromboxane A2 mediates increased pulmonary microvascular permeability following limb ischemia. *Circ Res* **64**: 1178–1189, 1989

29. Soong CV *et al.*: Endotoxaemia, the generation of the cytokines and their relationship to intramucosal acidosis of the sigmoid colon in elective abdominal aortic aneurysm repair. *Eur J Vasc Surg* **7**: 534–539, 1993

30. Corson RJ *et al.*: Lower limb ischaemia and reperfusion alters gut permeability. *Eur J Vasc Surg* **6**: 158–163, 1992

31. Roumen RM *et al.*: Intestinal permeability is increased after major vascular surgery. *J Vasc Surg* **17**: 734–737, 1993

32. Schneiderman J *et al.*: [Surgery for thoraco-abdominal aortic aneurysm]. *Harefuah* **120**: 179–181, 1991

33. Sandmann W *et al.*: [Surgical treatment of thoraco-abdominal and suprarenal aortic aneurysm]. *Zentralbl Chir* **113**: 1305–1314, 1988

34. von SL *et al.*: Perfusion with low systemic heparinization during resection of descending thoracic aortic aneurysms. *Eur J Cardiothorac Surg* **6**: 246–249, 1992

35. Jensen BF, Baekgaard N, Laustsen J: [Thoracoabdominal aortic aneurysms. Treatment, complications and early results]. *Ugeskr Laeger* **157**: 2008–2011, 1995

36. Tordoir JH *et al.*: Thoraco-abdominal aortic approach for the treatment of pararenal aneurysm. *Neth J Surg* **40**: 1–5, 1988

37. Ennker J *et al.*: [Surgery of abdominal aortic aneurysm – results in 502 patients]. *Langenbecks Arch Chir* **366**: 313–316, 1985

38. Wanebo HJ: Tumor necrosis factors. *Semin Surg Oncol* **5**: 402–413, 1989

39. Nolan JP, Camara DS: Intestinal endotoxins as co-factors in liver injury. *Immunol Invest* **18**: 325–337, 1989

40. Meyrick B, Johnson JE, Brigham KL: Endotoxin-induced pulmonary endothelial injury. *Prog Clin Biol Res* **308**: 91–99, 1989

41. Fletcher JR: Historical perspective of endotoxin effects on hemodynamics in animals. *Prog Clin Biol Res* **299**: 77–94, 1989

42. Frieling JT *et al.*: Circulating interleukin-6 receptor in patients with sepsis syndrome [see comments]. *J Infect Dis* **171**: 469–472, 1995

43. Pruitt JH, Copeland EB, Moldawer LL: Interleukin-1 and interleukin-1 antagonism in sepsis, systemic inflammatory response syndrome, and septic shock [editorial]. *Shock* **3**: 235–251, 1995

44. Rosenbloom AJ *et al.*: Leukocyte activation in the peripheral blood of patients with cirrhosis of the liver and SIRS. Correlation with serum interleukin-6 levels and organ dysfunction. *JAMA* **274**: 58–65, 1995

45. Ljunghusen O., *et al.*: Transient endotexemia during burn wound revision causes leukocyte beta 2 integrin up-regulation and cytokine release. *Inflammation* **19**: 457–468, 1995

46. Yentis SM: Cytokines and sepsis: time for reappraisal [editorial]. *Br J Anaesth* **74**: 119–120, 1995

47. Goldie AS *et al.*: Natural cytokine antagonists and endogenous antiendotoxin core antibodies in sepsis syndrome. The Sepsis Intervention Group. *JAMA* **274**: 172–177, 1995

Embolization from Abdominal Aortic Aneurysms

William W. Rose and Calvin B. Ernst

INTRODUCTION

Since the first successful repair of an abdominal aortic aneurysm (AAA) by Dubost on 29 March 1951, significant advances have been made in the management of this potentially lethal disease.[1] In Centers of Excellence the operative mortality for AAA repair is less than 5%.[2] Consequently, AAA repair has become a safe, widely performed and commonly accepted operation to prevent the disastrous complications of untreated AAA. The most common and feared complication is rupture which has a 90% mortality rate when considering both pre-hospital and operative deaths. A less common complication is peripheral macroembolization or microembolization from the AAA. Although infrequent, such embolic events, recognized either preoperatively or postoperatively, result in significant morbidity including digit or limb loss and renal failure.

This chapter summarizes contemporary clinical presentation and management of macroembolization and microembolization associated with AAA.

MACROEMBOLISM

Acute arterial ischaemia of an organ or extremity can be caused by thrombotic emboli (macroemboli), atheroemboli (micro- and macroatheroemboli), atherosclerotic thrombosis, vascular occlusion secondary to low flow or hypercoagulable states, arterial vasculopathies, trauma, iatrogenic injury, external compression syndromes, venous occlusive disease, or complications of vascular reconstruction. Thrombotic macroemboli account for more than 80% of acute arterial ischaemic episodes.[3] Of these embolic events, 85%–90% are caused by macroemboli originating in the heart. The remaining 5–10% of emboli come from uncommon nor-cardiac sources including arterial aneurysms, peripheral arterial atherosclerotic plaques, sites of vascular trauma, sites of malignant tumour invasion, the venous system (paradoxical emboli), and unknown sites.[3–5]

Infrarenal AAAs, along with femoral, popliteal, and subclavian artery aneurysms are the most common aneurysmal sources associated with arterial macroembolism.[6] Macroemboli from popliteal artery aneurysms may be clinically silent, but are symptomatic in approximately 25% of patients.[7] Emboli from femoral artery aneurysms occur in 5–10% of patients and from subclavian artery aneurysms in 33–68% of patients.[4,8,9]

The proportion of patients with AAAs presenting with emboli varies. In an analysis from Northwestern University, Baxter and his colleagues identified 15 (5%) of 302 patients who underwent AAA repairs and presented with distal embolization as the first manifestations of their AAAs.[10] Of these 15 patients, three had developed macroemboli. Lord and his colleagues reported on 133 patients undergoing AAA repair among whom 39 (29%) were found to have lower extremity emboli arising from the AAA mural thrombus.[11] In addition, Lord also noted that of 174 embolectomies for lower extremity ischaemia over a period of 4 years, in 16 patients (9%) the emboli were suspected to originate from AAAs.[11] In a study of 42 patients with radiographically documented non-cardiac lower extremity emboli, Kvilekval identified 10 patients (24%) in whom an AAA was the presumed embologenic source.[12]

Emboli arising from atherosclerotic plaques as well as those associated with AAA may be either macroscopic or microscopic. They are often collectively referred to as 'atheroemboli'. Macroscopic atheroemboli produce symptoms and signs identical to those thrombi originating from the heart or aneurysms. The pathophysiology, natural history, clinical presentation, and treatment of microscopic atheroemboli, however, are substantially different from those of macroemboli.

MACROEMBOLI FROM AAA

Arterial macroemboli originating from AAAs tend to lodge within the aortoiliac segment and less frequently in the lower legs. Macroemboli occluded the aortoiliac segment or the lower extremities in all 39 patients with AAAs in the study reported by Lord.[11] The Northwestern University study of 302 patients undergoing AAA repairs included three (1%) who presented with macroemboli, one to the popliteal artery and two to femoral–distal bypass grafts.[10]

CLINICAL PRESENTATION AND DIAGNOSIS

Typically, signs and symptoms of occlusion occur promptly and include the six Ps of acute arterial occlusion, pain, pallor, pulselessness, paresthesias, paralysis, and poikilothermia. In addition to arterial macroemboli, the differential diagnosis of acute limb ischaemia includes acute arterial thrombosis, aortic dissection, acute venous thrombosis, severe arterial spasm, neurologic disorders, and cardiogenic shock.

Doppler spectral waveform analysis and duplex imaging may provide additional useful information. A viable limb will have audible Doppler pulsatile flow signals and an ankle pressure greater than 30 mmHg. A threatened limb with reversible ischaemia lacks audible Doppler arterial signals although venous patency may be documented. Irreversibly ischaemic limbs have neither arterial nor venous flow signals.

The role of arteriography in acute peripheral ischaemia associated with AAA is controversial. The time needed to complete the arteriogram may prolong the period of ischaemia critically and, if the distal outflow tract is not opacified, clinically useful information is not provided. Arteriography may be valuable, however, if the diagnosis is unclear. Although arteriography is often used in patients suspected to have AAAs as the sources of macroemboli, arteriography may aggravate or precipitate the problem by catheter fragmentation of aneurysmal contents. Baxter reported a 20% incidence of arteriographic related emboli occurring among 15 patients who presented with distal embolization as their first manifestation of an AAA.[10]

That almost 50% of AAAs presenting with distal embolization were overlooked by arteriography and the diagnosis was only made by computed tomography (CT) scan emphasizes the shortcomings of arteriography in diagnosing AAAs. In addition, many AAAs associated with emboli are small. In the Northwestern University study patients who presented with emboli from AAA had aneurysms that ranged from 3.2 cm to 6.3 cm in diameter with a mean diameter of 4.3 cm.[10] Only three aneurysms had a diameter greater than 5 cm. Consequently, CT imaging appears to be the diagnostic study of choice for evaluating such small AAAs suspected of causing embolic phenomena. The CT criteria of emboli-prone AAAs include irregular lumen surfaces, multiple lumens, heterogeneity of the thrombus, calcification within the thrombus, and fissures extending from the lumen into the thrombus 10 (Fig. 1), Table 1. When such features are identified on preoperative CT images the surgeon should be

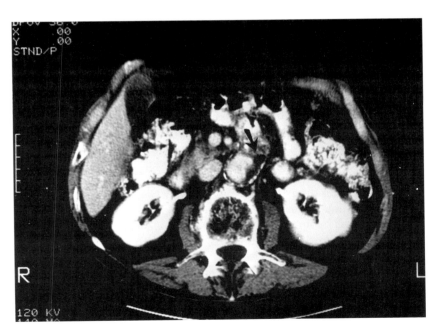

Fig. 1. Contrast-enhanced axial abdominal CT scan with soft tissue window from a patient with postoperative atheroembolism manifest by livido reticularis, ischaemic toes, and creatine phosphokinase levels of 600 000 IU/litre. The AAA exhibits an irregular aortic lumen, heterogeneous thrombus (arrow) and extensive calcifications.

Table 1.   CT Criteria of embolism-prone AAA

Irregular lumen surface
Multiple lumens
Heterogeneity of the thrombus
Calcification of the thrombus
Fissures from lumen into thrombus

sensitized to suspect operative embolic complications and take special technical precautions to minimize operative and postoperative embolic events.

MANAGEMENT

Heparin sodium therapy should be instituted as soon as the diagnosis of arterial macroembolism is made. Clot propagation is prevented, collateral circulation is maintained, and the risk of recurrent macroembolism is reduced.

Balloon catheter embolectomy through a groin incision is the optimal treatment for acute arterial macroembolism. Exposure and exploration of distal vessels may be required to remove retained distal thrombus. Thrombolytic therapy has been shown to be useful in patients with irretrievable clot in small peripheral vessels but such therapy is contraindicated in patients with an AAA.

Careful postoperative care and monitoring are required to manage patients' underlying medical conditions as well as expected complications of reperfusion. The consequences of ischaemic muscle reperfusion typically occur 12–24 hours after revascularization. These may be minimized by fasciotomy, adequate hydration, renal diuresis with mannitol, alkalinization of the urine with sodium bicarbonate, and insulin and glucose administration, if needed, to manage hyperkalaemia.

In patients with distal arterial embolization from AAA recurrent embolization may occur in up to 27%. Consequently, simultaneous or early staged aneurysm repair is recommended following clot extraction.[10,11] Whether or not concomitant AAA repair should be performed depends upon the patient's overall condition and the extent of extremity ischaemia. Finding mild ischaemia in a good risk patient, concomitant AAA repair may be safely performed after embolectomy. However, many patients will be better managed by first performing the embolectomy followed by AAA repair within a few days. It must be emphasized that such AAAs should be considered symptomatic and require urgent operation. In Lord's analysis, 11 of 39 patients underwent simultaneous aneurysm repair and embolectomy.[11] In five embolectomy was performed prior to aneurysmectomy and 15 patients underwent femoral–popliteal bypasses subsequent to repair of the AAA.

Among patients with an identified AAA source for macroemboli, the risk of operative repair is greater than for elective aneurysm repair. The Northwestern University group reported an operative mortality of 13%.[6,10] In addition, and in spite of taking special technical precautions to prevent embolization during AAA repair, 27% of patients had postoperative evidence of new emboli.

MICROEMBOLISM

Ischaemic events secondary to obstruction of small arterioles by microatheroemboli dislodged from aortic or peripheral aneurysms or ulcerated atheromatous plaques are colloquially referred to as 'trash foot', 'trash kidney', 'trash colon', or 'trash spinal cord'. Less than 5% of peripheral emboli causing acute ischaemia are atheroemboli.[13,14] Although an uncommon cause of acute arterial ischaemia, atheromatous embolization remains one of the most challenging diagnostic and therapeutic problems for vascular surgeons. The potential for devastating complications is significant because such atheroemboli may lead to limb loss, organ failure, visceral ischaemia, paralysis, or even death.

Spontaneous atheroembolization from an infrarenal AAA is a rare event.[6,10,11] Of the 15 patients who presented with distal embolic events among the 302 undergoing AAA repairs at Northwestern University, 12 (4%) had microatheroemboli.[10] Estes noted atheroembolism in three of 102 patients with AAAs which is typical of most reports.[15]

Other authors have studied the incidence of AAAs among patients with symptoms of atheroembolism. Among 62 patients treated for symptomatic microatheroemboli, Bauman and his co-workers documented AAAs in 12 (19%).[16,17] Keen and his colleagues identified 20 among 100 patients with AAAs in whom the AAA was suspected as the source of peripheral microatheroemboli.[18] Importantly, the mean diameter of the AAAs measured less than 4 cm.

PATHOPHYSIOLOGY

A sudden rupture of an atherosclerotic plaque causing showers of cholesterol-containing atheromatous debris characterizes the majority of episodes of microatheroembolism.[19] Microatheroemboli consist mainly of cholesterol crystals or fibrin and platelet aggregates. Histologic study documents cholesterol crystals and clefts within small arteries and arterioles with surrounding inflammatory cells including leukocytes and eosinophils. This acute arteritis persists for approximately 1–2 weeks and is replaced with infiltrating lymphocytes, monocytes, and foreign body giant cells eventuating in luminal occlusion.[4,20] If left untreated, recurrent microatheroemboli coupled with the reactive obliterative endarteritis culminates in tissue ischaemia, often with serious sequelae of renal failure, bowel infarction, and extremity tissue loss.

Microatheroembolism most often occurs spontaneously but may also occur following coughing, arteriographic catheter manipulation, blunt abdominal trauma, operative aortic manipulation, and also following systemic anticoagulation.[4,13,17,21] The propensity for spontaneous microatheroembolization will persist until the ulcerative plaque becomes covered with an overlying protective fibrin layer that may temporarily control recurrent episodes of embolization. That these microscopic atheroemboli recur, however, testifies to the instability of this fibrin shield. Anticoagulants are thought to aggravate the situation by preventing formation of a protective fibrin cap over the plaque or by causing intraplaque haemorrhage with plaque disruption.

Approximately 20% of patients presenting with atheroemboli have undergone previous invasive vascular procedures.[16,22,23] Operative manipulation and even 'atraumatic' clamping of atherosclerotic blood vessels can cause fragmentation of friable atheroma. This may result in distal embolization when the vessel cross-clamp is removed as well as retrograde embolization into visceral vessels secondary to aortic blood flow turbulence at the site of the proximal aortic clamp.

CLINICAL PRESENTATION AND DIAGNOSIS

Microscopic atheroemboli may remain clinically unrecognized in many patients.[19,24] The exact frequency of clinically silent atheroembolism is unknown although the autopsy incidence ranges from 1% to 12%.[24–27]

Clinical manifestations of symptomatic microatheroemboli include the blue toe syndrome with acute pain and cyanosis of the digits, as well as livido reticularis. The toe or a small area on the foot appears mottled, cyanotic, has slow capillary refill, and is tender. The discoloration is typically patchy and asymmetric. Livido reticularis may be manifest in the skin of the knees, thighs, or buttocks. Patients often complain of disabling myalgias. These symptoms usually resolve if embolization does not recur. With recurrent or persistent microatheroembolization, progression to ulceration and gangrene is not uncommon. Of clinical significance, proximal arterial pulses including pedal pulses, are usually palpable.

Clinically apparent atheroemboli from AAAs most often present with lower extremity symptoms. Kazmier and his colleagues described three patients with microatheroemboli from AAAs who presented with livido reticularis of the lower trunk and extremities and digital arterial occlusions with intact pedal pulse.[26] Eleven of 12 patients with AAAs reported by Baxter presented with focal digital ischaemia, the blue toe syndrome.[10] One patient complained of calf myalgia. This report also noted that ten of these patients presented with spontaneous atheroembolism and two developed their embolic events during aortography.

Duplex ultrasound of the abdominal aorta and femoral–popliteal segments should be performed to identify embologenic aneurysms. Ultrasound examination among patients with aneurysmal disease may document calcified and irregular plaques with absence of laminated thrombus. Friable or fungating plaques may also be observed within proximal arterial segments.[24] Aortography must be performed cautiously in such patients to avoid embolization secondary to catheter trauma. Biplane views of the aorta should be included to identify posterior ulcerating plaques. The use of CT scans is most helpful to define aortoiliac aneurysms and those aneurysms prone to embolization (Fig. 1, Table 1). Laboratory tests are rarely helpful; however, eosinophilia may be observed in up to 80% of patients with renal microatheroembolism.[28] Confirmation of cutaneous atheroembolism may be obtained by skin or muscle biopsies which document cholesterol crystal deposits in the small arterioles and capillaries.

MANAGEMENT

The natural history of microatheroemboli is one of recurrence with progressive tissue ischaemia and organ failure or limb loss, if left untreated. Anticoagulation may exacerbate the atheroembolic process and is, therefore, contraindicated once the diagnosis is made.[18] Following identification of the source of atheroemboli, treatment must include removal or exclusion of the embologenic focus. An AAA found to be the source of microatheroemboli should be treated urgently like any other symptomatic aneurysm. Appropriate preventive techniques should be used during operation to minimize intraoperative embolization.[29,30]

RESULTS

The operative mortality rate for surgical management of microatheroembolism was 4% among 100 patients reported by Keen and his co-workers.[18] This report included 20 patients with AAAs. The mortality rate was significantly higher when atheroma and intraluminal thrombi extended cephalad to the suprarenal aorta. This was related to the consequences of renal and visceral atheroemboli in addition to atheroemboli to the lower extremities. Baxter noted that among 15 patients with AAA identified as a source of their atheroemboli, eight (53%) eventually required amputation.[10] Renal failure secondary to recurrent atheroemboli from juxtarenal debris developed in five (33%) and the operative mortality was 13%.

EMBOLIZATION FOLLOWING ABDOMINAL AORTIC RECONSTRUCTION

Beyond macroembolization and microembolization as initial manifestations of AAAs, such embolic events may also occur during the operative and postoperative periods of aortic reconstruction.[6,29] Distal embolization of laminated thrombus or atheromatous debris from operative manipulation the aneurysm or proximal diseased aortic segment is an important cause of postoperative visceral and lower extremity ischaemia.[6,29,30,31]

Postoperative ischaemia of the legs has been reported in up to 10% of patients following AAA repair.[6,29–33] Approximately 50% of these events were recognized during or immediately following operation.[6,32,33] The Northwestern University group noted that of 15 patients who presented with preoperative embolization as the initial manifestation of their AAAs, four (27%) developed lower extremity embolic complications following AAA repair.[10] In addition, postoperative renal failure developed in five patients with four requiring chronic haemodialysis. Of the five patients with postoperative renal failure, three had posterior aortic thrombus extending above the level of the renal vessels that probably contributed to the operative embolization.

MANAGEMENT

Ischaemia resulting from macroemboli caused by loose fragments of aneurysmal thrombus is treated by prompt balloon catheter embolectomy. Such embolic episodes are usually recognized after the abdominal incision is closed and the surgical drapes are removed. Under such circumstances and provided the surgeon is confident that the iliac anastomosis is flawless, the embolus can almost always be removed through a groin incision by balloon-tipped catheter extraction. Thrombolytic therapy is contraindicated in the presence of a recently implanted aortoiliac prosthesis.

Microembolization without pulse deficits manifest by digital ischaemia, myositis, or livido reticularis should be treated expectantly using supportive measures primarily directed at preventing renal failure. Such measures include adequate hydration to ensure a brisk diuresis, administration of mannitol which may also provide an oxygen-free radical scavenger effect as well as diuresis, alkalinization of the urine to minimize tubular precipitation of myoglobin, and analgesia to control ischaemic digital pain and myalgia accompanying ischaemic myositis. Whether the vasodilatory effects of epidural anaesthesia, which is now often used during aortic reconstructive procedures, is helpful has not been studied. Should the rare episode of 'trash spinal cord' follow aortic reconstruction, supportive measures must be directed at minimizing the sequelae of paraplegia or paraparesis.

PREVENTION

Embolization during aortic reconstruction for AAA is most likely to occur during three stages of the operative procedure: during dissection and mobilization of the aneurysm and isolation of the proximal neck, during application of the aortic cross-clamp, and following removal of the aortic cross-clamp and restoration of blood flow (Fig. 2).

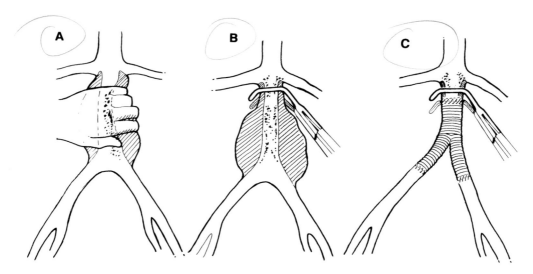

Fig. 2. Three stages of aortic reconstruction during which embolization is most likely to occur: (A) dissection and mobilization of the aneurysm, (B) application of the aortic cross-clamp, (C) removal of the aortic cross-clamp and restoration of blood flow.

It has been suggested that the incidence of operative embolization can be reduced by performing distal vascular clamping prior to placement of the proximal aortic clamp (Fig. 3). If the distal aorta or common iliac arteries are also diseased, distal clamps may be placed on internal iliac and external iliac vessels or on the common femoral vessels.[6,29,30] If atherosclerotic disease or thrombus, identified on preoperative aortography or CT imaging, extend proximally to the juxtarenal aorta, the renal arteries can be occluded temporarily prior to infrarenal, suprarenal, or supracoeliac cross-clamping to minimize the risk of renal embolization (Fig. 4). Particular attention should be exercised when aortographic or CT findings suggest aneurysmal morphology prone to peripheral embolization (Fig. 1, Table 1). Forewarned, the surgeon can place vascular clamps distally on relatively disease-free external iliac arteries before manipulating the AAA. When juxtarenal aortic disease is identified the proximal aortic clamp should be applied across the undiseased suprarenal or supracoeliac aorta during construction of the proximal aortic anastomosis. Such clamping of the minimally diseased aorta minimizes embolic events. Before constructing the proximal anastomosis, the aorta must be debrided and forcefully irrigated with saline solution to remove any residual debris. Finally, after completing the proximal anastomosis and before placing the final sutures in the distal anastomosis, the graft must be flushed by temporary release of the aortic clamp

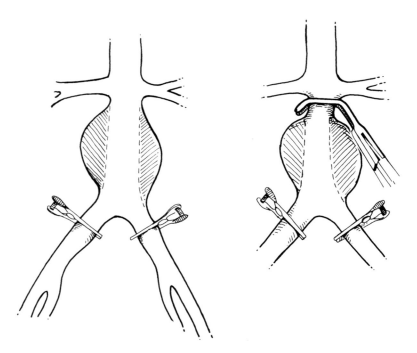

Fig. 3. Application of distal vascular clamps to the iliac vessels (left) prior to placement of the proximal aortic clamp (right) to minimize embolization in atheroembolic-prone AAA.

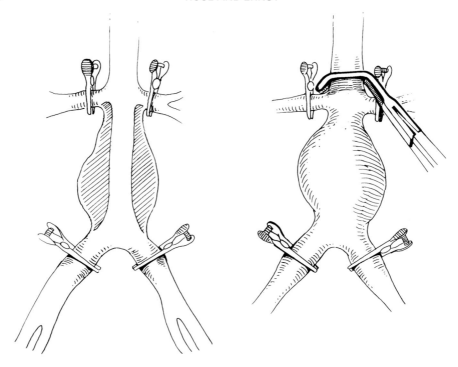

Fig. 4. Common iliac arteries occluded and temporary renal artery clamping (left) prior to applying suprarenal aortic clamp (right) to minimize renal atheroembolism when atherothrombotic disease is juxtarenal.

to wash any residual debris or thrombi from the prosthesis and proximal aorta (Fig. 5). Furthermore, the distal clamp should be similarly released to flush the iliofemoral system of any residual clot or debris.

Using preventive techniques for patients prone to operative embolization the incidence of such events following aortic reconstruction has been reported to be less than 1%.[29,30] This is in contrast to reports recording a frequency of distal embolization of 3–10% in similar patients.[6,32,33]

EMBOLIZATION ASSOCIATED WITH ENDOVASCULAR AORTIC GRAFTING

Transluminal endovascular grafting of AAAs appears to be an attractive alternative to conventional transabdominal or retroperitoneal aortic reconstruction.[34–38] Beyond the issue of long-term (greater than 5 years) durability of endovascular aortic grafting, the immediate morbidity and mortality will significantly impact acceptability and adoption of this innovative experimental technique. Just as arteriographic catheter fragmentation and dislodgment of aneurysmal thrombus or atheroembolism from diseased aortic segments can cause peripheral vascular

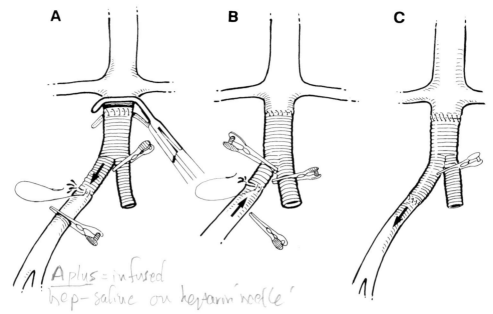

handwritten: A plus = infused
hep-saline on heparin noelle

Fig. 5. Graft flushing sequence to minimize operative embolization: (A) temporary release of the aortic clamp to flush residual debris or thrombi from the prosthesis and proximal aorta prior to completing the anastomosis. The proximal aorta flush manoeuvre can also be performed by temporarily releasing the clamp on the left limb of the prosthesis. (B) release of iliac clamp to retrograde flush the iliofemoral system prior to completing the anastomosis, (C) restoration of blood flow to the right leg with the left limb of the prosthesis still occluded.

occlusion, so can such manipulations coincident to placement of endovascular prostheses. Such embolic complications have been recognized among 3–10% of patients.[34-38] Parodi recorded three instances of embolization coincident to inserting an endovascular prosthesis resulting in three fatalities.[34] Of note, two patients in Parodi's study were admitted to the hospital with the 'blue toe syndrome'. This relatively low rate of embolic complications is a result of over-the-guidewire passage of current endovascular graft delivery systems, a manoeuvre that minimizes aneurysmal thrombus fragmentation.

Knowledge of the CT criteria of embolism-prone aneurysms should further refine selective criteria for successful endovascular grafting of AAAs and, just as with conventional AAA repairs, thereby minimize embolic complications.

REFERENCES

1. Dubost C, Allary M, Oeconomas N: Resection of an aneurysm of the abdominal aorta: Reestablishment of the continuity by a preserved human arterial graft with result after five months. *Arch Surg* **64**: 405–408, 1952

2. Ernst CB: Abdominal aortic aneurysm. *N Engl J Med* **328**: 1167–1172, 1993
3. Quiñones-Baldrich WJ: Acute arterial and graft occlusion: In: Moore WS (Ed) *Vascular Surgery: A Comprehensive Review*. Philadelphia: WB Saunders, 1993
4. Messina LM: Peripheral arterial embolism. In: Greenfield LJ (Ed) *Surgery: Scientific Principles and Practice*. Philadelphia: JB Lippincott, 1993
5. Kresowik TF: Paradoxical embolism. In: Ernst CB, Stanley JC (Eds) *Current Therapy in Vascular Surgery* 3rd edn. St Louis: Mosby, 1995
6. Keen RR, Yao JST: Aneurysms and embolization: Detection and management. In: Yao JST, Pearce WH (Eds) *Aneurysms: New Findings and Treatment*. Norwalk, Connecticut: Appleton and Lange, 1994
7. Lilly MP, Flinn WR, McCarthy WJ *et al.*: The effect of distal arterial anatomy on the success of popliteal artery aneurysm. *J Vasc Surg*, **7**:653–660, 1988
8. Graham LM, Zelenock CB, Whitehouse WM Jr *et al.*: Clinical significance of arteriosclerotic femoral artery aneurysms. *Arch Surg* **115**: 502–507, 1980
9. Mesh CL, Yao JST: Upper extremity bypass: Five-year follow-up. In: Yao JST, Pearce WH (Eds) *Long-Term Results in Vascular Surgery*. Norwalk, Connecticut: Appleton and Lange, 1993
10. Baxter BT, McGee GS, Flinn WR *et al.*: Distal embolization as a presenting symptom of aortic aneurysms. *Am J Surg* **160**: 197–201, 1990
11. Lord JW, Rossi G, Daliana M *et al.*: Unsuspected abdominal aortic aneurysms as the cause of peripheral arterial occlusive disease. *Ann Surg* **177**: 767–771, 1973
12. Kvilekval KHV, Yunis JP, Mason RA, Giron F: After the blue toe: Prognosis of noncardiac arterial embolization in the lower extremities. *J Vasc Surg* **17**: 328–353, 1993
13. Kempczinski RF: Atheroembolism. Kempczinski RF (Ed) *The Ischemic Leg*. Chicago: Year Book Medical Publishers, 1985
14. Kempczinski RF: Lower extremity arterial emboli from ulcerating atherosclerotic plaques. *JAMA* **241**: 807–810, 1979
15. Estes JE Jr: Abdominal aortic aneurysm: A study of one hundred and two cases. *Circulation* **2**: 258–264, 1950
16. Bauman DS, McGraw D, Rubin BG *et al.*: An institutional experience with arterial atheroembolism. *Ann Vasc Surg* **8**: 258–265, 1994
17. Baumann DS, Sicard GA: Atheroembolism. Callow AD, Ernst CB (Eds) *Vascular Surgery: Theory and Practice*. Stamford, Connecticut: Appleton and Lange, 1995
18. Keen RR, McCarthy WJ, Shireman PK *et al.*: Surgical management of atheroembolization. *J Vasc Surg* **21**: 773–781, 1995
19. Lie JT: Cholesterol atheromatous embolism: The great masquerader revisited. *Path Ann* **27**: 17–50, 1992
20. Gore I, McCombs HL, Lindquist RL: Observations on the fate of cholesterol emboli. *J Atheroscler Res* **4**: 527–535, 1964
21. Shah DM, Leather RP: Arterioarterial atherothrombotic microemboli of the lower limb. In: Veith FJ, Hobson RW, Williams RA, Wilson SE (Eds) *Vascular Surgery: Principles and Practice* 2nd edn. New York: McGraw-Hill, 1994
22. Fine MJ, Kapoor W, Falanga V: Cholesterol crystal embolization: A review of 221 cases in the English literature. *Angiology* **38**: 769–784, 1987
23. Kazmier FJ: Shaggy aorta syndrome and disseminated atheromatous embolization. In: Bergan JJ, Yao JST (Eds) *Aortic Surgery*. Philadelphia: WB Saunders, 1989
24. Kaufman JL, Shah DM, Leather RP: Atheroembolism and microthromboembolic syndromes: Blue toe syndrome and disseminated atheroembolism. In: Rutherford RB (Ed) *Vascular Surgery* 4th edn. Philadelphia: WB Saunders, 1995
25. Jenkins DM, Newton WD: Atheroembolism. *Am Surg* **57**: 588–590, 1991
26. Kazmier FJ, Sheps SG, Bernatz PE, Sayre GP: Livedo reticularis and digital infarcts: A syndrome due to cholesterol emboli arising from atheromatous abdominal aortic aneurysms. *Vasc Dis* **3**: 12–24, 1966
27. Maurizi CP, Barker AE, Trueheart RE: Atheromatous emboli: A postmortem study with special reference to the lower extremities *Arch Path* **86**: 528–534, 1968
28. Kasinath BS, Lewis EJ: Eosinophilia as a clue to the diagnosis of atheroembolic renal disease. *Arch Int Med* **147**: 1384–1385, 1987

29. Starr DS, Lawrie GM, Morris GC: Prevention of distal embolism during arterial reconstruction. *Am J Surg* **138**: 764–769, 1979

30. Imparato AM: Abdominal aortic aneurysm: Prevention of lower limb ischemia. *Surgery* **93**: 112–116, 1983

31. Iliopoulos JI, Zdon MJ, Crawford BG *et al.*: Renal microembolization syndrome: A cause for renal dysfunction after abdominal aortic reconstruction. *Am J Surg* **146**: 779–783, 1983

32. Strom JA, Bernhard VM, Towne JB: Acute limb ischemia following aortic reconstruction: A preventable cause of increased mortality. *Arch Surg* **119**: 470–473, 1984

33. Carballo RE, Towne JB: Acute limb ischemia following aortic reconstruction. In: Ernst CB, Stanley JC (Eds) *Current Therapy in Vascular Surgery* 3rd edn. St Louis: Mosby, 1995

34. Parodi JC: Endovascular repair of abdominal aortic aneurysms and other arterial lesions. *J Vasc Surg* **21**: 549–556, 1995

35. Moore WS, Rutherford RB: Transfemoral endovascular repair of abdominal aortic aneurysm: Results of the North American EVT phase I trial. *J Vasc Surg* **23**: 543–553, 1996

36. Blum U, Voshage G, Lammer J *et al.*: Endoluminal stent-grafts for infrarenal abdominal aortic aneurysms. *N Engl J Med* (in press)

37. Balm R, Eikelboom BC, May J *et al.*: Early experience with transfemoral endovascular aneurysm management (TEAM) in the treatment of aortic aneurysms. *Eur J Endovasc Surg* **11**: 214–220, 1996

38. Blum U, Voshage G, Lammer J *et al.*: Endoluminal stent-grafts for infrarenal abdominal aortic aneurysms. *N Engl J Med* **336**: 59–60, 1997

Inflammatory Response to Endovascular Treatment of Abdominal Aortic Aneurysms

Lars Norgren and Paul Swartbol

INTRODUCTION

Endovascular procedures are without doubt less invasive than corresponding open surgery, usually with a great impact on hospital stay and mobilization of the patients. On the other hand, endovascular treatment involves catheter manipulations inside lesser or greater parts of the vascular system with a possible subsequent endothelial injury. When excluding an aortic aneurysm, it is still left in place together with its mural thrombus, and manipulations with introducers and catheters are performed inside the aneurysm in the vicinity of, or even in, the mural thrombus. The biological responses to these manoeuvres might be different from those achieved during clamping and reperfusion, routine parts of open revascularizations. During endovascular procedures only very short-lasting ischaemic periods are induced, while on the other hand the endothelial cell injury might be pronounced, depending on the kind and magnitude of the procedure and on the size and configuration of introducers and catheters, for treatment of an aortic aneurysm no less than 18–24 F.

Despite the fact that endovascular procedures have been practised since the end of the 1960s it was not until the time when more extensive operations were performed, such as for aortic aneurysms, that investigators found that the biological reactions to this procedure might be different from those well known during and after open surgery; one example being a long-lasting postoperative fever.

INFLAMMATORY RESPONSE IN GENERAL

Cytokines

Sepsis, trauma and surgery are conditions giving rise to pronounced inflammatory responses. Cytokines, such as tumour necrosis factor (TNF)-α and interleukin (IL)-6 are proinflammatory mediators of the host response. It is well recognized that TNF-α infusions are able to reproduce cardiovascular collapse signs,[1] while IL-6 may induce fever and cause acute phase protein synthesis.[2]

In a study on patients undergoing cardiac operations, joint replacement or gastric operations respectively,[3] it was found that TNF-α concentrations were low, while IL-6 increased rapidly after surgery, followed by a delayed increase of C-reactive protein. The magnitude of the reaction was related to the severity of the surgical procedure. Low or zero values of TNF-α are generally found during uncomplicated surgery. In elective surgery or after trauma, IL-6 is detected 4–6 hours after the event without any close correlation to blood loss, fever, white cell count or duration of the surgical procedure.[4] It seems that TNF-α plays a limited role in the regulation of the acute phase response to trauma, while IL-6 variably does.

Increases of TNF-α are more frequently found together with IL-1β in the systemic inflammatory response syndrome (SIRS).[5] During more advanced surgical procedures such as liver transplantation, TNF-α and IL-6 increases have been recorded between the end of the anhepatic phase and the end of the procedure, closely correlated to subsequent infections.[6] It is also evident that endothelial cell pathophysiology plays a role in the development of SIRS and multiple organ failure, and that TNF-α and IL-6 are two of the cytokines frequently increasing in these conditions.[7] In patients in septic shock due to Gram-negative bacteria, survivors had lower levels of TNF-α than did non-survivors after a period of 10 days. However, TNF-α values did not strictly predict outcome.[8] Partly contradicting results were recorded in patients with multiple organ failure, caused by intra-abdominal infections,[9] where TNF-α levels were lower in those patients who did not survive, interpreted as an anergic immune status.

RESPONSES TO AORTIC ANEURYSM SURGERY

Cytokines

Compared with the response of inguinal hernia repair, elective aortic aneurysm surgery caused an IL-6 response which was exaggerated in association with subsequent major complications.[10] Comparing multiple trauma and ruptured aortic aneurysms and elective aortic aneurysms, it was found that non-survivors had after 6 hours significantly higher TNF-α levels than those who survived. Traumatized patients had significantly higher IL-6 levels while patients with ruptured abdominal aortic aneurysms (AAA) had higher TNF-α levels. The TNF-α response was recorded early in complicated cases. A close correlation between early and high levels of the cytokines and the development of multiorgan failure and acute respiratory disease syndrome (ARDS) was found.[11] In comparing elective and acute repair of aortic aneurysms it was found that both TNF-α and IL-6 were significantly higher in patients in shock and in those who subsequently died.[12] It has also been shown that a correlation exists between a sigmoid colon pH <7.0 after AAA repair and raised levels of TNF-α and IL-6.[13]

In the pathogenesis of atherosclerosis and of atherosclerotic abdominal aneurysms it seems that immunological mechanisms play an important role. Inflammatory white blood cells invade the vessel wall and release cytokines. It has thus been shown that the AAA wall produces IL-6.[14] Also TNF-α has been found in abdominal aneurysm tissues, which indicates in favour of an inflammatory aetiology to the aneurysm and also an involvement in tissue growth and neovascularization.[15–17]

Complement

The complement system is activated by various enzymes released from blood cells in different conditions, also surgical procedures. Aortic reconstructive surgery induces complement activation.[18–20] In a study from our group evaluating complement reactions during aortofemoral surgery utilizing two different graft materials, Dacron and expanded polytetrafluoroethylene (ePTFE),[20] it was found important to correct for haemodilution, which differs considerably between patients and during the course of surgery. A significant decrease of C1q and a corresponding increase of C5a were generally observed while terminal complexes remained unchanged. Until the third postoperative day insignificant differences were recorded between the two graft groups while later on patients receiving Dacron grafts showed significantly higher levels of C4 and C3 than those who had an ePTFE graft.

Responses to biomaterials

The response to any synthetic material inserted in the blood stream is a cascade of reactions concerning coagulation, activation of blood cells, release of various products, e.g. cytokines, and activation of the complement system.[20] Effects on acute thrombogenecity as well as on late graft failure due to intimal hyperplasia are expected. Recently, also variations in surface adhesion molecule expression have been discussed[21] but need to be further elucidated. *In vitro* and *in vivo* studies have focused on local and systemic responses to biomaterials.[10,22] Some inconsistency concerning the role of TNF-α in this situation is found,[10] which may be attributed to the laboratory methodology. Regularly C-reactive protein increases after vascular surgery, involving graft implantation or not. This reaction should therefore be interpreted as unspecific.

SIDE-EFFECTS AFTER ENDOVASCULAR SURGERY OF AORTIC ANEURYSMS

Little attention has been paid to specific cellular reactions after endovascular treatment of an aortic aneurysm; however, long-lasting fever has been recorded as has an increased level of C-reactive protein.[23] Technical complications such as haematoma, malplacement and migration of stented grafts, embolization and leakage have been registered in about one-third of the patients in the beginning of the endovascular era.[24] In a follow-up of 53 patients, local and vascular complications were found in 32% and systemic complications in 25%. The latter included renal insufficiency and cardiac problems such as myocardial infarction and cardiac arythmia.[25] In most patient materials a low incidence of macroembolization or microembolization is usually registered. Leakage, early or late, is a remaining problem with variations between the devices which are used.[26,27]

Guidelines for the development and use of endovascular prosthetic devices have been published, in the first place discussing technical evaluation. Concerning systemic side-effects only renal and haematological function studies are mentioned.[28]

In a prospective series of seven patients treated with an endoluminal procedure compared with seven patients treated conventionally for an aortic aneurysm, we recorded a decreased blood pressure during insertion of the endovascular device in the majority of cases.[29,30] There was a correlation to an increased level of TNF-α, occurring immediately post-implantation with a maximum 60 minutes later, and decreasing to zero values within 48 hours. In contrast, conventional surgery did not cause any TNF-α increase at all, while IL-6 increased in both groups, significantly more during open surgery, between 6 and 24 hours after clamping and implantation of the endovascular device, respectively (Fig. 1). The C-reactive protein increased in both groups with a similar pattern, demonstrating a peak at 48–72 hours postoperatively and with significantly higher values for the conventionally treated patients at 48 hours and at 7 days postoperatively.

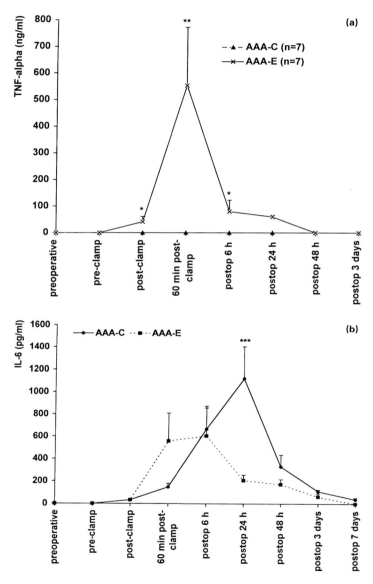

Fig. 1. Time course of TNF-α release (a) and of IL-6 release (b): 'pre-clamp' means immediately before balloon inflation or aortic clamping; 'post-clamp' means immediately after balloon deflation or declamping.

The body temperature was significantly higher in the conventionally treated patients 4–18 hours postoperatively. Thereafter, the endovascular patient group had a higher body temperature level, returning to normal with some variation, usually before the 6th postoperative day (Fig. 2).

Granulocyte-, leucocyte-, monocyte- and platelet counts showed that the white cells decreased, and monocytes were almost non-existent 60 minutes after the endovascular implantation. There was no corresponding finding during open surgery (Fig. 3). On the other hand, platelets showed the same pattern in both groups slightly decreasing until the 3rd postoperative day after which they increased.

Concerning complement proteins, there was less consumption of C1q, C4 and C3 in the endovascular patient group compared with conventional treatment. Increased C5a levels were recorded in the conventionally treated group while slight fluctuations were noticed during endovascular surgery. Terminal complexes did not vary between the groups.

The conclusions from this study were that endovascular aortic aneurysm repair induced a significant inflammatory response, mainly involving TNF-α and differing from the findings during open aneurysm repair. Conventional surgery induced responses which were more related to the extensive surgical trauma and a reperfusion injury. Partly contradicting this are results from another study[31] in which TNF-α was studied together with oxygen free radical production. In this study TNF-α was detected during conventional repair but was lower in the endovascular patient group.

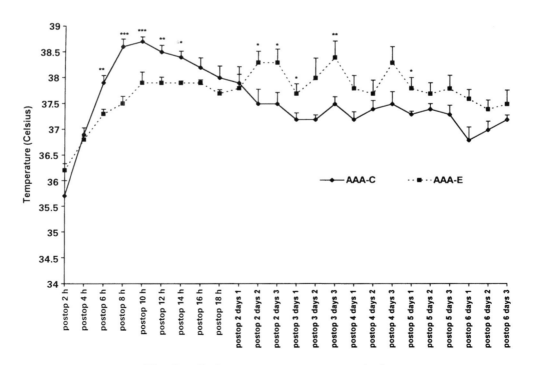

Fig. 2. Body temperature postoperatively.

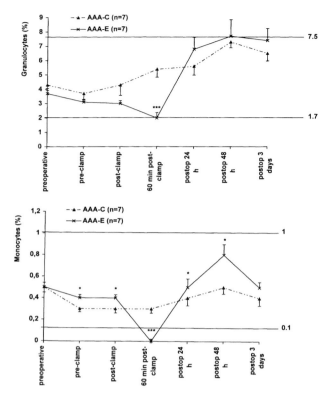

Fig. 3. Percentage granulocytes (upper curve) and monocytes (lower curve) preoperatively, during surgery and postoperatively

Production of oxygen free radicals was not significantly different between the two study groups. Differences between these two studies might be attributed to variations in blood sampling times and the methodology used for the analysis.

It may be that TNF-α and IL-6 induce tissue injury by alteration of surface adhesion molecules on white blood cells. To study surface adhesion molecule expression and as a follow-up to our clinical study, blood samples from the same patient groups were used to determine the response of white blood cells.[32] Monoclonal antibodies against the integrins CD11a, CD11b, CD11c, CD18 and L-selectin were used. The CD11b, CD11c and CD18 molecules on both granulocytes and monocytes were significantly upregulated 60 minutes after the endovascular procedure compared with conventional aneurysm repair (Fig. 4), and L-selectine molecules were by this time correspondingly cleaved off. A peak adhesion molecule expression 60 minutes after balloon deflation in the endovascular group correlated to the release of TNF-α. Whether the clinical correlate is tissue damage could not be stated as patients with complications and those without, had the same kind of cellular response, however, differing in magnitude.

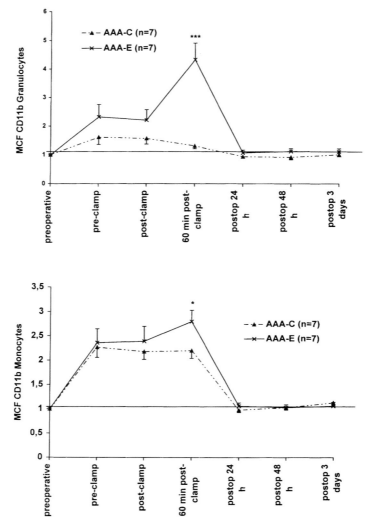

Fig. 4. Time course of plasma induced CD11b adhesion molecule expression on granulocytes and monocytes respectively.

The present findings with an extensive inflammatory response to endovascular procedures might have different reasons. One possibility is that the materials building up this stent-supported graft, woven polyester, platinum, nitinol wires and polyester sutures may cause inadvert reactions. In preliminary experiments regarding surface adhesion molecule expression, all components were, however, inert (Fig. 5). Another possibility is that manipulations inside the aortic aneurysm also touch the thrombus (Fig. 6), which first of all may induce micro- or macroembolization, but also cause release of toxic products and of cytokines. It is well known that bacteria, mainly *Staphylococcus epidermidis*, contaminate a

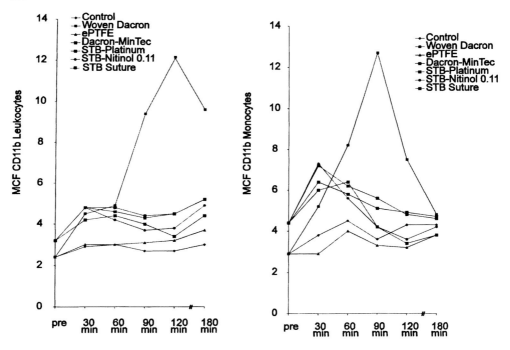

Fig. 5. CD11b adhesion molecule expression on leukocytes and monocytes incubated with various graft materials and components of the endovascular device.

proportion of aortic aneurysm thrombi, reported at from 5 to 25%.[33–37] Taking this low incidence into account it seems, however, less reasonable to assume that a bacteraemia explains our findings.

The thrombus is only partly built up by living cells, but has an ability to release cytokines such as TNF-α and IL-6 (preliminary results). Apparently, the thrombus also appears differently, being more or less organized. Using magnetic resonance imaging (MRI) and evaluating the signal intensity, good correlation was found between these findings and intraoperative characterization of the organization of the aortic aneurysm thrombus during open surgery.[38] In an ongoing study[39] we have shown that MRI performed pre- and postoperatively in patients undergoing endovascular treatment of aortic aneurysms is able to characterize remodelling of the thrombus by time. In some patients multiple layers of different age are seen (Fig. 7). Furthermore, this study has shown two cases of vertebral body infarction, none of these features being possible to evaluate on CT scan or angiography. One may speculate whether fresh thrombi are more prone to cause reactions and release of cytokines. A clinical impression is that in patients with aneurysms without or with only small thrombi, or when a non-touch technique has been possible, the adverse reactions, both blood pressure decreases and cellular responses, have been limited or absent.

The aim of treating aortic aneurysms is to reduce the risk of rupture, which means that a further growth should be prevented. Yet, little knowledge exists what happens

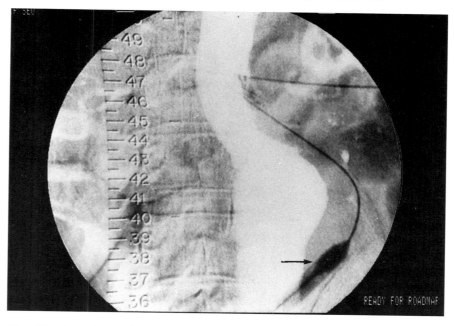

Fig. 6. The introducer (arrow) penetrating the thrombus during an endovascular procedure.

in the long run with an aortic aneurysm treated with an endovascular procedure. From most reports there seems to be a correlation between shrinkage of the aneurysm and absence of leakage. Leakage in this sense does not only mean the endovascular device not being tight enough to the native vessel proximally or distally, but also a leakage from open lumbar arteries or the inferior mesenteric artery. If leakage persists it has been shown that the aneurysm may grow. On the other hand, absence of leakage does not always mean that the aneurysm is reduced in size. Various methods may be used for the determination of aneurysm shrinkage, e.g. helical CT[40] or MRI.[39] Shrinkage and ingrowth of cells into the device have been shown during autopsy.[41] On the other hand, it has also been shown that late leakages at 12–18 months may develop, and the biology behind this is not known. Whether it implies growth of the aneurysmal neck, could probably not be excluded after 12–18 months.[42] In a recent publication it was shown that a paradoxic increase of the aortic neck diameter occurred both in patients whose aneurysm decreased and in those, where an increase was registered during a follow-up of 6 months or more.[43] The biology of the aneurysm *per se* may therefore be of great importance. It is well known that a lumbar aortic aneurysm has a reduced elastin content and also in patients with a family history, a decreased content of type III collagen.[44] The impact of inflammation and neovascularization should also be born in mind.[45] Whether β-blockers[46] or monoclonal antibodies to reduce surface adhesion molecule expression[47] could help reduce the risk of expansion should be further studied.

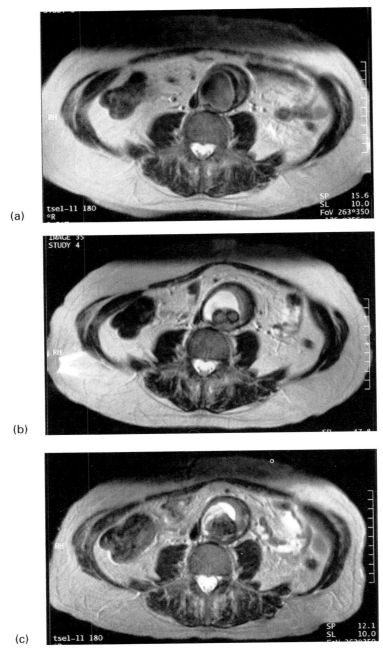

(a)

(b)

(c)

Fig. 7. T2-Weighted images of an aortic aneurysm preoperatively (a); 1 month postoperatively (b); and 6 months postoperatively (c). Preoperatively, there can be seen a low signal of an organized thrombus, while a fresh thrombus is seen at 1 month besides the organized part and finally remodelling of both the fresh and the organized thrombus is seen at 6 months.

To conclude, the development of an AAA involves inflammatory components. Whether these features and others involved in the growth of the aneurysm stop when an aneurysm is treated with an endovascular procedure, is not known. Inconsistently, it has also been shown that the endovascular procedure itself causes inflammatory responses different from those known from conventional aneurysm surgery. Correlation to complications seems reasonable, however, this kind of transient reactions occur also in non-complicated cases. Only time will show whether adverse reactions will appear later. Characterization of aneurysms which stop growing, shrink and disappear is of the greatest interest. Prospective studies, regular follow-up and, at the very best, randomized controlled studies of endovascular versus conventional treatment, will help answer these open questions.

ACKNOWLEDGEMENTS

We are grateful for contributions by the following colleagues from the Departments of Clinical Immunology, Interventional Radiology and Vascular Surgery: U. Albrechtsson, G. Danielsson, L. Engellau, T. Jonung, E. Ribbe, J. Thörne, L. Truedsson Z. Zdanowski.

REFERENCES

1. Warren RS, Starnes HF Jr, Gabrilove JL *et al.*: The acute metabolic effects of tumor necrosis factor administration in humans. *Arch Surg* **122:** 1396–1400, 1987
2. Marinkovic S, Jahreis GP, Wong GG, Baumann H: IL-6 modulates the synthesis of a specific set of acute phase plasma proteins *in vivo*. *J Immunol* **142:** 808–812, 1989
3. Kragsbjerg P, Holmberg H, Vikerfors T: Serum concentrations of interleukin-6, tumour necrosis factor-α, and C-reactive protein in patients undergoing major operations. *Eur J Surg* **161:** 17–22, 1995
4. Pullicino EA, Carli F, Poole S *et al.*: The relationship between the circulating concentrations of interleukin 6 (IL-6), tumor necrosis factor (TNF) and the acute phase response to elective surgery and accidental injury. *Lymphokine Res* **9:** 231–238, 1990
5. Dinarello CA: Interleukin-1. In: Thomson AW (Ed) *The Cytokine Handbook* pp. 31–56. San Diego: Academic Press Inc, 1992
6. Sautner T, Függer R, Götzinger P *et al.*: Tumour necrosis factor-α and interleukin-6: Early indicators of bacterial infection after human orthotopic liver transplantation. *Eur J Surg* **161:** 97–101, 1995
7. Wang X, Andersson R: The role of endothelial cells in the systemic inflammatory response syndrome and multiple system organ failure. *Eur J Surg* **161:** 703–713, 1995
8. Calandra T, Baumgartner JD, Grau GE *et al.*: Prognostic values of tumor necrosis factor/cachectin, interleukin-1, interferon-α, and interferon-gamma in the serum of patients with septic shock. Swiss-Dutch J5 Immunoglobulin Study Group. *J Infect Dis* **161:** 982–987, 1990
9. Hamilton G, Hofbauer S, Hamilton B: Endotoxin, TNF-a, interleukin-6 and parameters of the cellular immune system in patients with intraabdominal sepsis. *Scand J Infect Dis* **24:** 361–368, 1992
10. Baigrie RJ, Lamont PM, Kwiatkowski D *et al.*: Systemic cytokine response after major surgery. *Br J Surg* **79:** 757–760, 1992
11. Roumen RM, Hendriks T, van der Ven-Jongekrijg J *et al.*: Cytokine patterns in patients after major vascular surgery, hemorrhagic shock, and severe blunt trauma. Relation with

subsequent adult respiratory distress syndrome and multiple organ failure. *Ann Surg* **218:** 769–776, 1993

12.   Froon AHM, Greve JW, van der Linden CJ, Buurman WA: Increased concentrations of cytokines and adhesion molecules in patients after repair of abdominal aortic aneurysm. *Eur J Surg* **162:** 287–296, 1996

13.   Soong CV, Blair PH, Halliday MI *et al.*: Endotoxaemia, the generation of the cytokines and their relationship to intramucosal acidosis of the sigmoid colon in elective abdominal aortic aneurysm repair. *Eur J Vasc Surg* **7:** 534–539, 1993

14.   Szekanecz Z, Shah MR, Pearce WH, Koch AE: Human atherosclerotic abdominal aortic aneurysms produce interleukin (IL)-6 and interferon-gamma but not IL-2 and IL-4: the possible role for IL-6 and interferon-gamma in vascular inflammation. *Agents Actions* **42:** 159–162, 1994

15.   Newman KM, Jean-Claude J, Li H *et al.*: Cytokines that activate proteolysis are increased in abdominal aortic aneurysms. *Circulation* **90:** II224–227, 1994

16.   Szekanecz Z, Shah MR, Harlow LA *et al.*: Interleukin-8 and tumor necrosis factor-α are involved in human aortic endothelial cell migration. The possible role of these cytokines in human aortic aneurysmal blood vessel growth. *Pathobiology* **62:** 134–139, 1994

17.   Pearce WH, Sweis I, Yao JS *et al.*: Interleukin-1β and tumor necrosis factor-α release in normal and diseased human infrarenal aortas. *J Vasc Surg* **16:** 784–789, 1992

18.   De Mol Van Otterloo JCA, Van Bockel JH, Ponfoort ED *et al.*: The effects of aortic reconstruction and collagen impregnation of Dacron prostheses on the complement system. *J Vasc Surg* **16:** 774–783, 1992

19.   Pärsson H, Nässberger L, Norgren L: Inflammatory response to aorto-bifemoral bypass surgery. *Int Angiol* **4:** 483–491, 1996

20.   Swartbol P, Pärsson H, Truedsson L *et al.*: Aorto-bifemoral surgery induces complement activation and release of interleukin-6 (IL-6) but not tumor necrosis factor-alpha (TNFα). *J Cardiovasc Surg* **4:** 483–491, 1996

21.   Swartbol P, Truedsson L, Pärsson H, Norgren L: Surface adhesion molecule expression on human blood cells induced by vascular graft-materials *in vitro*. *J Biomed Mat Res* 1997 (in press)

22.   Cardona MA, Simmons RL, Kaplan SS: TNF and IL-1 generation by human monocytes in response to biomaterials. *J Biomed Mat Res* **26:** 851–859, 1992

23.   Blum U, Langer M, Spillner G *et al.*: Abdominal aortic aneurysms: preliminary technical and clinical results with transfemoral placement of endovascular self-expanding stent-grafts *Radiology* **198:** 25–31, 1996

24.   Parodi JC: Endovascular repair of abdominal aortic aneurysms. In: Chuter TAM, Donayre CE, White RA (Eds) *Endoluminal Vascular Prostheses* pp. 37–53. Boston: Little, Brown and Company, 1995

25.   May J, White GH, Yu W *et al.*: Surgical management of complications following endoluminal grafting of abdominal aortic aneurysms. *Eur J Vasc Endovasc Surg* **10:** 51–59, 1995

26.   Mialhe C, Amicabile C: Endovascular treatment of aneurysms of the subrenal aorta using the Stentor endoprosthesis. Preliminary series. *J Mal Vasc* **20:** 290–295, 1995

27.   Chuter TA, Wendt G, Hopkinson BR *et al.*: Transfemoral insertion of a bifurcated endovascular graft for aortic aneurysm repair: the first 22 patients. *Cardiovasc Surg* **3:** 121–128, 1995

28.   Veith FJ, Abbott WM, Yao JST *et al.*: Guidelines for development and use of transluminally placed endovascular prosthetic grafts in the arterial system. *J Vasc Surg* **21:** 670–685, 1995

29.   Norgren L, Albrechtsson U, Swartbol P: Side effect of endovascular grafting to treat aortic aneurysm *Br J Surg* **83:** 520–521, 1996

30.   Swartbol P, Norgren L, Albrechtsson L *et al.*: Biological responses differ considerably between endovascular and conventional aortic aneurysm surgery. *Eur J Vasc Endovasc Surg* **12:** 18–25, 1996

31.   Thompson MM, Nasim A, Sayers RD *et al.*: Oxygen free radical and cytokine generation during endovascular and conventional aneurysm repair. *Eur J Vasc Endovasc Surg* **12:** 70–75, 1996

32. Swartbol P, Norgren L, Pärsson H, Truedsson L: Endovascular abdominal aortic aneurysm repair induces significant alterations in surface adhesion molecule expression on donor white blood cells exposed to patient plasma. *Eur Soc Vasc Surg Venice* 1996 (abstract)

33. Steed DL, Higgins RS, Pasculle A, Webster MW: Culture of intraluminal thrombus during abdominal aortic aneurysm resection: significant contamination is rare. *Cardiovasc Surg* **1:** 494–498, 1993

34. Schwartz JA, Powell TW, Burnham SJ, Johnson G Jr: Culture of abdominal aortic aneurysm contents. An additional series. *Arch Surg* **122:** 777–780, 1987

35. McAuley CE, Steed DL, Webster MW: Bacterial presence in aortic thrombus at elective aneurysm resection: is it clinically significant? *Am J Surg* **147:** 322–324, 1984

36. Raso AM, Muncinelli M, Serra R *et al.*: Intraoperative microbiological monitoring in abdominal aortic aneurysms in elective surgery. A review of the literature and the authors' personal experience. *Minerva Cardioangiol* **40:** 375–381, 1992

37. van der Vliet JA, Kouwenberg PP, Muytjens HL *et al.*: Relevance of bacterial cultures of abdominal aortic aneurysm contents. *Surgery* **119:** 129–132, 1996

38. Castrucci M, Mellone R, Vanzulli A *et al*: Mural thrombi in abdominal aortic aneurysms: MR imaging characterization – useful before endovascular treatment? *Radiology* **197:** 135–139, 1995

39. Engellau L, Albrechtsson U, Norgren L: What does MRI add in the postoperative evaluation of endoluminally treated abdominal aortic aneurysms? (Personal series, to be published)

40. Rozenblit A, Marin ML, Veith FJ *et al.*: Endovascular repair of abdominal aortic aneurysm: value of postoperative follow-up with helical CT. *Am J Roentgenol* **165:** 1473–1479, 1995

41. Lundbom J, Hatlinghus S, Aadal P *et al.*: Autopsy findings in a patient with Stentor implant for abdominal aortic aneurysm. *J Endovasc Surg* **3:** 236, 1996

42. May J, White G, Yu W *et al.*: How durable is endoluminal aneurysm repair? Fate of the aneurysm sac and the patient after successful procedures. *J Endovasc Surg* **3:** 237, 1996

43. May J, White G, Yu W *et al.*: A prospective study of anatomico-pathological changes in abdominal aortic aneurysms following endoluminal repair: Is the aneurysmal process reversed? *Eur J Vasc Endovasc Surg* **12:** 11–17, 1996

44. Powell J, Greenhalgh RM: Cellular, enzymatic, and genetic factors in the pathogenesis of abdominal aortic aneurysms. *J Vasc Surg* **9:** 297–304, 1989

45. Thompson MM, Jones L, Nasim A *et al.*: Angiogenesis in abdominal aortic aneurysms. *Eur J Vasc Endovasc Surg* **11:** 464–469, 1996

46. Powell J: Does use of beta-blockers have any impact on the growth of aortic aneurysms? In: Greenhalgh RM, Fowkes FGR (Eds) *Trials and Tribulations of Vascular Surgery*. London: WB Saunders, 1996

47. Ricci MA, Strindberg G, Slaiby JM *et al.*: Anti-CD 18 monoclonal antibody slows experimental aortic aneurysm expansion. *J Vasc Surg* **23:** 301–307, 1996

Multiple Organ Dysfunction Syndrome in Abdominal Aortic Aneurysm Repair

Aires A. B. Barros D'Sa and Chee V. Soong

INTRODUCTION

Since the first report of abdominal aortic aneurysm (AAA) repair by Dubost in 1952,[1] the declining morbidity and mortality associated with this operation is attributable to advances in surgical and anaesthetic techniques, improved prosthetic design and better postoperative monitoring and management.[2-9] A return to normal life expectancy of good quality can be anticipated following this procedure even in those patients who spend prolonged periods in the intensive care unit and survive multiple organ dysfunction syndrome (MODS).[2,10-12]

The actual incidence of MODS following AAA repair is not well documented but probably contributes to about a quarter of all deaths resulting from surgery in both elective and emergency situations (Table 1).[12,13-15] The development of MODS following ruptured aneurysm repair may account for more than 90% of late deaths and when more than two organs fail the fatality rate may be 100%.[13] Dysfunction in isolated organs is much more common and even if self-limiting may contribute to fatality if the heart or kidneys are affected (Tables 2 and 3).[13,14,16-22] Following elective aneurysm repair, up to 50% of patients will develop some form of acute medical event requiring urgent attention.[23] In a series of patients presenting with ruptured aneurysm, cardiac complications occurred in more than 50%, renal failure in 20% and respiratory impairment in 10%.[24] In many cases organ dysfunction passes unnoticed and may be manifested only by biochemical changes. The impairment of one organ, however, may pose an additional strain on other organs and systems particularly those which have been previously compromised. If a combination of organs is impaired the prognostic risk of developing MODS is greater than the sum of their

Table 1. MODS as cause of death in aneurysm repair

	Elective %	Ruptured %
Meester et al.[13]	0	23
Søreide et al.[12]	20	21
Campbell et al.[14]	0	15
Lawrie et al.[15]	–	5

Table 2.   Isolated organ dysfunction as cause of death in patients operated for ruptured AAA

	Sepsis	Respiratory	Renal	Cardiac	Total %
Meester et al.[13]	5%	7%	4%	4%	49
Søreide et al.[12]	6%	—	—	6%	58
Meddings et al.[17]	—	3%	7%	3%	50
Fielding et al.[18]	2%	17%	17%	12%	43
Hicks et al.[19]	—	—	12%	25%	49
Campbell et al.[14]	5%	-	11%	5%	56
Lawrie et al.[15]	—	3%	3%	8%	20
Pedrini et al.[20]	—	—	2%	23%	40
Bickerstaff et al.[21]	—	4%	4%	4%	39

Table 3.   Complications following elective AAA repair

Complications	Bickerstaff et al.[21]	Campbell et al.[14]	Pedrini et al.[20]	Diehl et al.[22]
Cardiac	1	7	5	8
Respiratory	2	21	1	5
Renal	2	2	—	1
Limb ischaemia	1	5	—	—
Ileus	1	—	—	—
GI bleed	—	—	0.4	—
Mortality	7	6	6	5

individual risks taken together.[25] In a multicentre study of mortality following elective infrarenal aortic reconstruction, cardiac complications were the most common cause of death while MODS represented the 'final common pathway' leading to eventual demise in those who survived an initial adverse event.[26] The lack of clarity on the pathogenesis of organ dysfunction following AAA repair perhaps accounts for the number of varied theories which have been proposed.

FACTORS CONTRIBUTING TO MODS

Multiple factors are usually responsible for the development of MODS, the role played by each differing in importance when comparing outcomes in elective and ruptured cases. These include blood loss and transfusion, nutritional depletion, bowel ischaemia, endotoxaemia and impaired organ function and ischaemia-reperfusion injury.

Blood loss and blood transfusion

The volume of blood loss is of significance especially in patients in the ruptured group in whom the haemoglobin level at presentation was found to be a determinant predictive of mortality and the development of MODS.[27-29] Impairment of immune cell function may ensue 24 hours after haemorrhage and resuscitation with evidence of reduced capacity by the liver to eliminate absorbed bacteria and endotoxin from the portal blood.[30,31] Homologous blood transfusion may cause a reduction in lymphocyte count and function associated with an increased risk of postoperative infections.[32] Transfusion-related acute lung may result from the sequestration of activated granulocytes in the pulmonary parenchyma.[33] Even autologous blood can generate substantial numbers of activated leukocytes with evidence of increased expression of surface receptors.[34]

Nutritional depletion

All patients undergoing AAA surgery have to fast for a few days; those presenting with a ruptured aneurysm frequently languishing in the intensive care unit and dependent on their only source of nutrition, if administered at all, via the parenteral route. Much evidence now supports the superiority of enteral over parenteral nutrition especially as the latter is associated with gut mucosal atrophy and a reduction in IgA antibody secretion by the enterocytes which may in turn permit bacterial translocation through a disrupted mucosal barrier.[35-40] An increased acute phase response and tumour necrosis factor (TNF) production have also been observed in patients given total parenteral nutrition (TPN) and no enteral feeding.[41,42] In addition to the route of administration, the make-up of these feeds is just as vital. Diets which enhance the immune status of critically ill patients in intensive care units have been shown to reduce complications secondary to infection and shorter hospital stay.[43] Of all the components making up these feeds one amino acid, glutamine, has recently been the focus of much interest. In fact, this non-essential amino acid has been shown to be conditionally essential and a major nutrient of rapidly dividing cells such as the enterocytes and lymphocytes.[44,45] Glutamine supplements may be used to improve the phagocytic and immune function of macrophages and when added to TPN solutions will preserve intestinal mucosal morphology and its integrity.[46-49] In the critically ill, the supplementation of this amino acid in TPN solution has been found to preserve mucosal structure in the duodenum and reduce the loss of barrier function of the gut.[50] Other workers have demonstrated that its infusion into the lumen of gut may prevent a breach of the mucosal barrier function in septic states.[51] The reduction of glutamine levels in plasma of patients who have sustained trauma may provoke a depression of the immune state after major surgery.[52,53] Recently, a significant and persistent reduction in plasma glutamine concentration was observed following elective abdominal aortic aneurysm repair.[54] However, the effect of that fall in plasma glutamine concentration in this cohort of patients has not been properly evaluated.

Bowel ischaemia

As with many other clinical situations, the gut has been incriminated as the source of sepsis and of multiple organ failure.[55] The development of MODS may be caused by the egress of luminal contents and bacterial products across an ischaemic bowel wall. Transmural infarction of the bowel wall will allow direct peritoneal contamination and bacterial entry into the blood stream from the peritoneal cavity.[56] On the other hand, mild ischaemia may give rise to disruption of the bowel mucosa barrier with initial invasion of the portal venous system but a delay in systemic bacteraemia attributable to hepatic filtering (Fig. 1). The segment of bowel most commonly affected by ischaemia following AAA surgery is the left colon, the precarious blood supply to which may be compromised during aortic surgery. The main reason appears to be ligation of the inferior mesenteric artery but in some patients the iliac vessels are sacrificed or bypassed either because of aneurysmal involvement or occlusive disease. The collateral circulation to the bowel of these patients may prove inadequate particularly if atherosclerotic disease is also present. Hypovolaemia secondary to blood loss, inadequate fluid replacement or cardiac failure may further impair perfusion of the bowel. In addition, traction on the mesentery and eventration of small bowel may raise the plasma concentrations of prostaglandins and lead to haemodynamic disturbances.[57–60] All these factors may be individually insignificant but when they occur concomitantly, severe ischaemia of the bowel may follow.[61] Low blood flow states developing against a background of arterial constriction or occlusion of part of the mesenteric circulation may promote sufficient reduction in perfusion which precipitates intestinal ischaemia.[62]

Most reports on bowel ischaemia in patients undergoing aortic surgery dwell on the more severe types of presentation. However, many patients will suffer a milder reversible form which does not lead to macroscopic changes in the mucosa but which

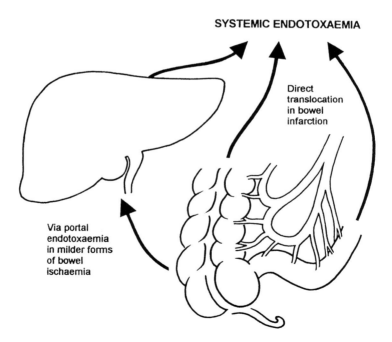

SYSTEMIC ENDOTOXAEMIA

Direct translocation in bowel infarction

Via portal endotoxaemia in milder forms of bowel ischaemia

Fig. 1.   The development of systemic endotoxaemia following different degrees of bowel ischaemia.

can produce microscopic mucosal injury characterized by epithelial lifting, disintegration of the lamina propria, haemorrhage and ulceration.[63] The mucosa at the tip of the villi is particularly prone to ischaemia due to the counter-current exchange mechanism of the vessels.[64] Shunting of blood during low flow states may lead to ischaemia affecting the tips of the villi only. This subclinical sequel to intestinal hypotension can produce an increase in mucosal permeability and permit the passage of luminal contents across the gut wall (Fig. 2).[65,66] It was proposed that the mucosal damage after temporary ischaemia occurred during re-establishment of normal blood flow instead of at the time of ischaemia. Parks and Granger[67] in 1986 demonstrated that the mucosal lesions following regional ischaemia were more pronounced during reperfusion compared with bowel subjected only to ischaemia.

The mechanism involved in this ischaemia-reperfusion injury is considered to be due to the generation of oxygen-derived free radicals via the xanthine oxidase system.[68] The free radicals generated can activate the arachidonic acid cascade with the production of thromboxanes and leukotrienes.[69,70] These byproducts are potent chemoattractants and can lead to the activation of neutrophils and to their sequestration in various body sites.[71] The accumulation of these neutrophils may lead to sludging of capillaries, no-reflow and a worsening of the insult.[72] This trapping of neutrophils in the microvasculature of the bowel following reperfusion injury may be minimized by pretreatment using allopurinol and superoxide dismutase;[73] neutrophil depletion prior to the insult itself reduces the ischaemia-reperfusion induced mucosal dysfunction.[74] An increase in intestinal permeability after abdominal aortic operations has been observed and the loss in mucosal barrier function may explain the higher incidence of infection by intestinal organisms and of mortality secondary to MODS in patients who develop evidence of ischaemic colitis following elective abdominal aortic surgery.[75,76]

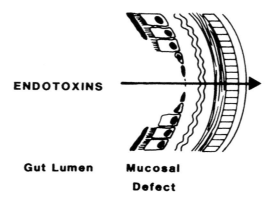

ENDOTOXINS

Gut Lumen　　**Mucosal**
Defect

Fig. 2. A breach in the mucosa leading to disruption of the barrier function and the development of endotoxaemia after mild ischaemia.

Endotoxaemia and organ impairment

Endotoxaemia may develop without bacteraemia if only bacterial byproducts and not the whole organism permeate the gut wall. Endotoxins are the lipopolysaccharide constituent of the membrane of Gram-negative bacteria and it is this component which has been held responsible for the septic shock syndrome.[77] In one report, endotoxins were detected in all patients with septic shock and eventual recovery was associated with their disappearance from peripheral blood.[78] A relationship was also demonstrated between the concentration of endotoxin and eventual outcome.[78,79]

Endotoxin can enhance monocyte phagocytosis, release of oxygen-derived free radicals, production of lysosomal enzymes, tumour cytotoxicity, microbial activity and expression of class II histocompatibility antigens.[80,81] It may also lead to the activation of neutrophils priming them to produce leukotrienes, thereby creating a vicious cycle.[82,83] That in turn can bring about increased lung vascular permeability and pulmonary oedema.[84–86] The endotoxaemia so produced can also lead to a further reduction of bowel mucosal blood flow compounding the ischaemic insult. Many workers have detected endotoxaemia in patients undergoing AAA repair and the presence of plasma endotoxin has been related to the development of colonic ischaemia.[87–91] Patients with ischaemia have been found to have significantly more organ dysfunction and greater endotoxaemia compared with those who had no evidence of bowel hypoperfusion. Unfortunately, the interpretation of data remains difficult as their presence in plasma even in septic patients is unpredictable.[79,91,92] There is also the theoretical possibility of environmental contamination of samples so that endotoxin measurements may be unreliable.[93]

It is now clear that endotoxin produces most of its effects via cytokine mediators. It have been suggested that endotoxin *per se* may not be too toxic but that it brings about certain changes via endogenous mediators which are generated mainly by the macrophage.[94–96] These polypeptide mediators including TNF, interleukin-1(IL-1) and interleukin-6(IL-6), are known to share and augment each other's multibiological effects.[97–99] Evidence now exists to suggest that TNF is one of the principal mediators of septic shock. Workers have shown that pre-treatment with a neutralizing monoclonal anti-TNF anti-serum prevents the lethal effect of endotoxin; TNF can activate polymorphonuclear leukocytes for enhanced phagocytosis and together with its ability to stimulate the release of neutrophil chemotactic factors will induce the sequestration of these cells in localized areas.[100,101] In the lung this inflammatory response will lead to an increase in permeability causing pulmonary oedema.[102] The detection of TNF in patients undergoing AAA repair has been sporadic and intermittent.[87,103,104] Like endotoxin, the finding of this peptide in the plasma even in septic patients may be unreliable and misleading; TNF was detectable in only 25 % of cases with sepsis in the intensive care unit.[105] Many reasons have been offered to explain the inconsistencies of TNF measurements and its detection in plasma. In view of its short half-life sudden bursts of its release may be missed unless sampling is performed at very short intervals. Also it has been suggested that circulating levels of certain cytokines may not correctly indicate their presence locally around the cells as they function primarily as paracrine and autocrine mediators.[106,107] This may explain its absence in the group of patients assessed earlier by Baigrie *et al.*[103] Nevertheless, significantly higher concentrations of this cytokine and greater organ impairment have been observed in patients with bowel ischaemia.[87] Plasma concentrations of TNF and IL-1 were found to be significantly higher in patients presenting with a ruptured AAA compared with those operated on electively and correlated well with the subsequent development of adult respiratory distress syndrome (ARDS) and MODS.[104] High concentrations of these cytokines were also observed following endovascular repair and were found to be associated with a drop in systemic blood pressure in patients undergoing the procedure.[108]

Like TNF, IL-1 is also a pyrogen, induces hypotension, activates and promotes adherence of neutrophils and causes an increase in acute phase protein synthesis.[109–111] By administering recombinant human IL-1 the septic syndrome can be reproduced which is attenuated by ibuprofen suggesting that the cytokine acts via the production of eicosanoids.[109,112] Although increased levels have been demonstrated in septic patients, no correlation between concentrations and outcome was observed.[113,114] By sampling both early and intensely workers have demonstrated a rise in IL-1 in patients undergoing elective AAA repair.[89,104] The elevation in concentration of this peptide was noted to peak at around 2 hours after the initiation of the surgical insult.[103]

The administration of endotoxin in healthy subjects can also give rise to an elevation of IL-6 concentrations.[115] In the intensive care unit, patients who developed septic shock have been observed to have significantly higher concentrations of IL-6 than those in non-septic patients.[116] The concentration on admission was found to be a useful prognostic indicator of eventual outcome and correlated with the actual duration of survival.[117] Its ability to predict outcome in patients with intra-abdominal sepsis was better than the APACHE II score.[118] In AAA surgery an association between the plasma levels of IL-6 and the development of complications has been observed.[103] As that rise seems to precede the development of these complications, its routine use to identify high risk patients in aortic surgery has been proposed. Production of IL-6 following elective surgery peaks between 4 and 48 hours and normally falls towards baseline afterwards, except in patients who develop bowel infarction, in which case production may be sustained and persistent.[87,89] The proposal that the colon may be driving the generation of this cytokine has been derived from results demonstrating a significant correlation between its peak levels and colonic perfusion.[87,119] In support of this proposition, Baigrie *et al.*[120] demonstrated an eight-fold greater concentration of IL-6 in the portal circulation than in the systemic. Unfortunately, the actual role of IL-6 in the pathogenesis of the septic syndrome and its contribution towards MODS remains unclear and some have suggested that it contributes very little to the development of endotoxic shock other than to upregulate the level of TNF receptors.[121]

Ischaemia-reperfusion and remote organ injury

The clamping and unclamping of the major vessels plus fluctuations in blood pressure may give rise to ischaemia-reperfusion injury affecting not only specific organs but also the entire host by a global effect. A fall in the concentration of (α-tocopherol, the major lipid phase anti-oxidant, in these patients has been detected following aortic surgery suggesting its consumption by free-radical induced lipid peroxidation.[122] More recently others have discovered that an increased plasma concentration of lipofuscin, a byproduct of lipid peroxidation, is associated with ARDS and MODS.[16] This acute but protracted deterioration in pulmonary function, characterized by hypoxaemia, reduced lung compliance and oedema of non-cardiac origin, may occur within hours of restoring blood flow to the lower limbs in aneurysm repair.[123] This pulmonary congestion may be modified by the administration of mannitol which further supports the view of the role played by oxygen-derived free radicals.[124] It has been shown that a higher number of activated neutrophils enter the lungs than leave them which allows the hypothesis that these cells are sequestrated within the lung parenchyma.[125] This trapping of activated neutrophils by the lungs has been associated with an increased level of plasma thromboxane produced. More recently, it has been shown that the revascularization of ischaemic limbs can give rise to increased bowel permeability[126] and increased production of thromboxane B2 which, when reduced, abrogated the increased mucosal damage – but the exact mechanism is not known.[126,127] Recent studies have clearly shown that reperfusion of the acutely ischaemic lower limb is accompanied by structural changes in the gut mucosa associated with increased systemic endotoxin concentrations and activation of the cytokine IL-6.[126,128] Similarly, ischaemia-reperfusion injury to the gut may cause damage to remote organs such as the liver and lungs.[129,130] The production of such a proinflammatory factor within the plasma which is stable to storage and transfer following ischaemia-reperfusion injury has been confirmed even though its identity remains unknown.[131]

SUMMARY

Dysfunction of the various organs, either in isolation or in combination, are common problems following surgery on the abdominal aorta, especially in those presenting with a ruptured aneurysm. Many aetiological factors have been implicated in their causation but the role played by each will no doubt differ in degree from patient to patient. The majority of patients undergoing aortic aneurysm surgery are elderly and frequently suffer other associated health problems such as ischaemic heart disease, diabetes, hypertension, cerebrovascular disease and chronic obstructive airways disease. Although the presence of these risk factors increases their susceptibility to specific related complications, it is also evident that these patients are particularly vulnerable to the effects of haemorrhage, nutritional deprivation, bowel ischaemia and ischaemia-reperfusion injury, the end-point of which is MODS (Fig. 3).

The majority of patients undergoing aortic surgery especially after aneurysm rupture suffer significant blood losses necessitating transfusions which cause specific harmful host responses. In addition, these patients, especially those who present as emergencies, will normally be deprived of nutrition for prolonged periods and consequently their nutritional reserves become depleted to a degree which renders them immunocompromised.

Hypotension is a common occurrence during aortic surgery affecting the patient in general or an organ in particular; restoration of adequate flow leads to

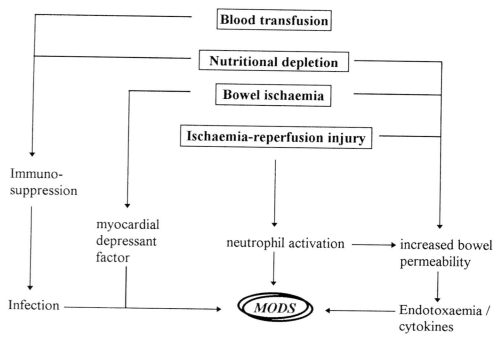

Fig. 3. Schematic representation of the role played by various factors in the development of MODS following AAA repair.

ischaemia-reperfusion injury of a degree reflecting the duration of preceding ischaemia. In this process oxygen-derived free radicals are produced which in turn generate byproducts which are potent neutrophil activators. The stimulation, infiltration and sequestration of these cells at local or remote sites will incur further damage to already injured cells. Whether the ischaemia is reversible or not, severe or mild, an increase in mucosal permeability of the bowel follows. The consequent permeation of luminal contents and bacterial products across the disrupted mucosal barrier gives rise to systemic endotoxaemia and the activation of the cytokine cascade, the resultant cytokine release causing damage via receptors attached to cell surfaces.

Unfortunately, the contribution made by each of these cascades cannot be easily comprehended and many questions remain unanswered. Even though gut ischaemia appears to play a pivotal role and causes MODS, the development of hypoxia and the low flow state associated with respiratory or cardiac failure can itself lead to injury of various organs. In a clinical situation it is difficult to ascertain which precedes the other. As humans are so complex it would be nearly impossible to dissect out the individual components which constitute the host response following abdominal aortic surgery or to identify their involvement in the development of MODS.

REFERENCES

1. Dubost C, Allary M, Oeconomos N: Resection of the abdominal aorta. *Arch Surg* **64:** 405–408, 1952
2. Crawford ES, Saleh SA, Babb III JW *et al.*: Infrarenal abdominal aortic aneurys. Factors influencing survival after operation performed over a 25 year period. *Ann Surg* **193:** 699–709, 1981
3. Creech O, Deterling CR, Edwards S *et al.*: Vascular prosthesis. Report of the committee for the study of vascular prosthesis of the society for vascular surgery. *Surgery* **41:** 62–80, 1957
4. Harrison JH, Swanson DS, Lincoln AF: A comparison of the tissue reactions to plastic materials - Dacron, Ivalon sponge, Nylon, Orlon and Teflon. *Arch Surg* **74:** 139–144, 1957
5. Creech O: Endoaneurysmorrhaphy and treatment of aortic aneurysms. *Ann Surg* **164:** 935–942, 1966
6. Makin GS. Changing fashions in the surgery of aortic aneurysms. *Ann R Coll Surg Engl* **65:** 308–310: 1983.
7. O'Toole DP, Quill D, Peyton M *et al.*: Radionuclide ventriculography and two dimensional echocardiography as predictors of left ventricular performance during aortic vascular surgery. *Eur J Vasc Surg* **2:** 329–332, 1988
8. Hessel EA: Introperative management of abdominal aortic aneurysms. *Surg Clin North Am* 69: 775–793, 1989
9. Kiell CS, Ernst CB: Advances in management of abdominal aortic aneurysm. *Adv Surg* **26:** 73–98, 1993
10. Gefke K, Schroeder TV, Thistd B *et al.*: Abdominal aortic aneurysm surgery: survival and quality of life in patients requiring prolonged postoperative intensive therapy. *Ann Vasc Surg* **8:** 137–143, 1994
11. SzilagyiDE, Smith RF, DeRusso FJ *et al.*: Contribution of abdominal aortic aneurysmectomy to prolongation of life. *Ann Surg* **164:** 634–638, 1966
12. Søreide O, Grimsgaard CHR, Myhre HO *et al.*: Time and course of death for 301 patients operated on for abdominal aortic aneurysm. *Age and Aging* **11:** 256–260, 1982
13. Meester RC, van der Graaf Y, Vos A, Eikelboom BC: Ruptured aortic aneurysm: early postoperative prediction of mortality using an organ system failure score. *Br J Surg* **81:** 512–516, 1994
14. Campbell WB, Collin J, Morris PS: The mortality of abdominal aortic aneurysm. *Ann Roy Coll Surg Engl* **68:** 275–278, 1986
15. Lawrie GM, Morris GC, Crawford S *et al.*: Improved results of operation for ruptured abdominal aortic aneurysms. *Surgery* **85:** 483–488, 1979
16. Roumen RMH, Hendriks T, de Man BM, Goris RJA: Serum lipofuscin as a prognostic indicator of adult respiratory distress syndrome and multiple organ failure. *Br J Surg* **81:** 1300–1005, 1994
17. Meddings RN, McCormick JStC, Mannam GC: Abdominal aortic aneurysm in south-west Scotland. *J R Coll Edinb* **36:** 6–10, 1991
18. Fielding JWL, Black J, Ashton F, Slaney G: Ruptured aortic aneurysms: postoperative complications and their aetiology. *Br J Surg* **71:** 487–491, 1984
19. Hicks GL, Eastland MW, DeWeese JA *et al.*: Survival improvement following aortic aneurysm resection. *Ann Surg* **181:** 863–869, 1975
20. Pedrini L, Mattioli R, Stella A *et al.*: Complications following the treatment of abdominal aortic aneurysms. *Ital J Surg Sci* **17:** 55–61, 1987
21. Bickerstaff LK, Hollier LH, van Peenen HJ *et al.*: Abdominal aortic aneurysms: The changing natural history. *J Vasc Surg* **1:** 6–12, 1984
22. Diehl JT, Cali RF, Hertzer NR, Beven EG: Complication of abdominal aortic reconstruction. *Ann Surg* **197:** 49–56, 1983
23. Campbell WB, Ballard PK, Goodman DA: Intensive care after abdominal aortic surgery. *Eur J Vasc Surg* 5: 665–668, 1991
24. Barros D'Sa AAB: Optimal travel distance before ruptured aortic aneurysm repair. In: Greenhalgh RM, Mannick JA (Eds) *The Cause and Management of Aneurysms*. London, Philadelphia: WB Saunders, 1990

25. Tilney NL, Bailey GL, Morgan AP: Sequential systems failure after rupture abdominal aortic aneurysms: An unresolved problem in postoperative care. *Ann Surg* **178**: 117–122, 1973

26. Galland RB: Mortality following elective infrarenal aortic reconstruction: a UK Joint Vascular Research Group Study. (Submitted for publication)

27. Bauer EP, Redaelli C, von Segesser LK, Turina MI: Ruptured abdominal aortic aneurysms: predictors for early complications and death. *Surgery* **114**: 31–35, 1993

28. Adachi Y, Matsumata T, Kuwano H *et al.*: A clinical analysis of multiple organ failure following elective surgery. *Surgery Today* **24**: 333–336, 1994

29. Hardman DT, Fisher CM, Patel MI *et al.*: Ruptured abdominal aortic aneurysms: who should be offered surgery? *J Vasc Surg* **23**: 123–129, 1996

30. Chaudry IH, Stephen RN, Harkema JM, Dean RE: Immunological alterations following simple haemorrhage. In: Faist E, Ninnemann JL, Green DR (Eds) *Immune Consequences of Trauma, Shock and Sepsis. Mechanisms and Therapeutic Approaches* pp. 363–373. Berlin: Springer, 1990

31. Ayala A, Perin MM, Chaudry IH: Increased susceptibility to sepsis following haemorrhage: defective Kupffer cell-mediated antigen presentation. *Surgical Forum* **40**: 102–104, 1989

32. Blumberg N, Heal JM: Effects of transfusion on immune function. Cancer recurrence and infection. *Arch Pathol Lab Med* **118**: 371–379, 1994

33. Reissman P, Manny N, Shapira SC *et al.*: Transfusion-related adult respiratory distress syndrome. *Israel J Med Sci* 29: 303–307, 1993

34. Connall TP, Zhang J, Kaupke CJ, Wilson SE: Leukocyte CD11b and CD18 expression are increased in blood salvaged for autotransfusion. *Am Surg* **60**: 797–800, 1994

35. Moore FA, Feliciano DV, Andrassy RJ *et al.*: Early enteral feeding, compared with parenteral, reduces post-operative septic complications. The results of a meta-analysis. *Ann Surg* **216**: 172–183, 1992

36. Moore EE, Jones TN: Benefits of immediate jejunostomy feeding after major abdominal trauma - a prospective randomised study. *J Trauma* **26**: 874–881, 1986

37. Burke DJ, Alverdy JC, Aoys E, Moss GS: Glutamine-supplemented total parenteral nutrition improves gut immune function. *Arch Surg* **24**: 1396–1399, 1989

38. Alverdy JC, Chi HS, Selivanov V *et al.*: The effect of route nutrient administration on the secretory immune system. *Current Surgery* **42**: 10–13, 1985

39. Alverdy JC, Chi HS, Sheldon GF: The effect of parenteral nutrition on gastrointestinal immunity; the importance of enteral stimulation. *Ann Surg* **202**: 681–684, 1985

40. Alverdy JC, Aoys E, Moss GS: Total parenteral nutrition promotes bacterial translocation from the gut. *Surgery* **104**: 185–190, 1988

41. Lowry SF: The route of feeding influences injury responses. *J Trauma* **30** (Suppl): S10–15, 1990

42. Fong Y, Marano MA, Bamber A *et al.*: Total parenteral nutrition and bowel rest modify the metabolism response to endotoxin in humans. *Ann Surg* 210: 449–457, 1989

43. Alexander JW: Immunoenhancement via enteral nutrition. *Arch Surg* **128**: 1242–1245, 1993

44. Newsholme EA, Newsholme P, Curi R *et al.*: A role for muscle in the immune system and its importance in surgery, trauma, sepsis and burns. *Nutrition* **4**: 261–268, 1988

45. Parry-Billings M, Evans J, Calider PC, Newsholme EA: Does glutamine contribute to immunesuppression after major burns. *Lancet* **336**: 523–525, 1990

46. Wallace C, Keast D: Glutamine and macrophage function. *Metabol Clin Exp* **41**: 1016–1020, 1992

47. Haque SM, Chen K, Usui N *et al.*: Alanyl-glutamine dipeptide-supplemented parenteral nutrition improves intestinal metabolism and prevents increased permeability in rats. *Ann Surg* **223**: 334–341, 1996

48. Li J, Langkamp-Henken B, Suzuki K, Stahlgren LH: Glutamine prevents parenteral nutrition-induced increases in intestinal permeability. *JPEN* **18**: 303–307, 1994

49. Tremel H, Kienle B, Weilemann LS *et al.*: Glutamine dipeptide-supplemented parenteral nutrition maintains intestinal function in the critically ill. *Gastroenterology* **107**: 1595–1601, 1994

50. van der Hulst RR, van Kreel BK, von Meyenfeldt MF *et al.*: Glutamine and the preservation of gut integrity. *Lancet* **341:** 1363–1365, 1993

51. Dugan ME, McBurney MI: Luminal glutamine perfusion alters endotoxin-related changes in ileal permeability of the piglet. *JPEN* **19:** 83–87, 1995

52. Stehle P, Zander J, Mertes N *et al.*: Effect of parenteral glutamine peptide supplements on muscle glutamine loss and nitrogen balance after major surgery. *Lancet* **i:** 231–233, 1989

53. Hammarqvist F, Wernerman J, Ali R *et al.*: Addition of glutamine to total parenteral nutrition after elective abdominal surgery spares free glutamine in muscle, counteracts the fall in muscle protein synthesis, and improves nitrogen balance. *Ann Surg* **209:** 455–461, 1989

54. Parry-Billings M, Baigrie RJ, Lamont PM *et al.*: Effects of major and minor surgery on plasma glutamine and cytokine levels. *Arch Surg* **127:** 1237–1240, 1992

55. Carrico CJ, Meakins JL, Fry D, Maier RV: Multiple-organ-failure syndrome. *Arch Surg* **121:** 196–208, 1986

56. Bennion RS, Wilson SR, Williams RA: Early portal anaerobic bacteraemia in mesenteric ischaemia. *Arch Surg* **119:** 151–155, 1984

57. Seltzer JL, Ritter DE, Starsnic MA, Marr AT: The haemodynamic response to traction on the abdominal mesentery. *Anesthesiology* **63:** 96–99, 1985

58. Gottlieb A, Skrinska VA, O'Hara P *et al.*: The role of prostacyclin in the mesenteric traction syndrome during anaesthesia for abdominal aortic reconstructive surgery. *Ann Surg* **209:** 363–367, 1989

59. Hudson JC, Wurm WH, OíDonnell TF Jr *et al.*: Hemodynamic and prostacyclin release in the early phases of aortic surgery: comparison of transabdominal and retroperitoneal approaches. *J Vasc Surg* **7:** 190–198, 1988

60. Hudson JC, Wurm WH, O'Donnell TF Jr *et al.*: Ibuprofen pretreatment inhibits prostacyclin release during abdominal exploration in aortic surgery. *Anesthesiology* **72:** 443–449, 1990

61. Fiddian-Green RG: Splanchnic ischaemia and multiple organ failure in the critically ill. *Ann Roy Coll Surg Engl* **70:** 128–134, 1988

62. Mathews JGW, Parks TG: Ischaemic colitis in experimental animal. Role of hypovolaemia in the production of the disease. *Gut* **17:** 677–684, 1976

63. Parks DA, Bulkley GB, Granger DN *et al.*: Ischaemic injury in the cat small intestine: role of superoxide radicals. *Gastroenterology* 82: 9–15, 1982

64. Jodal M, Haglund U, Lundgren O: Countercurrent exchange mechanisms in the small intestine. In: Shepard AP, Granger DN (Eds) *Physiology of the Small Intestinal Circulation* pp. 83–97. New York: Raven Press, 1984

65. Horton JW: Alterations in intestinal permeability and blood flow in a new model of mesenteric ischaemia. *Circ Shock* **36:** 134–139, 1992

66. Langer JC, Sohal SS: Increased mucosal permeability after intestinal ischaemia-reperfusion injury is mediated by local tissue factors. *J Ped Surg* **27:** 329–332, 1992

67. Parks DA, Granger DN: Contributions of ischaemic and reperfusion to mucosal lesion formation. *Am J Physiol* **250:** G749–753, 1986

68. McCord JM: Oxygen-derived free radicals in post-ischaemic tissue injury. *N Engl J Med* **312:** 159–163, 1985

69. Yamamoto S: Enzymes in the arachidonic acid cascade. In: Pace-Ascieak C, Granstrom E (Eds) *Prostaglandin and Related Substances* pp. 171–202. Amsterdam: Elsevier, 1983

70. Kaufman Jr RP, Klausner JM, Anner H *et al.*: Inhibition of thromboxane synthesis by free radical scavengers. *J Trauma* **28:** 458–464, 1988

71. Welbourn R, Goldman G, Kobzik L *et al.*: Neutrophil adhesion receptor CD18 mediates ischaemia-induced diapedesis. *FASEB J* **4:** 641, 1990

72. Schmid-Schönbein GW: Capillary plugging by granulocytes and the no-reflow phenomenon in the microcirculation. *Fed Proc* **46:** 2397–2401, 1987

73. Grisham MB, Hernandez LA, Granger DN: Xanthine oxidase and neutrophil infiltration in intestinal ischaemia. *Am J Physiol* **251:** G567–574, 1986

74. Kurtel H, Fujimoto K, Zimmerman BJ *et al.*: Ischaemia-reperfusion-induced mucosal dysfunction: Role of neutrophils. *Am J Physiol* **261:** G490–496, 1991

75. Roumen RMH, van der Vliet JA, Wevers RA, Goris RJ: Intestinal permeability is increased after major vascular surgery. *J Vasc Surg* **17**: 734–437, 1993

76. Fiddian-Green RG, Gantz NM: Transient episodes of sigmoid ischaemia and their relation to infection from intestinal organisms after abdominal aortic operations. *Crit Care Med* **15**: 835–839, 1987

77. Rietscel ET, Schade U, Jensen M *et al.*: Bacterial endotoxin: chemical structure, biological activity and role in septicaemia. *Scand I Infect Dis* **31**(Suppl): 8–24, 1982

78. McCartney AC, Banks JG, Clements GB *et al.*: Endotoxaemia in septic shock: Clinical and post-mortem correlations. *Int Care Med* **9**: 117–122, 1983

79. Danner RL, Elim RJ, Hosseini JM *et al.*: Endotoxaemia in human septic shock. *Chest* **9**: 169–75, 1991

80. McLeish KR, Wellhausen SR, Dean WL: Biochemical basis of HLA-DR and CR modulation on human peripheral blood monocytes by lipopolysaccharide. *Cellular Immunol* **108**: 242–248, 1987

81. Appel SH, Wellhausen SR, Montgommery R *et al.*: Experimental and clinical significance of endotoxin-dependent HLA-DR expression in monocytes. *J Surg Res* **47**: 39–44, 1989

82. Grisham MB, Everse J, Janssen HF: Endotoxaemia and neutrophil activation *in vivo*. *Am J Physiol* **254**: H1017–1022, 1988

83. Doefler ME, Danner RL, Shelhamer JH, Parillo JE: Bacterial lipopolysaccharides prime human neutrophils for enhanced production of leukotriene B4. *J Clin Invest* **83**: 970–977, 1989

84. Brigham KL, Bowers RE, Haynes J: Increased sheep lung vascular permeability caused by E.coli endotoxin. *Circ Res* **45**: 292–297, 1979

85. Heflin AC Jr, Brigham KL: Prevention by granulocyte depletion of increased vascular permeability of sheep lung following endotoxaemia. *J Clin Invest* **68**: 1253–1260, 1981

86. Smedley LA, Tonnesen MG, Sandhaus RA, Rowlands BI, Barros D'Sa AAB: Neutrophil mediated injury to endothelial cells. Enhancement by endotoxin and essential role of neutrophils elastase. *J Clin Invest* **77**: 175–179, 1986

87. Soong CV, Blair PHB, Halliday MI *et al.*: Endotoxaemia, the generation of the cytokines and their relationship to intramucosal acidosis of the sigmoid colon in elective abdominal aortic aneurysm repair. *Eur J Vasc Surg* **7**: 534–539, 1993

88. Soong CV, Blair PHB, Halliday MI, Barros D'Sa AAB: Bowel ischaemia and organ impairment in elective abdominal aortic aneurysm surgery. *Br J Surg* **81**: 965–968, 1994

89. Roumen RMH, Frieling JTM, van Tits HWHJ, van der Vliet JA, Goris RJA: Endotoxaemia after major vascular operations. *J Vasc Surg* **18**: 853–857, 1993

90. Welch M, Douglas JT, Smyth JV, Walker MG. Systemic endotoxaemia and fibrinolysis during aortic surgery. *Eur J Vasc Endovasc Surg* **9**: 228–232, 1995

91. Caridis DT, Reihold RB, Woodruff PWH, Fine J: Endotoxaemia in man. *Lancet* **ii**: 1381–1386, 1972

92. Fink PC, Lehr L, Urbascheck RM, Kozak J: Limulus amoebocyte lysate test for endotoxaemia investigations with a femtogram sensitive spectrophotometric assay. *Clin Worchenschir* **59**: 213–218, 1981

93. Watson RWG, Redmond HP, McCarthy J *et al.*: Endotoxin regulates early host response to surgery. *Br J Surg* **81**: 757, 1994

94. Michalek SM, Moore RN, McGhee JR, Rossenrtreich DL, Mengenhagen SE: The primary role of lymphoreticular cells in the mediation of host responses to bacterial endotoxin. *J Infect Dis* **141**: 55–63, 1980

95. Beutler B, Cerami A: Cachectin: More than a tumour necrosis factor. *N Engl J Med* **316**: 379–385, 1987

96. Beutler B: Cachectin in tissue injury, shock and related states. *Crit Care Clin* **5**: 353–367, 1989

97. Beutler B, Milsark IW, Cerami AC: Passive immunization against cachectin/tumour necrosis factor protects mice from lethal effects of endotoxin. *Science* **229**: 869–871, 1985

98. Dinarello CA: The biology of interleukin 1 and comparison to tumour necrosis factor. *Immunol Lett* **16**: 227–232, 1987

99. Le J, Vilcek J: Interleukin-6: A multifunctional cytokine regulating immune reactions and the acute phase protein response. *Lab Invest* **61**: 588–602, 1989

100. Shalaby MR, Aggarwal BB, Rinderknecht E *et al.*: Activation of human polymorphonuclear neutrophils functions by interferon-gama and tumour necrosis factor. *J Immunol* **135**: 2069–2073, 1985
101. Streiter RM, Remick DG, Ward PA *et al.*: Cellular and molecular regulation of tumour necrosis factor-alpha production by pentoxyfylline. *Biochem Biophys Res Comm* **155**: 1230–1236, 1988
102. Welbourn R, Goldman G, OíRiordan M *et al.*: Role of tumour necrosis factor as mediator of lung injury following lower torso ischaemia. *Am J Physiol* **70**: 2645–2649, 1991
103. Baigrie RJ, Lamont PM, Kwiatkowski D *et al.*: Systemic cytokine response after major surgery. *Br J Surg* **79**: 757–760, 1992
104. Roumen RMH, Hendriks T, van der Ven-Jongekrijg J *et al.*: Cytokine patterns in patients after major vascular surgery, hemorrhagic shock, and severe blunt trauma. *Ann Surg* **218**: 769–776, 1993
105. Debets JMH, Kampmeijer R, van der Linden MPMH *et al.*: Plasma tumour necrosis factor and mortality in critically ill septic patients. *Crit Care Med* **17**: 489–494, 1989
106. Metcalf D: The leukaemia inhibitory factor (LIF). *Int J Cell Cloning* **9**: 95–108, 1991
107. Poo WJ, Conrad L, Janeway CA Jr: Receptor directed focusing of lymphokine release by helper T cells. *Nature* **332,** 378–380, 1988
108. Swartbol P, Norgren L, Albrechtsson U *et al.*: Biological responses differ considerably between endovascular and conventional aortic aneurysm surgery. *Eur J Vasc Endovasc Surg* **12**: 18–25, 1996
109. Weinberg JR, Wright DJM, Guz A: Interleukin-1 and tumour necrosis factor cause hypotension in the conscious rabbit. *Clin Sci* **75**: 251–255, 1988
110. Pohlman TH, Stannes KA, Beatty PG *et al.*: An endothelial cell surface factor(s) induced *in vitro* by lipopolysaccharide, interleukin-1, and tumour necrosis factor-alpha increases neutrophil adherence by Cdw-18-dependent mechanism. *J Immunol* **136**: 4548–4553, 1986
111. Rosenblum MG, Donato NJ: Tumour necrosis factor alpha: a multifaceted peptide hormone. *Crit Rev Immunol* **9**: 21–44, 1989
112. Danis VA, Kulesz AJ, Nelson DS, Brooks PM: Cytokine regulation of human monocyte interleukin-1 (IL-1) production *in vitro*. Enhancement of IL-1 production by interferon (IFN) gamma, tumour necrosis factor-alpha, IL-2 and IL-1, and inhibition by IFN-alpha. *Clin Exp Immunol* **80**: 430–443:, 1990
113. Cannon JG, Tompkins RG, Gelfland JA *et al.*: Circulating interleukin-1 and tumour necrosis factor in septic shock and experimental endotoxin fever. *J Infect Dis* **161**: 79–84, 1990
114. Cannon JG, Stanford GG, Corsetti JR *et al.*: Plasma concentrations of interleukin-1 and tumour necrosis factor in a small group of patients with sepsis syndrome. *Crit Care Med* **17**: S58, 1989
115. Fong Y, Moldawer LL, Marano M *et al.*: Endotoxaemia elicits increased circulating β2-IFN/IL-6 in man. *J Immunol* **142**: 2321–2324, 1989
116. Hack CE, De Groot ER, Felt-Bersma RJF *et al.*: Increased plasma levels of interleukin-6 in sepsis. *Blood* **74**: 1704–1710, 1989
117. Calandra T, Gerain J, Heumann D *et al.*: High circulating levels of interleukin-6 in patients with septic shock: Evolution during sepsis, prognostic value, and interplay with other cytokines. *Am J Med* **91**: 23–29, 1991
118. Patel RT, Deen KI, Youngs D *et al.*: Interleukin-6 is a prognostic indicator of outcome in severe intra-abdominal sepsis. *Br J Surg* **81**: 1306–1308, 1994
119. Green M, Hickney NC, Crowe A *et al.*: Interleukin-6 production by the colon is a response to sigmoid ischaemia. *Br J Surg* **81**: 615, 1994
120. Baigrie RJ, Lamont PM, Whiting S, Morris PJ: Portal endotoxin and cytokine response during abdominal aortic surgery. *Am J Surg* **166**: 248–251, 1993
121. Libert C, Vink A, Coulie P *et al.*: Limited involvement of interleukin-6 in the pathogenesis of lethal septic shock as revealed by the effect of monoclonal antibodies against interleukin-6 or its receptor in various murine models. *Eur J Immunol* **22**: 2625–2630, 1992
122. Murphy ME, Kolvenbach R, Aleksis M, Hansen R, Sies H: Antioxidant depletion in aortic cross clamping ischaemia: increase of the plasma (α-tocopheryl quinone/(α-tocopherol ratio. *Free Radical Biol Med* **13**: 95-100, 1992

123. Fantini GA, Conte MS: Pulmonary failure following lower torso ischaemia: clinical evidence for a remote effect of reperfusion injury. *Am Surg* **61**: 316–319, 1995
124. Paterson IS, Klausner JM, Goldman G, et al. Pulmonary oedema after aneurysm surgery is modified by mannitol. *Ann Surg* **210**: 796–801, 1989
125. Paterson IS, Klausner JM, Mannick JA, Hechtman HB: The lung traps activated neutrophils following aneurysm repair. *Br J Surg* **80**: 519, 1993
126. Corson RJ, Paterson IS, OíDwyer ST *et al.*: Lower limb ischaemia and reperfusion alters gut permeability. *Eur J Vasc Surg* **6**: 158–163, 1992
127. Corson RJ, Fisher M, Ward I *et al.*: Thromboxane antagonism prevents hind limb ischaemia / reperfusion induced gut damage. *Br J Surg* **80**: 1464–1465, 1993
128. Yassin MMI, Barros DíSa AAB, Parks G *et al.*: Mortality following lower limb ischaemia-reperfusion: a systemi inflammatory response? *World J Surg* **20**: 961–967, 1996
129. Poggetti RS, Moore FA, Moore EE *et al.*: Simultaneous liver and lung injury following gut ischaemia is mediated by xanthine oxidase. *J Trauma* **32**: 723–728, 1992
130. Poggetti RS, Moore FA, Moore EE *et al.*: Liver injury is a reversible neutrophil-mediated event following gut ischaemia. *Arch Surg* **127**: 175–179, 1992
131. Paterson IS, Smith FCT, Tsang GMK, Hamer JD, Shearman CP: Reperfusion plasma contains a neutrophil activator. *Am Vasc Surg* **7**: 68–75, 1993

PERIPHERAL VASCULATURE

Thrombus as a Prognostic Indicator in Popliteal Aneurysms

Shane T. R. MacSweeney

INTRODUCTION

The popliteal artery is the most common site of peripheral arterial aneurysm.[1] Those affected are overwhelmingly male and often elderly.[2,3] The limb threatening potential of popliteal aneurysm has been recognized for centuries but early attempts at surgical treatment were accompanied by prohibitive rates of gangrene and exsanguinating haemorrhage.[4] John Hunter's technique of ligation of the healthy superficial femoral artery well above the aneurysm sac was described in 1786 and had an improved outcome,[4,5] but although surgical treatment of popliteal aneurysm has been feasible for over 200 years it continues to provoke controversy.

Popliteal aneurysms may present with a wide variety of symptoms, including a pulsatile mass, compression of surrounding structures, venous thrombosis and aneurysm rupture, but thrombosis and embolization resulting in ischaemia remain by far the most common complications.[2,6–14]

Thrombus may be encountered in popliteal aneurysms in one of three settings; the acutely ischaemic limb, the chronically ischaemic limb and the asymptomatic aneurysm. These situations will be dealt with in turn.

POPLITEAL ANEURYSM CAUSING ACUTE ISCHAEMIA: THE IMPACT OF THROMBOLYSIS

Popliteal aneurysm may result in acute ischaemia by distal embolization, thrombosis of the aneurysm sac, or both. The combination of an acutely thrombosed popliteal aneurysm and an obliterated distal vasculature is difficult to treat by conventional methods. Historically, acute limb ischaemia resulting from popliteal aneurysm has carried a poor prognosis with amputation rates of 28–69%.[10,15–17]

Thrombolysis, has the potential to improve outcome by clearing the thrombosed aneurysm and the distal arterial circulation, converting an emergency operation with poor runoff into an urgent elective repair with good runoff.

Hoelting, retrospectively reviewed 24 patients who presented with acute limb ischaemia complicating popliteal aneurysm. Four patients underwent primary amputation (17%). Nine patients were treated with preoperative urokinase infusion. An angiographically demonstrated improvement in runoff was seen in all nine patients, lysis was partial in three and complete in six in whom ischaemic symptoms resolved fully. All patients subsequently underwent bypass grafting and exclusion with no limb loss and no graft occlusions in the short- or long-term (mean follow-up

5.2 years). Of 11 patients treated by surgery alone, all had residual clot in the runoff vessels on postoperative angiography, four developed early graft occlusions, one of which lead to amputation.[18] Browse described thrombolysis in eight patients with thrombosed popliteal aneurysms with complete clearance in seven and partial clearance in one, with all bypass grafts remaining patent at 1 year.[19] Carpenter reported complete clearance in six and partial clearance in one of seven patients treated with lysis.[13] Similar results have been achieved by others.[20,21] In nine patients with ischaemic complications (seven rest pain, two claudication) detailed by Bowyer, thrombolysis was impossible for technical reasons in one, one patient died of haemorrhagic complications, lysis failed in two and was successful in five (56%), mean time to lysis was 32 hours.[22] Similar results were reported by Ramesh in 12 patients with acute thrombosis with complete lysis in six, partial lysis in one and failure in five.[23]

Some patients with acute ischaemia will present with neurological deficit and will be unable to tolerate the delay imposed by preoperative thrombolysis. Intraoperative thrombolysis in combination with catheter embolectomy provides an effective method in this group. In six patients undergoing intraoperative lysis angiographic success was demonstrated in all five who had angiograms performed, all limbs were salvaged and all grafts remained patent at a minimum of 6 months follow-up.[24]

Retrospective reports of successful lysis of acutely thrombosed popliteal aneurysms can present an overoptimistic picture. In a prospective multicentre study, 16 of 23 popliteal aneurysms presenting with acute ischaemia in which thrombolysis was employed had a successful outcome. Three of these were treated by long-term anticoagulation alone following complete clearance by lysis and the remainder by exclusion and bypass. Seven patients (30%) required amputation following failed lysis and surgery.[25]

Thrombolysis carries a 15% risk of minor haemorrhage, a 5% risk of serious haemorrhage and a 1% risk of stroke which is fatal in 50%.[26] Lysis may cause acute limb deterioration due to embolization; this is more common in patients with popliteal aneurysm (13%) than in patients with other causes of thrombosis (2%).[27] Massive distal embolization may be limb threatening. This complication may be reduced by using lysis only to clear the runoff vessels without attempting to clear the aneurysm itself.[27] (Fig. 1). However, the presence of a thrombosed popliteal aneurysm often goes unrecognized until it is unmasked by thrombolysis[28] (Fig. 2).

Despite the lack of randomized controlled studies, thrombolysis is clearly a useful technique in the management of acute ischaemia complicating popliteal aneurysm. In a few patients it may remove the need for any form of surgery[25] although others have reported that anticoagulation does not prevent thromboembolic complications.[29] More usually it is used to improve runoff as an adjunct to exclusion and bypass. Thrombolysis allows limb salvage in some patients who otherwise would be predicted to require amputation. It is well recognized that arterial runoff is also an important determinant of long-term graft patency,[2,30–32] although good results can be achieved with saphenous vein despite decreased runoff.[33] This would suggest that thrombolysis probably also improves the long-term results of bypass surgery in those with acute ischaemia.

Despite modern treatment methods, acute ischaemia complicating popliteal aneurysm remains a dangerous limb-threatening problem.[23,34] Some will require primary amputation because of advanced ischaemia at the time of presentation,[3,18,25,34]

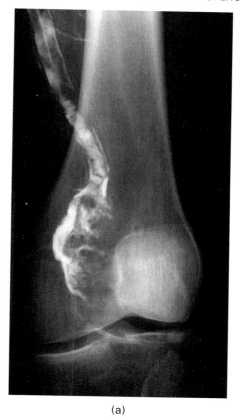
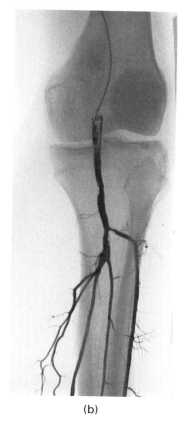

(a)   (b)

Fig. 1. Initial (a) and follow-up (b) angiograms in a patient presenting with an acutely thrombosed popliteal aneurysm, showing clearance of the runoff vessels. The risk of acute deterioration can be minimized by restricting lysis to the runoff vessels, avoiding the large volume of thrombus within the aneurysm sac, as seen here.

in others failed revascularization will require amputation. Even in those for whom limb salvage is successful, morbidity is high; 36% will have postoperative complications and 10% long-term vascular or neurological impairment.[34]

POPLITEAL ANEURYSM CAUSING CHRONIC ISCHAEMIA

Chronic ischaemia may be associated with a thrombosed aneurysm or a patent aneurysm with varying degrees of occlusion of the runoff vessels. Patients with popliteal aneurysm are at high risk of occlusive atherosclerotic peripheral vascular disease and it may be impossible to distinguish between occlusion of crural and pedal vessels due to embolization or atherosclerosis.[32] Raptis has argued that embolization from popliteal aneurysm is unlikely because angiography may demonstrate distal vessel occlusion in the presence of a patent aneurysm with no evidence of intraluminal

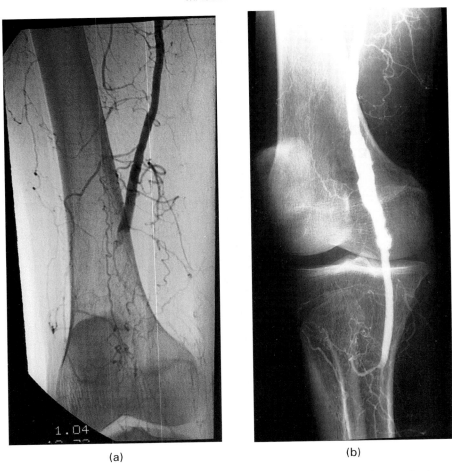

(a)   (b)

Fig. 2.   (a). Initial angiogram in a patient with acute ischaemia showing occlusion at the level of the adductor hiatus, thrombolysis revealed an unsuspected popliteal aneurysm with poor runoff (b).

thrombus – and histology of tibial vessels from limbs amputated as a result of popliteal aneurysm has shown typical atherosclerotic plaques.[35] However, only 10% of patients presenting with popliteal aneurysm have normal distal arterial anatomy. This represents far more extensive distal disease than would be predicted purely on the basis of atherosclerosis.[32] The presence of intraluminal thrombus and a patent popliteal aneurysm was associated with one or no patent crural vessels in 8 of 13 (62%) of cases.[32] While some distal disease must be due to atherosclerosis, if chronic embolization is accepted as an entity then prognosis should be worse in patients with a patent popliteal aneurysm, particularly those with intraluminal thrombus, than in those with a chronically thrombosed aneurysm. Occlusion of the runoff vessels, whatever the cause, is associated with a worse prognosis as slow flow through a dilated artery with a poor runoff predisposes to thrombosis.[29,35]

  In summary, chronic ischaemia due to distal occlusion with a patent aneurysm is a potentially unstable situation with a high risk of further deterioration and should be treated aggressively whereas chronic ischaemia due to thrombosis of the aneurysm sac is more likely to be stable and can be treated according to the severity of symptoms.[8,12]

ASYMPTOMATIC POPLITEAL ANEURYSM

The management of asymptomatic popliteal aneurysm remains controversial. Traditionally regarded as 'a sinister harbinger of sudden catastrophe',[36] an aggressive management policy of early surgical intervention has been advocated.[2,8,9,16,17,30,31,34,36-38] However, many of the series upon which these conclusions are based are retrospective analyses of patients collected over decades, during which diagnostic and management techniques have changed significantly. Recently, this aggressive approach has been challenged by those who advocate a more selective policy.[22,39,40] They argue that some popliteal aneurysms remain asymptomatic for long periods, that prophylactic surgery carries considerable morbidity and expense and that newer treatment modalities reduce the threat from acute complications.

Analysis of data on the natural history of asymptomatic aneurysms treated conservatively is further complicated because often no distinction is made between those who did not have surgery because they were considered too high an operative risk, had small aneurysms or refused an operation. Complication rates would be expected to differ in these groups. Most of the asymptomatic aneurysms in these series were discovered in those with a symptomatic contralateral aneurysm and might be expected to have a worse prognosis than those with aneurysms detected as truly incidental findings. Based on these highly selected series, asymptomatic popliteal aneurysms have an ischaemic complication rate of 0–23.8% per annum (mean 9.8%) over a mean follow-up of 46 months (range 17–72 months).[2,3,6,11,12,16,29,36,37,40,41]

Michaels and Galland used a mathematical model to analyse criteria for elective popliteal aneurysm surgery. They concluded that elective surgery was better than conservative treatment after 16 months assuming a 14% per annum risk of complications. Operative mortality, limb loss and 5-year graft patency rates for asymptomatic and symptomatic patients were 0.4% vs 4.7%, 0.8% vs 18.2% and 80% vs 65% respectively.[42] Unfortunately this approach is critically dependent on the numerical assumptions which are made, and reliable data on complication rates are lacking for the reasons outlined above. However, despite recent advances including thrombolysis, it is clear that results of treatment of acute ischaemia complicating popliteal aneurysm are not good enough to justify an expectant policy for all patients with asymptomatic popliteal aneurysm and that conversely, the morbidity and cost of elective repair and risks of conservative treatment are not such as to justify routine repair of all popliteal aneurysms on diagnosis. Several attempts have been made to identify those at high and low risk of complications.

Schellack et al. managed 26 high surgical risk elderly patients considered to have mainly 'small' aneurysms conservatively with an 8% complication rate and no limb loss over 37 months.[6] Collin reported that of seven high-risk patients with small asymptomatic aneurysms treated conservatively all died of unrelated causes without developing complications.[40] Those with popliteal aneurysms have a reduced life expectancy, particularly 'high-risk' patients and are both more likely to die from intercurrent disease without complications from their aneurysm and to develop postoperative complications from elective repair.[2,11,16,36,37,40]

Some have suggested that aneurysm size is unrelated to risk of thrombosis[9,10] or even that small aneurysms are more likely to thrombose.[38] However, Lowell et al. found that three factors predicted the development of complications in those with

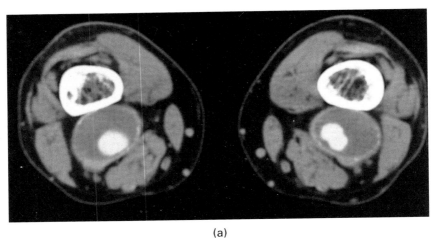

(a)

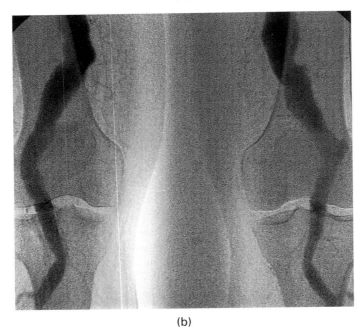

(b)

Fig. 3. (a). CT scan showing bilateral large popliteal aneurysms, the lumen is shown enhanced by contrast with the remainder of the aneurysm sac filled with thrombus. (b). Angiogram of the same patient showing distortion of the popliteal artery. Elongation causes the artery to buckle between fixed branching points.

asymptomatic aneurysms, diameter larger than 2cm, one or fewer patent crural vessels, and intraluminal thrombus. In limbs that developed complications one of these factors was present in 92% and two in 58% compared with 38% and 8% respectively in those that did not.[3] Dawson found that 86% of asymptomatic patients with one or both ankle pulses absent at presentation developed symptoms within 3 years compared with 36% in those with normal ankle pulses. Previous abdominal aortic aneurysm surgery was also associated with complications, 83% vs 40% at 3 years, although in some of these cases thrombosis occurred as a direct result of the aortic procedure. Increasing popliteal aneurysm diameter was associated with complications with no aneurysm under 2cm causing symptoms and all of those greater than 4cm doing so, however the data were incomplete. The presence of thrombus was not recorded.[29]

Comparison of the morphological features of popliteal aneurysms presenting with thrombosis with those that did not revealed thrombosis to be more common when there was distortion within the aneurysm, large size and distortion above or below the aneurysm (Fig. 3). A combination of distortion and diameter greater than 3cm was present in 13 of 15 thrombosed aneurysms.[23] No analysis of the role of thrombus within the aneurysm prior to occlusion was possible in this study. Several authors have stated that thrombus within the aneurysm sac indicates an increased risk of complications and is an indication for elective repair.[32,34,43] This risk is not quantified. It would seem self-evident that if two otherwise identical aneurysms were detected, one with thrombus and the other without, then the one with thrombus would be more likely to embolize, particularly if the thrombus was floating (Fig. 4).

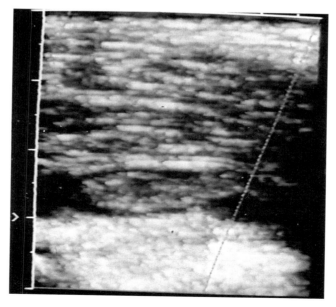

Fig. 4. Duplex scan showing the lumen of an aneurysmal popliteal artery full of loose thrombus, which had already led to embolization.

The various risk factors identified in these studies are interdependent. Thrombus within the aneurysm sac is more common in larger aneurysms.[25,44] Aneurysmal dilatation involves lengthening as well as widening of the artery. Lengthening causes the artery to buckle between fixed branching points and become distorted.[45] Absent distal pulses may reflect previous embolization arising from intraluminal thrombus. An asymptomatic aneurysm containing intraluminal thrombus is therefore also likely to be larger, more distorted and have fewer patent runoff

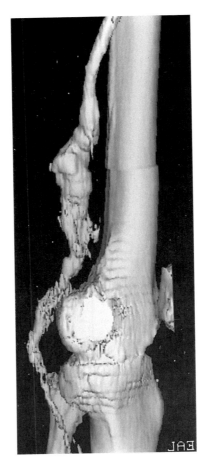

Fig. 5. Three-dimensional spiral CT reconstruction of a popliteal aneurysm showing that the aneurysm is confined to the suprageniculate popliteal artery. This aneurysm is potentially suitable for endovascular repair; most are not.

vessels. It seems clear that while the presence of intraluminal thrombus is associated with a worse prognosis, in the absence of prospective studies it is impossible to quantify the risk accurately or to distinguish the component due to thrombus from other associated risk factors.

The relative risks and benefits of elective and emergency repair may also change with the advent of successful endovascular techniques.[46] However, in our experience most patients with popliteal aneurysms are unsuitable for endovascular repair because of concern about the long-term effects of placing a stent graft across the knee joint (Fig. 5). Perhaps in the longer term, better understanding of the environmental and genetic mechanisms involved in the pathogenesis of popliteal aneurysm in the individual patient may allow improved prediction of prognosis.[44]

REFERENCES

1. Lawrence PF, Lorenzo-Rivero S, Lyon JL: The incidence of iliac, femoral, and popliteal artery aneurysms in hospitalized patients. *J Vasc Surg* **22:** 409–415, 1995
2. Anton GE, Hertzer NR, Beven EG et al.: Surgical management of popliteal aneurysms. Trends in presentation, treatment, and results from 1952 to 1984. *J Vasc Surg* **3:** 125–134, 1986
3. Lowell RC, Gloviczki P, Hallett JW Jr et al.: Popliteal artery aneurysms: the risk of nonoperative management. *Ann Vasc Surg* **8:** 14–23, 1994
4. Schechter DC, Bergan JJ: Popliteal aneurysm: a celebration of the bicentennial of John Hunter's operation. *Ann Vasc Surg* **1:** 118–126, 1986
5. Home E: An account of Mr Hunter's method of performing the operation for the popliteal aneurifm. *London Med J* **7:** 391–406, 1786
6. Schellack J, Smith RB, Perdue GD: Nonoperative management of selected popliteal aneurysms. *Arch Surg* **122:** 372–375, 1987
7. Hardy JD, Tompkins WC, Hatten LE, Chavez CM: Aneurysms of the popliteal artery. *Surg Gynecol Obstet* **140:** 401–404, 1975
8. Guvendik L, Bloor K, Charlesworth D: Popliteal aneurysm: sinister harbinger of sudden catastrophe. *Br J Surg* **67:** 294–296, 1980
9. Szilagyi DE, Schwartz RL, Reddy DJ: Popliteal arterial aneurysms. Their natural history and management. *Arch Surg* **116:** 724–728, 1981
10. Bouhoutsos J, Martin P: Popliteal aneurysm: a review of 116 cases. *Br J Surg* **61:** 469–475, 1974
11. Wychulis AR, Spittell JA Jr, Wallace RB: Popliteal aneurysms. *Surgery* **68:** 942–952, 1970
12. Roggo A, Brunner U, Ottinger LW, Largiader F: The continuing challenge of aneurysms of the popliteal artery. *Surg Gynecol Obstet* **177:** 565–572, 1993
13. Carpenter JP, Barker CF, Roberts B et al.: Popliteal artery aneurysms: current management and outcome *J Vasc Surg* **19:** 65–72, 1994
14. Kotval PS, Shah PM, Babu SC et al.: Popliteal vein compression due to popliteal artery aneurysm: effects of aneurysm size. *J Ultrasound Med* **14:** 805–811, 1995
15. Graham AR, Lord RS, Bellemore M, Tracy GD: Popliteal aneurysms. *Aust N Z J Surg* **53:** 99–103, 1983
16. Vermilion BD, Kimmins SA, Pace WG, Evans WE: A review of one hundred forty-seven popliteal aneurysms with long-term follow-up. *Surgery* **90:** 1009–1014, 1981
17. Reilly MK, Abbott WM, Darling RC: Aggressive surgical management of popliteal artery aneurysms. *Am J Surg* **145:** 498–502, 1983
18. Hoelting T, Paetz B, Richter GM, Allenberg JR: The value of preoperative lytic therapy in

limb-threatening acute ischemia from popliteal artery aneurysm. *Am J Surg* **168:** 227–231, 1994

19. Browse DJ, Torrie EP, Galland RB: Early results and 1-year follow-up after intra-arterial thrombolysis. *Br J Surg* **80:** 194–197, 1993
20. Taylor LM Jr, Porter JM, Baur GM *et al.*: Intraarterial streptokinase infusion for acute popliteal and tibial artery occlusion. *Am J Surg* **147:** 583–588, 1984
21. Garramone RR Jr, Gallagher JJ Jr, Drezner AD: Intra-arterial thrombolytic therapy in the initial management of thrombosed popliteal artery aneurysms. *Ann Vasc Surg* **8:** 363–366, 1994
22. Bowyer RC, Cawthorn SJ, Walker WJ, Giddings AE: Conservative management of asymptomatic popliteal aneurysm. *Br J Surg* **77:** 1132–1135, 1990
23. Ramesh S, Michaels JA, Galland RB: Popliteal aneurysm: morphology and management. *Br J Surg* **80:** 1531–1533, 1993
24. Thompson JF, Beard J, Scott DJ, Earnshaw JJ: Intraoperative thrombolysis in the management of thrombosed popliteal aneurysm. *Br J Surg* **80:** 858–859, 1993
25. Varga ZA, Locke-Edmunds JC, Baird RN: A multicenter study of popliteal aneurysms. Joint Vascular Research Group. *J Vasc Surg* **20:** 171–177, 1994
26. Berridge DC, Makin GS, Hopkinson BR: Local low dose intra-arterial thrombolytic therapy: the risk of stroke or major haemorrhage. *Br J Surg* **76:** 1230–1233, 1989
27. Galland RB, Earnshaw JJ, Baird RN *et al.*: Acute limb deterioration during intra-arterial thrombolysis. *Br J Surg* **80:** 1118–1120
28. Lancashire MJ, Torrie EP, Galland RB: Popliteal aneurysms identified by intra-arterial streptokinase: a changing pattern of presentation. *Br J Surg* **77:** 1388–1390, 1990
29. Dawson I, Sie R, van Baalen JM, van Bockel JH: Asymptomatic popliteal aneurysm: elective operation versus conservative follow-up. *Br J Surg* **81:** 1504–1507, 1994
30. Shortell CK, Deweese JA, Ouriel K, Green RM: Popliteal artery aneurysms: a 25-year surgical experience. *J Vasc Surg* **14:** 771–776, 1991
31. Farina C, Cavallaro A, Schultz RD *et al.*: Popliteal aneurysms. *Surg Gynecol Obstet* **169:** 7–13, 1989
32. Lilly MP, Flinn WR, McCarthy WJ *et al.*: The effect of distal arterial anatomy on the success of popliteal aneurysm repair. *J Vasc Surg* **7:** 653–660, 1988
33. Hagino RT, Fujitani RM, Dawson DL *et al.*: Does infrapopliteal arterial runoff predict success for popliteal artery aneurysmorrhaphy? *Am J Surg* **168:** 652–656, 1994
34. Halliday AW, Taylor PR, Wolfe JH, Mansfield AO: The management of popliteal aneurysm: the importance of early surgical repair. *Ann Roy Coll Surg Engl* **73:** 253–257, 1991
35. Raptis S, Ferguson L, Miller JH: The significance of tibial artery disease in the management of popliteal aneurysms. *J Cardiovasc Surg* **27:** 703–708, 1986
36. Gifford RW, Hines EA, Janes JM: An analysis and follow-up of one hundred popliteal aneurysms. *Surgery* **33:** 284–293, 1953
37. Dawson I, van Bockel JH, Brand R, Terpstra JL: Popliteal artery aneurysms. Long-term follow-up of aneurysmal disease and results of surgical treatment. *J Vasc Surg* **13:** 398–407, 1991
38. Inahara T, Toledo AC: Complications and treatment of popliteal aneurysms. *Surgery* **84:** 775–783, 1978
39. Quraishy MS, Giddings AE. Treatment of asymptomatic popliteal aneurysm: protection at a price. *Br J Surg* **79:** 731–732, 1992
40. Hands LJ, Collin J: Infra-inguinal aneurysms: outcome for patient and limb. *Br J Surg* **78:** 996–998, 1991
41. Whitehouse WM Jr, Wakefield TW, Graham LM *et al.*: Limb-threatening potential of arteriosclerotic popliteal artery aneurysms. *Surgery* **93:** 694–699, 1983
42. Michaels JA, Galland RB. Management of asymptomatic popliteal aneurysms: the use of a Markov decision tree to determine the criteria for a conservative approach. *Eur J Vasc Surg* **7:** 136–143, 1993
43. Muller RC, Striffeler H, Stirnemann P: [Popliteal aneurysm]. [German] *Schweiz Med Wochenschr J Suisse Med* **123:** 2390–2393, 1993
44. MacSweeney STR, Skidmore C, Turner RJ *et al.*: Unravelling the familial tendency to

aneurysmal disease: Popliteal aneurysm, hypertension and fibrillin genotype. *Eur J Vasc Endovasc Surg* **12:** 162–166, 1996

45. Dobrin PB: Mechanics of normal and diseased blood vessels. *Ann Vasc Surg* **2:** 283–294, 1988

46. Marin ML, Veith FJ, Panetta TF *et al.*: Transfemoral endoluminal stented graft repair of a popliteal artery aneurysm. *J Vasc Surg* **19:** 754–757, 1994

Popliteal Artery Thrombosis Caused by Popliteal Entrapment Syndrome

Lewis J. Levien

SUMMARY

Popliteal artery entrapment syndrome is a common cause of claudication symptoms in young adults under 40 years of age. If left untreated, the condition may progress to popliteal artery occlusion in these young patients who usually have no other risk factors for atherosclerotic disease. The disorder appears more common than previously suspected.

In 41 patients 73 limbs with this syndrome have been treated, and on the basis of the experience gained from this series of patients and a review of the recorded literature, we have attempted to correlate the known embryology of the popliteal structures with the development of the popliteal entrapment syndrome types I to IV. A functional type of entrapment possibly associated with hypertrophy of an abnormally laterally placed medial head of gastrocnemius has been postulated and is now termed type VI entrapment.

The aggressive natural history and destructive nature of a significant popliteal entrapment mechanism upon the popliteal artery is stressed. Based upon this aggressive natural history, it is recommended that all symptomatic patients in whom a popliteal artery entrapment syndrome is diagnosed, should have surgical intervention. This intervention should consist of myotomy or division of the offending entrapment mechanism if deterioration of the artery has not yet resulted. In the presence of aneurysm formation, arterial thrombosis or other evidence of popliteal artery degeneration, a myotomy and replacement of the diseased popliteal artery with a vein graft is the preferred method of treatment .

In normal individuals, forced plantar and dorsiflexion may result in obstruction to flow in otherwise normal popliteal arteries. The significance and natural history of this finding in an otherwise asymptomatic person is not clear. At present there is no evidence in favour of offering such individuals any form of surgical intervention.

INTRODUCTION

The development of the sudden onset of severely limiting claudication or, in more severe instances, critical ischaemia of a leg in an otherwise healthy athletic young person, is for the individual concerned a catastrophic event. In our series of patients presenting with isolated unilateral or bilateral limb ischaemia under the age of 50 years, the majority of patients have been found on further investigation to have some form of popliteal artery entrapment as the cause of the lower limb arterial occlusion.[1,2] This chapter is based on our experience with 73 instances of popliteal artery entrapment syndrome encountered and treated in 41 patients. Of these, in 18 limbs the presentation was one of sudden onset of severe limiting claudication, or of critical ischaemia.

The original description of the popliteal entrapment syndrome described the type I entrapment,[3] which is now recognized to be the least frequently clinically encountered form of this disease.[4-6] The medial deviation of the popliteal artery in the popliteal fossa that is expected with the type I entrapment, is usually not seen in the other more common types. In patients who present with isolated popliteal thombosis, angiographic demonstration of the entrapment mechanism is often not feasible. Surgery usually consists of a vein graft bypass to the infragenicular patent distal popliteal or tibial arteries, resulting in failure to expose at surgery the offending entrapment. In individuals with symptoms of claudication in whom the pathology has not yet progressed to occlusion, the presence of full and normal peripheral pulses in the resting position, may falsely reassure the clinician that no significant vascular pathology exists.[7] For these reasons, we believe that the diagnosis of popliteal entrapment is frequently overlooked in young individuals who present with lower limb occlusive vascular disease.

As will be emphasized in this chapter, it would appear that all forms of clinically symptomatic popliteal artery entrapment can progress to total occlusion of the popliteal artery with the consequent development of a critically threatened limb. On the other hand, the recognition of the presence of a popliteal artery entrapment before irreversible changes have occurred within the entrapped popliteal vessels, permits a return to normality by simple surgical division of the offending structures. It therefore behoves the physician dealing with vascular disease to be familiar with all the forms and presentations of this varied syndrome.[5]

TYPES OF ENTRAPMENT

The original description of a popliteal artery entrapment followed its recognition by a medical student during a postmortem dissection. Anderson Stuart[3] described an abnormal popliteal artery passing medial to the medial head of the gastrocnemius muscle. This is now termed the classical or type I popliteal entrapment[8] and implies a marked medial deviation of the popliteal artery in the popliteal fossa, both anatomically and on angiogram as demonstrated in Fig. 1(I).

In the type II entrapment, the popliteal artery is medially displaced to a degree, but the medial head of gastrocnemius attaches to the lateral aspect of the medial femoral condyle or intercondylar area . The artery therefore lies on the medial aspect of an abnormally placed medial head as demonstrated in Fig. 1(II).

Should an abnormal additional slip of muscle tissue occur arising from either the medial or lateral femoral condyles, if this abnormal additional slip of the medial head of the gastrocnemius muscle lies posterior to the popliteal vessels, it will form the mechanism for a type III entrapment as demonstrated in Fig. 1(III).

A type IV entrapment occurs when the popliteal artery lies deep to the popliteus

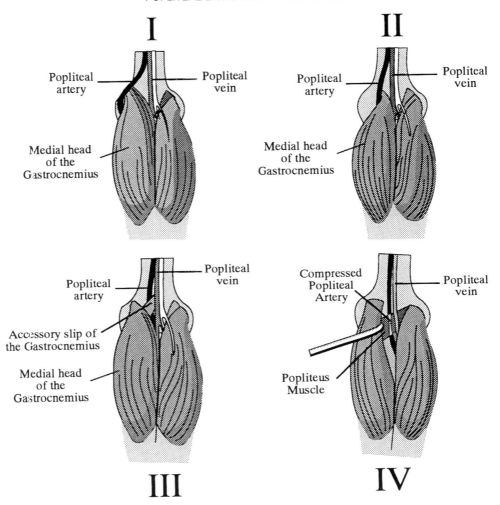

Fig. 1.   The anatomy of the popliteal artery entrapment syndrome types I–IV.

muscle or some other abnormal fibrous band[9] in the popliteal fossa (Fig. 1(IV)). When the entrapment mechanism includes or surrounds the popliteal vein as well as the artery, Rich[8] has termed this a type V entrapment. Any of the types of entrapment with the exception of the type I, may include the tibial nerve resulting in neurological parasthesiae in addition to claudication as the presenting symptom.

We and others have observed a type of popliteal artery entrapment occurring in the apparent absence of an anatomic abnormality.[10,11] In such individuals the exact nature of the entrapment mechanism remains unexplained. It has been postulated that a hypertrophic medial head of gastrocnemius impinges upon the medial and posterior aspect of the popliteal artery,[12,13] and can cause physiological occlusion of the artery in extreme plantar flexion. Others have postulated and advanced evidence for the entrapment occurring as a result of compression of the distal popliteal artery as it passes through the soleal muscle sling.[23] Up to one-third of apparently normal individuals may display the phenomenon of reduced or abolished popliteal artery blood flow with extremes of plantar flexion against resistance.[10] We subscribe to the postulate that this may be due to acquired hypertrophy of a somewhat laterally inserted muscular belly of the medial head of gastrocnemius. It is proposed that this 'functional' type of popliteal entrapment should be termed type VI. When symptomatic, this type VI entrapment has been complicated by deterioration and ultimately total occlusion of the popliteal artery in three cases in our series, confirming that the type VI entrapment, when symptomatic, may not be a benign entity.

Table 1.   Analysis of types of popliteal artery entrapment syndrome and associated numbers of patients presenting with popliteal artery occlusion

Type	Total no.	Popliteal artery patent	Popliteal artery occluded resulting in severe ischaemia
I	5	1	4
II	12	7	5
III	21	17	4
IV	10	8	2
VI	25	22	3

EMBRYOLOGY

The anatomy of the various types of popliteal artery entrapment can be explained as a form of developmental anomaly. In lower order animals, the medial head of the gastrocnemius muscle arises proximally from the posterior aspect of the fibula and lateral tibia. During development in the human, as the limb rotates medially and the knee extends, the medial head of the gastrocnemius muscle migrates to its definitive attachment on the posterior surface of the medial femoral condyle.[14]

The embryological popliteal artery is the continuation of the primitive axial or ischiadic artery.[15,16] The proximal portion of the popliteal artery is derived from the axial artery and develops in continuity with the developing femoral artery. The primitive distal popliteal axial artery, lying deep to the forming popliteus muscle, disappears at about the 20–22 mm stage of the embryo, and the definitive distal popliteal artery forms from new vessels *after* the medial head of the gastrocnemius has migrated medially.[14,17] The medial head of gastrocnemius migrates through the popliteal fossa at about the same time as the transformation of the arterial structures.[18,21]

Should the definitive distal popliteal artery have formed prior to the migration, the newly formed artery may be swept medially to form a type I entrapment with the definitive artery now lying medial to the normally placed medial head of the gastrocnemius muscle. Alternatively, a well-formed distal popliteal artery may arrest the migration of the medial head resulting in a type II entrapment with the medial head of the gastrocnemius now more laterally placed than normal. Lesser abnormalities may occur if mesodermal remnants of the medial head persist posterior to the popliteal artery, constituting a type III popliteal entrapment formed either by mature skeletal muscle or fibrous and tendinous bands. Should the axial artery persist as the definitive distal popliteal artery, it will course deep to the popliteus muscle in its primitive position, resulting in a type IV entrapment. We have postulated that in some individuals a more lateral attachment of the muscular portion of the medial head of the gastrocnemius to the posterior aspect of the medial femoral condyle, may predispose such individuals to an acquired type of entrapment which is more likely to manifest should they undergo muscle hypertrophy consequent on regular lower limb exercise.

PATHOLOGY

The pathology of popliteal artery entrapment is presumably similar to any other form of chronic extrinsic recurrent arterial compression. Repetitive chronic trauma results in a degenerative process totally dissimilar to atheromatous change, in that the artery is affected from the outside. In evaluating arteries removed from patients who have undergone popliteal artery thombosis secondary to popliteal entrapment syndrome, we have recognized three stages in the progression of this disease process.[19]

In stage 1 the pathology is characterized by adventitial thickening and fibrosis with neovascularization in the adventitial portion of the popliteal artery with relatively few changes in the medial or intimal layers.

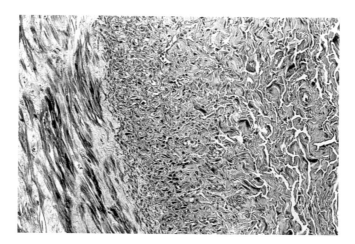

Fig. 2a. Stage 1 of the pathology. A medium power view of the adventitial neovascularisation. Note the intact media.

As the disease progresses, fragmentation of the external elastic lamina, replacement of the medial muscle by collagen and invasion of the media by new vessels and fibrosis characterizes stage 2 of this progressive pathological process. With progressive loss of the medial muscle and elastic tissue, the damaged artery becomes predisposed to aneurysmal change. In five of our 16 cases presenting with popliteal artery thrombosis secondary to popliteal entrapment syndrome, aneurysmal change was documented in association with the thrombosed segment.

In stage III the degenerative process results in almost total destruction of the media

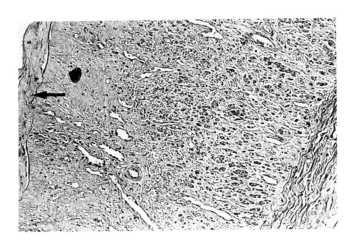

Fig. 2b. Stage 2. A medium power view of transmedial neovascularization, with relative sparing of the intima (arrow).

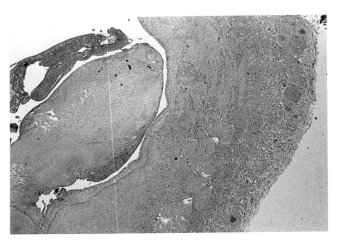

Fig. 2c. Low power view of the full thickness of the wall of a popliteal artery which has undergone thrombosis. This demonstrates progression to stage 3 disease with disruption of the media, neovascularization and proliferation of the intima with consequent overlying thrombus formation.

and replacement by fibrous tissue. Degenerative changes of the intima become manifest. Finally, degenerative changes of the intima with extensive fibrosis, and destruction of the internal elastic lamina render the artery liable to thrombosis. Once this stage has been reached, the entire arterial wall has been extensively damaged and largely replaced by fibrous tissue. It is therefore suggested that the occurrence of thrombosis should be regarded as evidence that the artery is no longer salvageable, and should be replaced by vein grafting. Thrombectomy, endarterectomy, thrombolysis and other less radical forms of therapy can therefore be expected to have a poorer medium-term patency than replacement of the thrombosed or aneurysmal segment with a vein graft.

CLINICAL PRESENTATION

Although originally thought to be rare, popliteal entrapment syndrome is now recognized as being more frequently a cause of vascular symptoms in young individuals than previously suspected.[20] Incidences between 0.17[12] and 3.5%[21] have been suggested. Previous reports indicate a marked sex difference favouring males[4,5] but this may have been a sampling error. In the present series the male:female ratio was 4:3.

In patients where the arterial pathology has not yet progressed to thrombosis and occlusion, the presentation is most frequently with claudication-like symptoms,[4,22] Typically, patients describe a progressive limitation of exercise tolerance, limited by calf and foot pain, blanching and numbness, relieved by rest. Often a single episode of strenuous exercise precipitates the development of claudication symptoms which then become progressive. Parasthesiae, presumably due to tibial nerve compression, may be present.[23] In most cases the symptoms are initially unilateral, despite the frequent presence of bilateral entrapment.

When the popliteal artery undergoes thrombotic occlusion, the presentation is that of severe limiting claudication or critical ischaemia with rest pain. Only one patient in our series lost a limb. She was demonstrated to have a hypercoagulable state with hyperactive platelets as demonstrated by increased reactivity to collagen, ADP and adrenaline. Two further patients who required emergency revascularization after

Table 2. The demographics of 73 limbs treated for popliteal entrapment syndrome

Total limbs	73
Presenting with claudication	55
Presenting with severe or critical ischaemia (occlusion)	18
Aneurysmal change	5
Venous obstruction	6
Limb loss	1
Right side	37
Left side	36

thrombosis were demonstrated likewise to have hypercoagulable states (one AT III deficiency, and one hyperactive platelets demonstrating increased sensitivity to collagen and adrenaline), suggesting that an immediate threat to the limb will result from localized popliteal artery disease only in those patients who have some additional factor which will adversely affect the otherwise healthy distal circulation. A small proportion of patients will present with or have associated venous obstruction of the popliteal vein due to the entrapment mechanism.[24,6]

Up to one-third of individuals may physiologically occlude their popliteal arteries with forced plantar flexion or dorsiflexion of the foot. In such individuals, the ankle pulses will diminish or be abolished with these manoeuvres. The significance of this finding in the asymptomatic individual remains uncertain.

INVESTIGATION

In young patients who present with vascular claudication symptoms, particularly in the absence of other specific risk factors for the development of atheromatous disease, the diagnosis of popliteal entrapment syndrome should be strongly considered. The reduction or abolishment of ankle pulses with dorsiflexion or plantar flexion against resistance strongly supports, but is probably not diagnostic of this condition.[10,13,20,23,25] In the 57 limbs presenting with claudication, all cases tested demonstrated reduction of ankle perfusion pressure with flexion manoeuvres against resistance.

Duplex Doppler with colour flow imaging,[26–28] CT scanning,[29] MRI scanning and MRI angiography[30] have all been used to confirm the diagnosis of popliteal entrapment syndrome. In the cases managed in the present series, these investigations were utilized only when required to exclude popliteal adventitial cystic disease.[31] Conventional contrast angiography was the preferred method of investigation for confirmation of the diagnosis.

In cases other than types I and II, no medial deviation of the popliteal artery may be seen in the resting position on angiogram. It is imperative that the patient be allowed to exert maximal dorsiflexion and plantar flexion against resistance in order to demonstrate popliteal artery abnormality in the other types of popliteal entrapment.[32]

MANAGEMENT

Recommendations for the management of popliteal entrapment syndrome have been to offer all patients in whom this condition is diagnosed some form of operative intervention.[4] This advice is based upon the experience that the major proportion of patients presenting with the syndrome had already developed popliteal artery occlusion.[7] Balanced against this is the excellent natural history that can be expected with a simple myotomy or release of the entrapment mechanism if the diagnosis is made prior to extensive arterial degeneration.

However, we and others have demonstrated that a substantial proportion of normal individuals occlude their popliteal artery with extreme plantar flexion.[10,23] There appears to be little doubt that all type I to IV anatomic entrapments should be released if diagnosed prior to arterial occlusion, and that a posterior approach to the popliteal artery offers the clearest anatomic display of the abnormal entrapment mechanism. Less certainty exists as to the correct form of management of the 'functional' or type VI entrapment. On the basis of the present series, it is recommended that symptomatic patients with positive non-invasive evidence of entrapment with flexion stress, be offered myotomy of the muscular portion of the medial head of the gastrocnemius muscle. For this purpose the medial approach is used. This policy has resulted in uniformly successful relief of symptoms in all 21 of the patients offered this procedure.

In patients who have progressed to thrombosis and occlusion of the popliteal artery, attempts to reopen the artery by Fogarty balloon catheter or thrombolysis may initially be successful, but the advanced nature of the degenerative pathology in the artery predicts for a poor medium-term patency.[9] In such circumstances, replacement of the occluded popliteal artery with an autologous vein graft remains the procedure of choice. For this purpose a medial approach is preferred in the patient with documented occlusion or aneurysm disease, in order to allow harvesting of the long saphenous vein and to facilitate exposure of the distal patent popliteal vessels.

REFERENCES

1. Hamming JJ, Vink M: Obstruction of the popliteal artery at early age. *J Cardiovasc Surg* **6:** 516, 1965
2. Levien LJ: Unpublished data
3. Stuart TPA: Note on a variation in the course of the popliteal artery. *J Anat Physiol* **13:** 162, 1879
4. Fowl RJ, Kempczinski RF, Whelan TJ: Popliteal artery entrapment. In: Rutherford RB (Ed) *Vascular Surgery*. Philadelphia, London: WB Saunders, 1995
5. Love JW, Whelan TJ: Popliteal artery entrapment syndrome. *Am J Surg* **109:** 620–624, 1995
6. Insua JA, Young JR, Humphries AW: Popliteal artery entrapment syndrome. *Arch Surg* **101:** 771–775, 1970
7. Persky JM, Kempczinski RF, Fowl RJ: Entrapment of the politeal artery. *Surg Gynecol Obstet* **173 :** 84, 1991
8. Rich NM, Collins GJ, McDonald PT *et al*.: Politeal vascular entrapment – its increasing interest. *Arch Surg* **114:** 1377–1384, 1979
9. Haimovici H, Sprayregen S, Johnson F: Popliteal artery entrapment by fibrous band. *Surgery* **72:** 789–792, 1972
10. Erdoes LS, Devine JJ, Berhard BM *et al*.: Popliteal vascular compression in a normal population. *J Vasc Surg* **20:** 978–986, 1994
11. Verhoeven ELG, Lucarotti ME, Campbell WB: Vanishing popliteal entrapment. *Euro J Vasc Endo Vasc Surg* **9:** 244–246 , 1995
12. Bouhoutsos J, Daskalakis E: Muscular abnormalities affecting the popliteal vessels. *Br J Surg* **68:** 501–506, 1981
13. Rignault DP, Pailler JL, Lunely F: The 'functional' popliteal artery syndrome. *Int Angiol* **4:** 341, 1985
14. Colborn GL, Lumsden AB, Taylor BS, Skandalakis JE: The surgical anatomy of the popliteal artery. *Am Surg* **60:** 238–246, 1994

15. Senior HD: The development of the arteries of the human lower extremities. *Am J Anat* **25**: 55–95, 1919

16. Senior HD: The development of the human femoral artery, a correction. *Am J Anat* **17**: 271–279, 1920

17. Carter A E, Eban R: A case of bilateral developmental abnormality of the popliteal arteries and gastrocnemius muscles. *Br J Surg* **51**: 518–522, 1964

18. Bardeen CR: Development and variation of the nerves and the musculature of the inferior extremity and of the neighbouring regions of the trunk in man. *Am J Anat* **6**: 259–390, 1907

19. Levien L J: In preparation.

20. Clanton TO, Solcher BW: Chronic leg pain in the athlete. *Clin Sports Med* **13**: 743–759, 1994

21. Gibson MHL, Mills JG, Johnson GE, Downs AR: Popliteal entrapment syndrome. *Ann Surg* **185**: 341–348, 1977

22. Darling RC, Buckley CJ, Abbott WM, Raines JK: Intermittent claudification in young athletes: popiteal artery entrapment syndrome. *J Trauma* **14**: 543–552, 1974

23. Turnipseed WD, Pozniak M: Popliteal entrapment as a result of neurovascular compression by the soleus and plantaris muscles. *J Vasc Surg* **15**: 285–294, 1992

24. Gherkin TM, Beebe HG, Williams DM *et al.*: Popliteal vein entrapment presenting as deep venous thrombosis and chronic venous insufficiency. *J Vasc Surg* **18**: 760–766, 1993

25. Chernoff DM, Walker AT, Khorasani R *et al.*: Asymptomatic functional popliteal artery entrapment: demonstration at MR imaging. *Radiology* **195**: 176–180, 1995

26. Akkersdijk WL, de Ruyter JW, Lapham R *et al.*: Colour duplex ultrasonagraphic and provocation of popliteal artery compression. *Eur J Vasc Endovasc Surg* **10**: 342–345, 1995

27. MacSweeny STR, Cuming R, Greenhalgh RM: Colour doppler ultrasonographic imaging in the diagnosis of popliteal artery entrapment syndrome. *Br J Surg* **81**: 822–823, 1994

28. Di Marzo L, Cavallaro A, Sciacca V *et al.*: Diagnosis of popliteal artery entrapment syndrome: the role of duplex scanning. *J Vasc Surg* **13**: 434–438, 1991

29. Rizzo RJ, Flinn WR, Yao JST *et al.*: Computed tomography for evaluation of arterial disease in the popliteal fossa. *J Vasc Surg* **11**: 112–119, 1990

30. Fujiwara H, Sugano T, Fujii N: Popliteal artery entrapment syndrome: accurate morphological diagnosis utilizing MRI. *J Cardiovasc Surg* **33**: 160–162, 1992

31. Bergan JJ: Adventitial cystic disease of the popliteal artery. In: Rutherford RB (Ed) *Vascular Surgery.* Philadelphia, London: WB Saunders, 1995

32. Greenwood LH, Yrizarry JM, Hallett JW: Popliteal artery entrapment: importance of the stress run-off for diagnosis. *J Cardiovasc Intervent Radiol* **9**: 93–99, 1986

Inflammatory Responses to Claudication – Do they Matter?

U. J. Kirkpatrick and C. N. McCollum

INTRODUCTION

Intermittent claudication is the most common symptom of disease affecting the peripheral arteries. The prevalence of claudication is low under the age of 50 years at 1.0–1.5% in men but rises substantially in the elderly with quoted prevalence up to 20–25% in those over 85.[1,2]

The prognosis for the legs in patients with claudication is good, with only 1–10% requiring reconstructive surgery and very few coming to amputation.[3] Claudication is a strong predictor of subsequent mortality which more than doubles that in non-claudicants.[4-6] The majority of claudicants die from associated cardiovascular events, in particular stroke and myocardial infarction, with this high mortality risk only partly explained by the expected association of peripheral vascular disease with coronary artery disease due to the generalized nature of atherosclerosis.[7-9]

Explanations for the excess mortality in claudicants

Ongoing research involving claudicants has sought to explain the excess mortality in this group of patients. Patients with intermittent claudication may have a transient but repeated ischaemia-reperfusion injury each time they walk as the leg muscles become ischaemic with exercise followed by a reperfusion injury during recovery on resting.[10]

An alternative explanation for the excess mortality seen in claudicants relates to changes in blood levels of potassium. Plasma potassium and adrenalin concentrations increase during exercise and decrease rapidly shortly after exercise. It has been proposed that this rapid alteration in potassium after exercise may facilitate arterial thrombosis when there is pre-existing arterial disease.[11]

A further explanation may be damage to the normal regulatory sympathetic drive following repeated ischaemia-reperfusion injury. In animal studies, ischaemia-reperfusion injury impairs the sympathetic neuronal uptake mechanisms, thus allowing certain agonists to exert a more potent contractile effect on the vasculature.[12]

Benefit of exercise in claudicants

The initial clinical status provides no prognostic clue to subsequent progress.[13] Supervised exercise programmes have more than doubled walking distance in claudicants within 12 weeks, possibly due to an improvement in skeletal muscle oxidative metabolism.[14] Studies involving moderate-to severe claudication have shown that exercise training results in a greater improvement in walking distance at 1 year than percutaneous transluminal angioplasty and this effect is greatest in patients with superficial femoral artery disease.[15] These studies clearly justify our current advice to patients; that they should take regular exercise.

Biochemical changes in atherosclerosis

There are a number of biochemical markers which are elevated in those with widespread atherosclerosis. The Edinburgh Artery Study has shown that patients with peripheral artery disease have higher levels of blood viscosity, haematocrit, fibrinogen, uric acid and plasma leucocyte elastase.[16] Tissue plasminogen activator inhibitor, P-selectin, β-thromboglobulin, prostacyclin biosynthesis and von Willebrand factor (vWF) are all also raised in patients with widespread atherosclerotic disease.[17–19] Initial blood viscosity, fibrinogen level and cross-linked fibrin degradation products may correlate with disease progression.[13,20] The multiple haemostatic abnormalities seen in atherosclerosis resemble the non-specific, haematological stress-syndrome response to acute and chronic inflammatory disorders and may only represent a non-specific secondary response.[21]

Exercise-induced biochemical changes in claudicants

Biochemical changes are known to occur in claudicants after exercise: plasma thromboxane rises within 15 minutes following exercise, total antioxidant concentrations fall and lipid peroxide levels rise after exercise.[22–25] The high cardiovascular mortality rate of claudicants has been linked to increases in urinary microalbumin excretion as a reflection of a repetitive systemic microvascular injury.[10] However, less than 50% of claudicants show a rise in urinary microalbumin after exercise.[26] The apparent systemic injury seen in claudication even led some authors to suggest that exercise may exacerbate this injury and that early surgical intervention may ameliorate this effect.[27] Claudicants demonstrate a higher resting state of neutrophil activation than controls and this systemic level of neutrophil activation increases further and significantly after exercise.[28,29]

A STUDY ON REPEATED EXERCISE

To distinguish whether claudicants have a distinct reperfusion injury of skeletal muscle after exercise they must at least be compared with controls who have some likelihood of atherosclerotic disease and are matched for age, smoking history and hypertension. If there is underlying coronary artery disease, then exercise may induce an ischaemia-reperfusion injury of the myocardium, and these changes may predominate over any ischaemia-reperfusion injury of skeletal muscle.

The relative importance of white cell and platelet products is unclear; although white cell involvement is considered necessary for an ischaemia-reperfusion injury, platelet activation may be more important in precipitating arterial thrombosis and the resulting increased cardiovascular morbidity and mortality. It is known that P-selectin is an adhesion molecule which is a constituent of the membrane of the platelet α granules but is also a component of the membrane of the Weibel–Palade bodies of endothelial cells and is released on cellular activation. We have measured soluble P-selectin as a reflection of platelet activation.[30,31]

This study aimed to evaluate the effect of a second exercise challenge and examine whether biochemical changes were cumulative. This reflects more closely the repeated exercise that patients with intermittent claudication experience in their normal daily activity.

Subjects

Thirty-four patients aged > 40 years with a diagnosis of chronic stable intermittent claudication and an ankle brachial pressure index (ABPI) less than 0.8 in at least one leg were recruited from our vascular outpatient clinic. Ethical committee approval and informed consent were obtained. No patient had received medication with a significant antiplatelet, anticoagulant or haemorheological modifying component including all non-steroidal anti-inflammatory drugs within the previous 2 weeks.

Twelve control patients with ABPIs greater than 1.0 were recruited, matched for age, sex, history of hypertension, smoking history, and cardiac history. These controls were recruited from patients attending an abdominal aortic aneurysm screening programme or from relatives of claudicants already in the study.

Study protocol

All patients attended the department in the 2 weeks preceding the study day so that ABPI could be measured and they were familiar with the treadmill. On the study day, patients arrived by taxi in the morning having starved from midnight the night before and then rested for at least one hour on a couch before an initial blood sample was taken by direct venepuncture with a 19G needle. Patients then walked on the treadmill at 3.2km/h and 10% gradient to their maximum ability until stopped by pain. Serial blood samples were taken by direct venepuncture from the antecubital fossa at 5, 15 and 30 minutes post-exercise. The patients then performed a further identical exercise challenge 30 minutes following the first exercise with blood samples being taken at 5 and 15 minutes post-exercise.

Control patients followed the same protocol but walked on the treadmill for a set time of 5 minutes.

Sample assays

Full blood count and the assay for neutrophil hydrogen peroxide generation were performed immediately following sampling. Neutrophil hydrogen peroxide production was measured by a flow cytometric technique.[32] Soluble P-selectin was measured by a standard ELISA assay as were levels of vWF using commercial antiserum.[33]

Statistical analysis

Results have been analysed by repeated measures analysis of variance (ANOVA). Log transformation was performed on non-parametric data. Mann-Whitney testing has been used for comparison between claudicants and controls. Results are expressed as the mean ± SEM.

RESULTS

In claudicants, the white cell count increased from 7.37±0.35 to 8.29±0.37 ×10^9/l at 5 minutes after exercise (p<0.01) and rapidly returned to baseline within 15 minutes following exercise (Fig. 1). The same pattern of response occurred after each exercise in both claudicants and controls, but the initial count in controls was only 5.86±0.34 ×10^9/l. The circulating white cell count was significantly higher in patients with claudication compared with controls throughout the experiments (p<0.02).

The response of circulating platelets to exercise was similar in both claudicants and controls with a peak value attained within 5 minutes of exercise (Fig. 2); claudicants had a mean level of 245±14 ×10^9/l platelets at rest and this increased to 259±16 ×10^9/l at 5 minutes after exercise (p<0.05). The mean resting platelet count in controls was 226±28 ×10^9/l.

There was no overall significant change in neutrophil hydrogen peroxide generation after exercise in either claudicants or controls (p=0.35 and p=0.90 respectively, ANOVA). However, there was a correlation between resting neutrophil activation and the ABPI (r = −0.395, p=0.02) in patients with claudication (Fig. 3).

The endothelial cell marker, vWF, showed a cyclical pattern with a peak occurring 15 minutes after cessation of exercise (Fig. 4). However, this only occurred in the

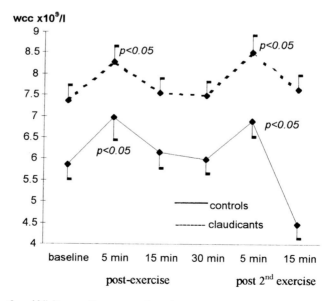

Fig. 1. White cell count (wcc) changes during exercise in claudicants and controls.

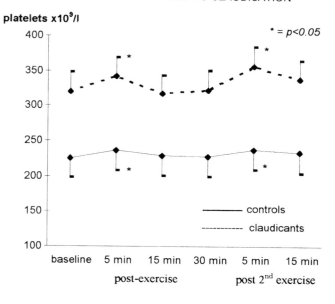

Fig. 2. Changes in platelet count following exercise in claudicants and controls.

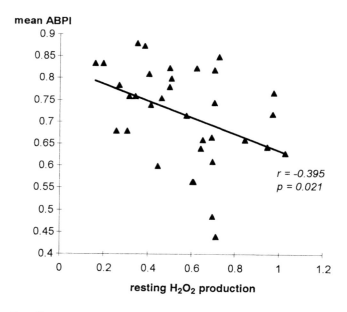

Fig. 3. Correlation between ankle brachial pressure index (ABPI) and resting neutrophil hydrogen peroxide generation.

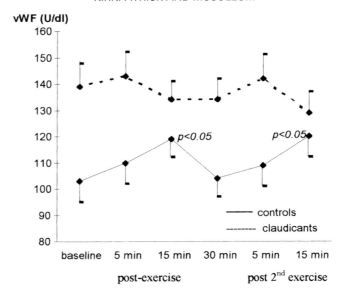

Fig. 4. von Willebrand factor (vWF) following exercise in claudicants and controls.

control patients. At rest the plasma levels of vWF in controls were 103±8U/dl and this increased to 119±7U/dl at 15 minutes after exercise (p<0.01). The same pattern was repeated following the second exercise. Claudicants had higher levels of plasma vWF throughout (p<0.03) but did not show a consistent pattern of response to exercise (p>0.1 ANOVA).

Soluble P-selectin was 320±28 ng/ml initially and peaked at 342±27 ng/ml and 357±28 ng/ml at 5 minutes after first and second exercises respectively in claudicants; this reached statistical significance following the second exercise only (Fig. 5). In control subjects initial levels of sP-selectin were 274±40 ng/ml and there was no consistent pattern of change after exercise (p=0.6 ANOVA).

DISCUSSION

The increase in platelet and white cell count after exercise was the expected physiological response. The leucocytosis induced by exercise has been shown to be biphasic with an immediate transient increase in circulating white blood cells followed by a delayed response over 2 hours after cessation of exercise;[34] the initial leucocytosis may be an effect of adrenalin on leucocyte demargination, while the action of cortisol on the bone marrow causes the delayed leucocytosis.[34] Exercise-induced release of radiolabelled erythrocytes, platelets and granulocytes from the spleen has a reciprocal time-course to the corresponding cell count in peripheral blood and the lung fields.[35]

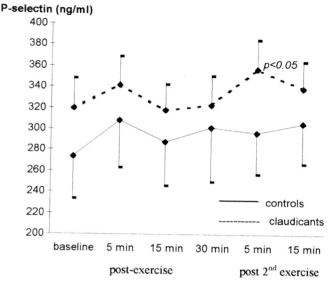

Fig. 5.   Changes in soluble P-selectin during exercise in claudicants and controls.

The results show a peak level of vWF at 15 minutes after exercise in control subjects despite their smaller numbers. A possible explanation for this may be that the endothelium of patients with atherosclerosis was activated and no longer able to generate the normal response to exercise. Indeed the levels of vWF were consistently higher in the claudicant group compared with controls. In a previous study, patients with peripheral vascular disease had higher levels of vWF and the markers of endothelial cell damage correlated with the severity of hypoxia measured by oximeter as percutaneous oxygen saturation.[36] The correlation between resting neutrophil activation and ABPI suggests that biochemical markers may be used to delineate the severity of peripheral vascular disease.

The progressive increase in soluble P-selectin after exercise in patients with intermittent claudication may indicate platelet activation in claudicants and hence explain the high associated cardiovascular morbidity and mortality in such patients. The P-selectin expression in plasma was also significantly increased in patients with unstable angina, and immediately after exercise in patients with proven cardiac disease.[37,38] Given that peak P-selectin levels occur within 5 minutes of exercise and peak vWF levels occur at 15 minutes after exercise, the endothelium may not be the source of P-selectin here. However, the responses of both soluble P-selectin and platelet count followed the same pattern after exercise. It is possible that soluble P-selectin levels depend on the numbers of circulating platelets. However, P-selectin changes in the control group did not approach statistical significance (p=0.56) despite clear-cut changes in platelet numbers. The P-selectin changes may be specific to claudicants.

Claudicants represent a heterogeneous group of patients with a wide range of arterial disease in terms of severity and location. Patients with superficial femoral artery disease show greater improvement in supervised exercise programmes than patients with aorto-iliac disease[15] and biochemical changes may also vary depending on the level of disease. Claudicants may have a clinical history of previous cardiac disease while others may have undiagnosed disease, and the effect of a subclinical ischaemia-reperfusion of the myocardium may be an influence. The question of whether the inflammatory events that accompany exercise in claudicants influence the rate of subsequent myocardial infarction and stroke merits further research.

REFERENCES

1. Dormandy J, Mahir M, Ascady G et al.: Fate of the patient with chronic leg ischaemia. *J Cardiovasc Surg* **30:** 50–57, 1989
2. Hale WE, Marks RG, May FE et al.: Epidemiology of intermittent claudication: evaluation of risk factors. *Age Ageing* **17:** 57–60, 1988
3. Dormandy JA. Natural history of intermittent claudication. *Hospital Update* **17:** 314–320, 1991
4. Kannel WB, McGee DL: Update on some epidemiologic features of intermittent claudication: the Framingham study. *J Am Geriatr Soc* **33:** 13–18, 1985
5. Jonason T, Ringqvist I: Mortality and morbidity in patients with intermittent claudication in relation to the location of the occlusive atherosclerosis in the leg. *Angiology* **36:** 310–314, 1985
6. Jelnes R, Gaardsting O, Hougard Jensen K: Fate in intermittent claudication: outcome and risk factors. *Br Med J* **293:** 1137–1140, 1986
7. O'Riordain DS, O'Donnell JA: Realistic expectations for the patient with intermittent claudication. *Br J Surg* **78:** 861–863, 1991
8. Reunanen A, Takkunen H, Aromaa A: Prevalence of intermittent claudication and its effect on mortality. *Acta Med Scand* **211:** 249–256, 1982
9. Bainton D, Sweetnam P, Baker I, Elwood P: Peripheral vascular disease: consequence for survival and association with risk factors in the Speedwell prospective heart disease study. *Br Heart J* **72:** 128–132, 1994
10. Tsang GMK, Sanghera K, Gosling P et al.: Pharmacological reduction of the systemically damaging effects of local ischaemia. *Eur J Vasc Surg* **8:** 205–208, 1994
11. Lin H, Young DB: Interaction between plasma potassium and epinephrine in coronary thrombosis in dogs. *Circulation* **89:** 331–338, 1994
12. Sobey CG, Sozzi V, Woodman OL: Ischaemia/reperfusion enhances phenylephrine-induced contraction of rabbit aorta due to impairment of neuronal uptake. *J Cardiovasc Pharmacol* **23:** 562–568, 1994
13. Dormandy JA, Hoare E, Khattab AH et al.: Prognostic significance of rheological and biochemical findings in patients with intermittent claudication. *Br Med J* **4:** 581–583, 1973
14. Hiatt WR, Regensteiner JG, Hargarten ME et al.: Benefit of exercise conditioning for patients with peripheral arterial disease. *Circulation* **81:** 602–609, 1990
15. Perkins JMT, Collin J, Creasy TS et al.: Exercise training versus angioplasty for stable claudication. Long and medium term results of a prospective, randomised trial. *Eur J Vasc Endovasc Surg* **11:** 409–413, 1996
16. Lowe GDO, Fowkes FGR, Dawes J et al.: Blood viscosity, fibrinogen, and activation of coagulation and leukocytes in peripheral arterial disease and the normal population in the Edinburgh Artery Study. *Circulation* **87:** 1915–1920, 1993
17. Blann AD, Dobrotova M, Kubisz P, McCollum CN: Von Willebrand factor, soluble P-selectin, tissue plasminogen activator and plasminogen activator inhibitor in atherosclerosis. *Thromb Haemost* **74:** 626–630, 1995
18. Cella G, Zahavi J, De Haas HA, Kakkar VV: b-Thromboglobulin, platelet production time and platelet function in vascular disease. *Brit J Haematol* **43:** 127–136, 1979

19. Fitzgerald GA, Smith B, Pedersen AK, Brash AR: Increased prostacyclin biosynthesis in patients with severe atherosclerosis and platelet activation. N Engl J Med **310**: 1065–1068, 1984

20. Fowkes FGR, Lowe GDO, Housley E et al.: Cross-linked fibrin degradation products, pregression of peripheral arterial disease, and risk of coronary heart disease. Lancet **342**: 84–86, 1993

21. Stuart J, George AJ, Davies AJ et al.: Haematological stress syndrome in atherosclerosis. J Clin Pathol **34**: 464–467, 1981

22. Khaira HS, Nash GB, Bahra PS et al.: Thromboxane and neutrophil changes following intermittent claudication suggest ischaemia-reperfusion injury. Eur J Vasc Endovasc Surg **10**: 31–35, 1995

23. Edwards AT, Blann AD, Suarez-Mendez VJ et al.: Systemic responses in patients with intermittent claudication after treadmill exercise. Br J Surg **81**: 1738–1741: 1994

24. Khaira HS, Maxwell SRJ, Shearman CP: Antioxidant consumption during exercise in intermittent claudication. Br J Surg **82**: 1660–1662, 1995

25. Shearman CP, Gosling P, Gwynn BR, Simms MH: Systemic effects associated with intermittent claudication. A model to study biochemical aspects of vascular disease? Eur J Vasc Surg **2**: 401–404, 1988

26. Matsushita M, Nishikimi N, Sakurai T et al.: Urinary microalbumin as a marker for intermittent claudication. Eur J Vasc Endovasc Surg **11**: 421–424, 1996

27. Hickey NC, Gosling P, Baar S et al.: Effect of surgery on the systemic inflammatory response to intermittent claudication. Br J Surg **77**: 1121–1124, 1990

28. Hickman P, Hill A, McLaren M et al.: Exercise induces activation in claudicants but not in age-matched controls [abstr]. Br J Surg **80**: 1472, 1993

29. Eyers PS, Lardi A, Wood JA, McCollum CN: Exercise primes neutrophils in patients with intermittent claudication [abstr]. Br J Surg **81**: 1799–1826, 1994

30. Wagner DD: The Weibel-Palade body: the storage granule for von Willebrand factor and P-selectin. Thromb Haemost **70**: 1–5, 1993

31. McEver RP, Beckstead JH, Moore KL et al.: GMP-140, a platelet a-granule membrane protein, is also synthesized by vascular endothelial cells and is localized in Weibel-Palade bodies. J Clin Invest **84**: 92–99, 1989

32. Bass DA, Parce JW, Dechatelet LR et al.: Flow cytometric studies of oxidative product formation by neutrophils: A graded response to membrane stimulation. J Immunol **130**: 1910–1917, 1983

33. Short PE, Williams CE, Picken AM, Hill FGH: Factor VIII related antigen: an improved immunoassay. Med Lab Sci **39**: 351–355, 1982

34. McCarthy DA, Perry JD, Melsom RD, Dale MM: Leucocytosis induced by exercise. Br Med J **295**: 636, 1987

35. Allsop P, Peters AM, Arnot RN et al.: Intrasplenic blood cell kinetics in man before and after brief maximal exercise. Clin Sci **83**: 47–54, 1992

36. Blann AD, Seigneur M, Adams RA, McCollum CN: Neutrophil elastase, von Willebrand factor, soluble thrombomodulin and percutaneous oxygen in peripheral atherosclerosis. Eur J Vasc Endovasc Surg **12**: 218–222, 1996

37. Ikeda H, Takajo Y, Ichiki K et al.: Increased soluble form of P-selectin in patients with unstable angina. Circulation **92**: 1693–1696, 1995

38. Pan YZ, Wu BM, Hong XS: The clinical significance of platelet activation during exercise-induced myocardial ischaemia. Chung Hua Nei Ko Tsa Chih **33**: 106–108, 1994

Buerger's Disease

Jesse E. Thompson

INTRODUCTION

In 1879 Felix von Winiwater, one of Theodor Billroth's surgical assistants in Vienna, reported an inflammatory disorder of the blood vessels of the lower extremity which he termed 'endarteritis obliterans'.[1] This report stemmed from a detailed study of the amputated right leg of a 57-year-old man with 'spontaneous gangrene'. Winiwater noted the involvement of both arteries and veins.[2]

In 1908, 29 years later, Leo Buerger, working at the Mount Sinai Hospital in New York City, described the same disease, a condition occurring in young men with progressive vascular insufficiency of the extremities leading to gangrene and amputation. From clinical observations and detailed pathologic study of 11 amputated lower extremities Buerger renamed the disease 'thromboangiitis obliterans' (TAO).[3] An even more detailed description appeared in Buerger's book published in 1924.[4] He believed it to be distinct from arteriosclerosis.[2] Over the next several decades, many cases of lower extremity gangrene at any age from any cause were diagnosed as TAO.[5]

As a result of overdiagnosis of TAO and confusion with arteriosclerosis obliterans (ASO), skepticism arose as to the very existence of Buerger's disease as a separate clinical entity. Wessler et al.[6] at the Beth Israel Hospital in Boston were the chief opponents of Buerger's disease and maintained that it was indistinguishable from arteriosclerosis, systemic embolization or idiopathic peripheral arterial thrombosis. Subsequent studies, however, have shown that TAO is a specific entity distinct from ASO based on clinical, arteriographic and histopathologic findings.[5,7–10] Today we know Buerger's disease as a disorder found predominantly in young male smokers. Buerger did not mention cigarette smoking in his original article. It was not until 1918 that Meyer first suggested that TAO was related to tobacco usage.[2]

EPIDEMIOLOGY

Buerger's disease was originally thought to occur almost exclusively in Ashkenazim Jews. However, this reflected the patient population Buerger was treating at Mount Sinai Hospital in New York City. The disease affects all races and ethnic groups and has a worldwide distribution although there is a greater prevalence in Japan, India, Southeast Asia, Israel and Eastern Europe than in Western Europe and North America.[5,10] Accurate statistics are difficult to obtain. DeBakey and Cohen[11] in their study of Buerger's disease in the US Army in World War II gave an estimated incidence of 7 per 100 000 white males aged 20–44 years. Shionoya estimates the incidence to be 5 per 100 000 in Japan.[12] In patients presenting with peripheral vascular disorders the reported proportion with a diagnosis of Buerger's disease is 0.75% in North America, 0.25% in the UK, 3.3% in Poland, 80% in Israel, and 16–66% in Korea and Japan.[12,13]

While predominantly a disease of men, Buerger's disease does occur in women; Shionoya reported an incidence of 2% in Japan. Although the annual incidence of TAO in North America has declined over the years, there has been a relative increase among women (8–23%), attributable to the increased prevalence of smoking in young women.[2,13–15]

AETIOLOGY

The cause of Buerger's disease is unknown. It has been suggested that it is an infectious disorder, but no organisms of any sort have ever been identified in acute Buerger's lesions.[2,13] Smoking is almost invariably associated with the onset of TAO, its progression and remission. Cotinine, the major urinary metabolite of nicotine, is a marker for the level of smoking activity.[16] Studies demonstrate a close relationship between levels of active smoking and the course of Buerger's disease. True non-smokers practically never develop the disease. The role of passive smoking is still inconclusive.[16] Papa et al.[17] studied patients with Buerger's disease for cellular and humoral sensitivity to tobacco glycoprotein (TGP) antigen using healthy smokers and healthy non-smokers as controls. Patients with Buerger's disease and healthy smokers had the same rate of cellular response to TGP. If TGP has an immunologic role in TAO additional factors may be operative.

The prevailing notion is that an autoimmune mechanism is probably involved in Buerger's disease. Gulati et al.,[18] using homogenized human arteries as antigens, found antiarterial antibodies; immunoglobulins IgM, IgG, and IgA; and C3 components in the diseased vessels of TAO patients. Adar et al.[19] found a higher degree of cell-mediated sensitivity and antibodies to types I and III collagen, constituents of human arteries, in TAO patients than in controls. Hada et al.[20] observed the stimulation index to types I and IV collagen and cell-mediated reactivity to type V collagen, elastin and laminin to be higher in TAO patients than controls. Increase in complement factor C4 has also been reported.[12]

A genetic predisposition may also be a factor in the aetiology. Human leucocyte antigen (HLA) typing shows significantly higher frequencies of A1, A9, AW24, B5, B8, BW10, BW40, BW54, CW1, DR2, DR4 and lower frequencies of DR9, DRW6, and DRW52 in patients with Buerger's disease compared with those who do not have the disease.[10,12,17] Findings are not consistent, however, and others have not been able to confirm these results.[13]

Other factors which may be involved in aetiology include the presence of anti-phospholipid antibody,[21] deficiency of protein S,[22] and increased platelet response to serotonin.[23] It has also been suggested that Buerger's disease is a result of a hypercoagulable state but studies have been inconclusive.[24,25]

The aetiology of Buerger's disease remains obscure but a genetic predisposition and autoimmune mechanisms in combination with tobacco usage and other factors may induce the disease in susceptible individuals.

PATHOLOGY

Buerger's disease is a segmental inflammatory occlusive disorder which involves predominantly the medium-size and small arteries of both lower and upper extremities. Involvement of visceral vessels has also been described.[10] All three layers of the vessel wall are affected by the inflammatory process, but the normal architecture of the wall is preserved. Thrombosis of the lumen occurs in the involved segments. Whether the thrombosis comes first, followed by the inflammatory response, or vice versa, is not known. There are three stages: acute, intermediate and chronic. In the acute stage the thrombus is cellular and contains lymphocytes, fibroblasts and giant cells. Microabscesses consisting of polymorphonuclear leucocytes and giant cells are also found in the thrombus. The inflammatory process can extend into the periarterial tissues to involve the associated vein and nerve. The intermediate stage is one of healing.

In the third or chronic stage the occluding thrombus is well organized and recanalization may be evident. The artery and vein and adjacent nerve may be bound together in a firm cord. The general architecture of the vessel wall is still well preserved including the internal elastic lamina. The pathological changes in the involved veins are quite similar to those in the affected arteries. Superficial phlebitis in Buerger's disease is histologically similar to idiopathic venous thrombosis.[2,10,12]

DIAGNOSTIC CRITERIA

No single test is pathognomonic for the diagnosis of Buerger's disease, which remains primarily a clinical one. Arteriographic and histopathologic criteria are supportive and laboratory data are largely exclusive. Shionoya's clinical criteria are (1) smoking history, (2) onset before the age of 50, (3) infrapopliteal arterial occlusive lesions, (4) either upper limb involvement or phlebitis migrans, and (5) absence of arteriosclerotic risk factors other than smoking. The clinical diagnosis is made when all five requirements are met.[12]

Mills and Porter,[13] have proposed their diagnostic criteria (Table 1) divided into major and minor categories and they have emphasized factors to be excluded, which require a considerable number of laboratory examinations.

Arteriography should be employed regularly, if not routinely, especially if a bypass operation is being considered. Multiple segmental occlusions of distal infrapopliteal arteries are characteristic of Buerger's disease with the occlusions being tapered or abrupt; normal arterial segments are interspersed with the occluded segments. The distal vessels have a corkscrew appearance while the collateral vessels around the occlusions have a tree-root or spider-leg configuration (Fig. 1). The aortic,

Table 1. Diagnostic criteria of Buerger's disease

Major criteria

Onset distal extremity ischaemic symptoms before 45 years of age
Tobacco abuse
Exclusion of:
    Proximal embolic source (cardiac, TOS, ASO, aneurysm)
    Trauma and local lesions (entrapment, adventitial cyst)
    Autoimmune disease
    Hypercoagulable state
    Atherosclerosis
       Diabetes
       Hyperlipidaemia
       Renal failure
       Hypertension
Undiseased arteries proximal to popliteal or distal brachial level
Objective documentation of distal occlusive disease by:
    Arteriography
    Histopathology, rare

Minor criteria

Migratory superficial phlebitis
Raynaud's syndrome
Upper extremity involvement
Instep claudication

Modified from ref. 13, with permission.

iliac, and femoral vessels are not usually involved unless thrombosis from below progresses centrally.[14]

Histopathological confirmation is not essential and is not usually feasible in the acute stage. If a specimen from an acute lesion is available, the findings are confirmatory. Findings in amputated specimens are usually of the chronic stage and are non-specific.[2]

DIFFERENTIAL DIAGNOSIS

Buerger's disease must be differentiated from a number of other disorders, the principal being atherosclerosis obliterans in young individuals. Clinical, angiographic and pathologic features carefully observed nowadays can distinguish the two disorders in most cases.[10] Other clinical differential diagnoses are shown in Table 2. Appropriate studies to exclude these disorders must be carried out. Vascular laboratory tests such as thigh, calf, ankle and toe pressures are helpful in diagnosis.[10,14]

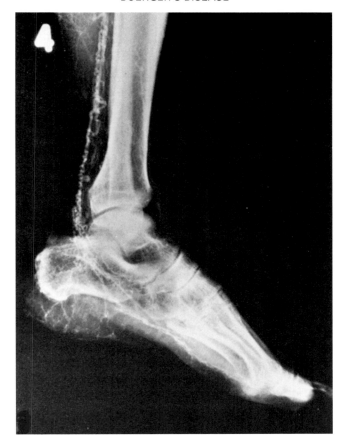

Fig. 1. Arteriogram in Buerger's disease. The posterior tibial, peroneal, and anterior tibial arteries are occluded. Corkscrew type collaterals are seen. (From ref. 35, with permission.)

CLINICAL PRESENTATION

The typical Buerger's disease patient is a male smoker under the age of 40 who presents with lower extremity rest pain, digital ulceration or gangrene. Claudication when present is usually confined to the instep. Two limbs are usually involved at the initial presentation and frequently three or all four are affected. Pulses proximal to the ankle and wrist are ordinarily present and normal. Pedal and wrist pulses are usually absent. The upper extremity is involved in a third to half the patients and is the primary seat in 10–20%. Raynaud's phenomena, paresthesias and superficial thrombophlebitis are present in about a third of the patients.[13] Dependent rubor may also be present. Phlebitis involves the smaller veins of the foot or ankle and does not usually involve the greater or lesser saphenous veins.[12,26,27]

Table 2. Differential diagnoses for Burger's disease

Atherosclerotic disease	*Autoimmune disease*
In situ thrombosis	Scleroderma
Emboli	Systemic lupus erythematosus
Arterial origin	Rheumatoid arthritis
Cardiac origin	Mixed connective tissue disease
Risk factors	
Hyperlipidaemia	*Vasculitides*
Hypertension	Polyarteritis
Diabetes mellitus	Giant cell arteritis
	Takayasu's arteritis
Upper extremity	Hypersensitivity angiitis
Innominate artery stenosis	
Subclavian stenosis/aneurysm	*Haematologic disorders*
Thoracic outlet syndrome	Polycythemia
Occupational injury	Thrombocytosis
	Dysproteinaemias
Popliteal artery lesions	Hypercoagulable states
Entrapment	
Adventitial cystic degeneration	
Aneurysm	
Embolus or thrombosis *in situ*	
Trauma	

Modified from ref. 10, with permission.

CLINICAL COURSE

Buerger's disease characteristically has remissions and exacerbations, intimately related to smoking activity. Gangrene of the toes is common, requiring amputation. Progression into the suprapopliteal segments may occur, even into the aorto-iliac area, resulting in major amputations below or above the knee. In the upper extremity, involvement of the brachial artery rarely follows involvement of forearm arteries. Amputation of fingers may be required but not of the hand or arm. If the patient with Buerger's disease completely abstains from smoking, the disease process may be halted, lesions will heal, the clinical course will be uneventful and benign, and a good prognosis may be expected. If the patient continues to smoke, progression is inexorable and amputations will be the inevitable result.[12,27]

TREATMENT

Total abstinence from tobacco is the only way of arresting the progression of Buerger's disease; any therapy, medical or surgical, will be ineffective if tobacco usage continues. The disease has been reported in pipe smokers and in those using chewing tobacco and snuff.[13] When the patient first presents with Buerger's disease, various measures must be instituted in addition to the admonition to cease smoking.

Local measures include nail removal to drain infections, gentle saline cleansing of ulcerations, avoidance of tissue-toxic agents, and gentle debridement. Conservatism and patience are the orders of the day at this point. Analgesics may be necessary for pain control.[12,13] The pain is frequently excruciating due to ischaemia of the sensory nerves and the incorporation in fibrous tissue of the artery, vein and nerve. With severe pain epidural anaesthesia with an inlying catheter may be used. Alcohol in the form of whisky or brandy has been given to deaden pain and promote vasodilatation. Antibiotics are necessary to control infection. Anticoagulants, especially heparin, have been employed to retard proximal thrombosis. A number of drugs have been used in Buerger's disease: thrombolytic agents, prostaglandins, prostacyclin, antiplatelet agents, anti-malarials, typhoid vaccine, pyrogens, steroids, vasodilators, calcium channel blockers, α-adrenergic blockers and haemorrheologic agents such as pentoxifylline.[12,13,26] Hyperbaric oxygen has also been employed. None of these methods of treatment has been particularly effective except prostaglandin and prostacyclin. In a recent randomized study of iloprost (an analogue of prostacyclin) versus aspirin, iloprost resulted in ulcer healing or pain relief in 85% of 58 patients versus 17% of 65 patients taking aspirin. There was a 6% amputation rate in the iloprost group compared with 18% in the aspirin group.[28] In an earlier study in 1980 Eastcott, using prostaglandin PGE1, reported ulcer healing in 54.5% of 11 patients with Buerger's disease.[5]

Surgical treatment becomes necessary if conservative medical measures fail to improve the situation and the patient continues to smoke. Surgical measures include sympathectomy, peripheral sensory nerve crushing, arterial reconstruction, and amputation. In various reports, about 50% of Buerger's disease patients have undergone lumbar sympathectomy with removal of ganglia L2 and L3. In the occasional cases where thoracic sympathectomy has been employed, ganglia T2, T3 and the lower third of the stellate ganglion are removed. The rationale for sympathectomy is to provide vasodilatation, which increases skin circulation and hopefully promotes healing of ulcers.[12,13,26,27]

Sensory nerve interruption has been employed over the years occasionally to relieve intractable pain.[29]

Thromboendarterectomy has little or no place in the management of Buerger's disease because of the underlying process and the arteries involved. Postoperative occlusion is very common. The principal reconstructive manoeuver used is bypass grafting. The rare cases of suprapopliteal occlusion are the best cases for bypass. In Shionoya's series from Japan bypasses were performed in 44 (17%) of 255 patients with Buerger's disease.[12] The life table patency of the infrainguinal grafts (11%) was 56% at 1 year, 48% at 2 years and 32% at 10 years. In Sayin's series of 16 bypasses in Istanbul, the 1–7 year patency was 62.5%.[30]

A recent report from Japan cited 15 bypasses to the plantar arteries with a 60% patency rate. All grafts remained patent in those who stopped smoking during the short follow-up period.[31]

Such results of grafting are inferior to those for atherosclerotic occlusions. However, even short-term patency for several months may allow local debridement of necrotic tissue, healing of ulceration, and avoidance of major amputation.

In a report from the UK, Hodgson et al. reported a case of acute Buerger's disease in which streptokinase and heparin were used to lyse the thrombus, followed by balloon angioplasty to dilate the stenosed area. The patient had a good result with no recurrence at 2 years of follow-up.[32]

For those patients who continue smoking heavily the result is usually amputation, first of the digits and finally of the lower extremities. Hand or arm amputation is rare. Table 3 displays the results of therapy in several selected series. The differences in amputation rates in America and the UK compared with those in Japan and the Middle East are quite striking, as are the sizes of the series. Although Shionoya reports only a 2.7% incidence of major leg amputations, he states that digital gangrene or ulceration occurred in 72% of his patients, and amputation of a finger or toe was frequently required.[12,26]

Table 3.   Surgical treatment in Buerger's disease

Reb.	No. of patients	Sympathectomy	Bypass grafts	Amputations		
				Minor	Major	Total
Eastcott (1984)[5]	81	37 46%	0	14 17%	18 22%	32
Pairolero et al. (1984)[33]	12	12 100%	0	NA	NA	8
Mills et al. (1987)[14]	26	12 46%	6 23%	10 38%	8 31%	18
Olin et al. (1990)[15]	89	23 26%	0	23 26%	16 18%	39
Sayin et al. (1993)[30]	216	203 94%	16 7.4%	29 13%	4 1.85%	33
Shionoya (1995)[12]	255	130 51%	44 17.2%	NA	7 2.7%	7

SURVIVAL

Despite the grim outlook for the extremities in Buerger's disease, the long-term survival of these patients is quite good. In fact several studies show that the survival is the same as that of an age-matched normal population and far above that of patients with generalized atherosclerotic disease, being 98% at 5 years and 94% at 10 years in contrast to a 5-year survival of 76% for atherosclerosis[8,10,33,34] This reflects the distribution of disease mainly in the extremities, sparing largely the coronary, cerebral, renal and visceral arteries. Involvement of these vessels has been documented in only a few patients, almost all as single case reports.[2,10,12] A unique case of Buerger's disease in a saphenous vein arterial graft has been reported.[2]

REFERENCES

1.   Von Winiwater F: Ueber eine eigenthümliche form von endarteriitis und endophlebitis mit gangrän des fusses. *Arch Klin Chir* **23:** 202–226, 1879

2. Lie JT: Thromboangiitis obliterans (Buerger's disease) revisited. *Path Ann* **23:** 257–291, 1988
3. Buerger L: Thromboangiitis obliterans: A study of the vascular lesions leading to presenile spontaneous gangrene. *Am J Med Sci* **136:** 567–580, 1908
4. Buerger L: *The Circulatory Disturbances of the Extremities: Including Gangrene, Vasomotor and Trophic Disorders* 628 pp. Philadelphia: WB Saunders, 1924
5. Eastcott HHG: Buerger's disease. In: Bergan JJ, Yao JST (Eds) *Evaluation and Treatment of Upper and Lower Extremity Disorders* pp. 483–497. Orlando: Grune & Stratton, 1984
6. Wessler S, Si-Chun M, Gurewich V, Freiman DG: A critical evaluation of thromboangiitis obliterans. The case against Buerger's disease. *N Engl J Med* **262:** 1149–1160, 1960
7. McKusick VA, Harris WS, Ottesen OE *et al.*: Buerger's disease: a distinct clinical and pathologic entity. *J Am Med Assoc* **181:** 5–12, 1962
8. McPherson JR, Juergens JL, Gifford RW Jr: Thromboangiitis obliterans and arteriosclerosis obliterans. Clinical and prognostic differences. *Ann Int Med* **59:** 288–296, 1963
9. Greenhalgh RM: On Buerger's disease: A recognizable syndrome. In: Bergan JJ, Yao JST (Eds) *Gangrene and Severe Ischemia of the Lower Extremities* pp. 139–155. New York: Grune & Stratton Inc, 1978
10. Blebea J, Kempczinski RF: Buerger's disease. In: White RA, Hollier LH (Eds) *Vascular Surgery: Basic Science and Clinical Correlations* pp. 169–176. Philadelphia: JB Lippincott, 1994
11. DeBakey ME, Cohen BM: *Buerger's Disease, A Follow-up Study of World War II Army Cases* pp. 1–143. Springfield, IL: CC Thomas, 1963
12. Shionoya S: Buerger's disease (thromboangiitis obliterans). In: Rutherford RB (Ed) *Vascular Surgery* 4th edn, pp. 235–244. Philadelphia: WB Saunders, 1995
13. Mills JL, Porter JM: Buerger's disease: A review and update. *Semin Vasc Surg* **6:** 14–23, 1993
14. Mills JL, Taylor LM Jr, Porter JM: Buerger's disease in the modern era. *Am J Surg* **154:** 123–129, 1987
15. Olin JW, Young JR, Graor RA *et al.*: The changing clinical spectrum of thromboangiitis obliterans (Buerger's disease). *Circulation* **82** (Suppl IV): IV3–IV8, 1990
16. Matsushita M, Shionoya S, Matsumoto T: Urinary cotinine measurements in patients with Buerger's disease. Effects of active and passive smoking on the disease process. *J Vasc Surg* **14:** 53–58, 1991
17. Papa M, Bass A, Adar R *et al.*: Autoimmune mechanisms in thromboangiitis obliterans (Buerger's disease): The role of tobacco antigen and the major histocompatibility complex. *Surgery* **111:** 527–531, 1992
18. Gulati SM, Madhra K, Thusoo TK *et al.*: Autoantibodies in thromboangiitis obliterans (Buerger's disease). *Angiology* **33:** 642–651, 1982
19. Adar R, Papa MZ, Halpern Z *et al.*: Cellular sensitivity to collagen in thromboangiitis obliterans. *N Engl J Med* **308:** 1113–1116, 1983
20. Hada M, Sakihama T, Kamiya K *et al.*: Cellular and humoral immune responses to vascular components in thromboangiitis obliterans. *Angiology* **44:** 533–540, 1993
21. Casellas M, Perez A, Cabero I *et al.*: Buerger's disease and antiphospholipid antibodies in pregnancy. *Ann Rheuma Dis* **52:** 247–248, 1993
22. Athanassiou P, McHale J, Dikeou S: Buerger's disease and protein S deficiency: Successful treatment with prostacyclin. *Clin Exp Rheum* **13:** 371–375, 1995
23. Pietraszek MH, Choudbury NA, Koyane K *et al.*: Enhanced platelet response to serotonin in Buerger's disease. *Throm Res* **60:** 241–246, 1990
24. Choudbury NA, Pietraszek MH, Hachiya T *et al.*: Plasminogen activators and plasminogen activator inhibitor 1 before and after venous occlusion of the upper limb in thromboangiitis obliterans. *Thromb Res* **66:** 321–329, 1992
25. Cutler DA, Runge MS: 86 years of Buerger's disease – what have we learned? *Am J Med Sci* **309:** 74–75, 1995
26. Shionoya S: Buerger disease: diagnosis and management. *Cardiovasc Surg* **1:** 207–214, 1993
27. Colburn MD, Moore WS: Buerger's disease. *Heart Dis Stroke* **2:** 424–432, 1993

28. Fiessinger JN, Schäfer M for the TAO Study: Trial of iloprost versus aspirin treatment for critical limb ischemia of thromboangiitis obliterans. *Lancet* **335:** 555–557, 1990

29. White JC, Smithwick RH, Simeone FA: *The Autonomic Nervous System* pp. 479–483. New York: Macmillan, 1952

30. Sayin A, Bozhurt AK, Tuzun H *et al*.: Surgical treatment of Buerger's disease: Experience with 216 patients. *Cardiovasc Surg* **1:** 377–380, 1993

31. Sasajima T, Kubo Y, Izumi Y *et al*.: Plantar or dorsalis pedis artery bypass in Buerger's disease. *Ann Vasc Surg* **8:** 248–257, 1994

32. Hodgson TJ, Gaines PA, Beard JD: Thrombolysis and angioplasty for acute lower limb ischemia in Buerger's disease. *Cardiovasc Intervent Radiol* **17:** 333–335, 1994

33. Pairolero PC, Joyce JW, Skinner CR *et al*.: Lower limb ischemia in young adults: Prognostic implications. *J Vasc Surg* **1:** 459–464, 1984

34. Ohta T, Shionoya S: Fate of the ischemic limb in Buerger's disease. *Br J Surg* **75:** 259–262, 1988

35. Neiman HL, Yao JST: *Angiography of Vascular Disease* p. 139. New York: Churchill Livingstone, 1985

Takayasu's Disease and Giant Cell Arteritis

Michael Horrocks

INTRODUCTION

Arteritis is a complex and underestimated clinical entity that may present in many ways. Because of the diversity of clinical features and the overlapping of the syndromes associated with arteritis, different classifications have been developed. The simplest classification is to divide cases into those with giant cell arteritis and those with non-giant cell arteritis.

Giant cell arteritis has two distint clinical entities which are pathologically similar in that both involve arteries of medium and large size and are characterized by infiltration with giant cells. The two clinical entities are temporal arteritis and Takayasu's arteritis.

The non-giant cell varieties of arteritis encompass a variety of relatively uncommon diseases which may be associated with other systemic autoimmune diseases such as systemic lupus erythematosis, periarteritis nodosa, etc. These diseases generally result in organ dysfunction because of ischaemia and this is commonly amenable only to medical treatment.

Rarely, non-giant cell arteritis may manifest as acute vascular occlusions and these may be complicated by the presence of circulating anticoagulants. Such cases may present with spontaneous arterial or venous thrombosis giving rise to emergency admissions. Occasionally, non-giant cell arteritis may also present with rupture of small aneurysms most commonly found in the gastrointestinal tract.

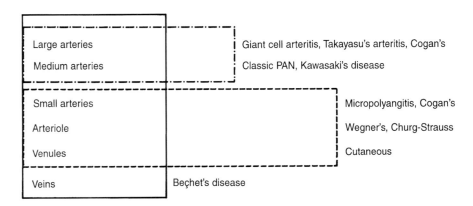

Fig. 1. Classification of vasulitis based on pathology.

GIANT CELL ARTERITIS

Giant cell arteritis is a systemic granulomatous pan-arteritis which can affect any medium or large size artery but most frequently affects the medium sized extracranial arteries. Temporal arteritis was first described in 1932 by Horton who subsequently described its histological and clinical characteristics.[1] The first reported case of blindness caused by temporal arteritis appeared in 1938 and has become the most commonly feared complication. Although any medium or large sized artery can be involved, the great vessels are the most commonly involved. Stenoses are usually peripherally located in these vessels and the aorta itself is usually spared. Extracranial lesions occur in less than 10% of patients and blindness can usually be prevented by early steroid therapy. The pan-arteritis with giant cells is sporadic and may not always be seen on biopsy.

The natural history of temporal arteritis is fairly typical. Classically middle-aged or elderly women develop a flu-like illness with pyrexia, headache, aching muscles and weight loss. These symptoms may persist for a few weeks and then spontanously subside. In the second or third week of illness they may develop pain on eating and may notice associated headache and tenderness over the temporal artery. These symptoms often settle down within a few weeks although joint discomfort may persist.

Some weeks after the initial onset of the symptoms the patients may develop visual symptoms with eye muscle weakness, amaurosis fugax and occasionally optic nerve neuritis giving rise to blindness. Blindness is said to occur in up to 50% of untreated patients and throughout this time the erythrocyte sedimentation rate remains raised, usually elevated above 40 mm/Hg. Occasionally, bilateral arm or even leg pain may develop some weeks after the onset of symptoms, but the natural history is that arterial narrowing only rarely progresses to complete occlusion of the vessel.

In rare instances the disease may follow an accelerated course and following a flu-like illness the patient may proceed to complete blindness or even death from dissection of the thoracic aorta within days of the onset of the symptoms. More commonly the disease progresses in phases and may be missed because of the rather vague symptoms that develop, particularly in the more elderly patients who cannot recall a flu-like illness and may just have malaise, anorexia and weight loss.

Diagnosis

The diagnosis is initially suspected following the typical clinical history. Temporal artery biopsy remains the principle method of diagnosis in the presence of a raised sedimentation rate. It is best to do the biopsy before starting steroids although the pathological findings will not be obscured within the first few days of steroid treatment. The presence of giant cell infiltration may only be present in a few of the specimens examined by the pathologist and so a generous biopsy (up to 7cm) may be taken. It has been advocated that if one side is negative and there is a high index of clinical suspicion, then biopsy should be considered from the other side.

Large vessel complications

In 1938 Jennings described aortic and extracranial large vessel involvement in giant cell arteritis and since then much of the information related to large vessel involvement is based on autopsy studies in asymptomatic patients or on isolated case reports.[2] In one series of 72 cases, Lie reported involvement of the ascending aorta, aortic arch, subclavian, axilary and femoropopliteal arteries.[3] Nine of his patients underwent major limb amputation and in 18 patients their death was directly attributable to extracranial giant cell arteritis. Death was reported as a ruptured abdominal aortic aneurysm in six, aortic dissections in six, stroke in three and myocardial infarction in three. All these patients had histologically proven giant cell arteritis. There were 51 women and 21 men and all but one were Caucasian.

Large vessel disease should be suspected in the presence of aortic insufficiency, bruits over the large arteries or diminished or absent pulses causing claudication or limb ischaemia. Radiological features showed the typical long segments of smooth contour arterial stenoses alternating with segments of normal calibre or small fusiformed dilatations. The vessels principally involved are the subclavian, axillary and brachial arteries and in a few of the lesions there may be tapered occlusion of the affected large arteries with a distinct absence of plaque or ulceration as seen in atherosclerosis. Computed tomography (CT) or magnetic resonance imaging (MCI) may be helpful in demonstrating aneurysms of the aorta or aortic dissection.

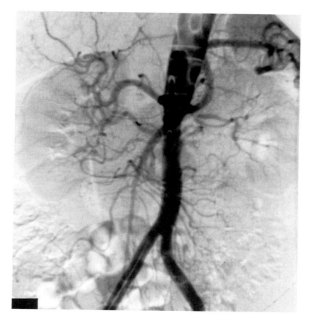

Fig. 2. The lumbar arteriogram of a woman aged 60 with a 3-year history of arteritis subsequently proven on biopsy to be temporal arteritis. The angiogram shows a tight stenosis of the left renal artery subsequently successfully treated by angioplasty.

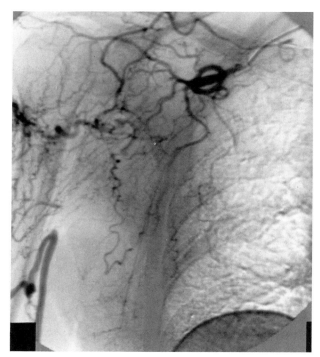

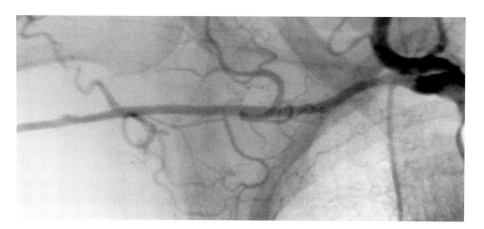

Figs 3 and 4. These figs show the right axillary artery of the same patient before and after recanalization angioplasty. This procedure required an open brachial arteriotomy in order to pass the guidewire, the conventional approach having failed. She also underwent successful recanalization angioplasty of a similar lesion on the left and both have remained patent for more than 12 months.

Treatment

The management of acute giant cell arteritis is to give prednisolone 60 mg daily for 1 week which is then reduced to 45 mg/day for 30 days. Thereafter the dose should be reduced by 5 mg every 2 weeks until the dose reaches 10 mg/day. Prednisolone is then reduced by 1 mg every 2 weeks with the patient being monitored by sedimentation rate or by C-reactive protein concentration levels.[4] Kyle suggests that sedimentation rate can be safely used to monitor disease activity rather than using C-reactive protein.[5]

Surgery is rarely necessary for temporal arteritis but may be indicated in threatened limb loss, severe hypertension or incapacitating intermittent claudication. Surgical therapy should not really be undertaken before trial of steroids as ischaemic symptoms often improve after the use of steroids.[6] Endarterectomy or bypass grafting in the acute phase of the disease usually results in rapid occlusion of the operated vessels and is best delayed until the acute phase settles.

Results of angioplasty and surgery in this group of conditions suggests that short lesions may well be treated successfully by angioplasty and that bypass operations, provided it is to a non-affected part of the artery, can be very successful.

Summary

Aortic and extracranial giant cell arteritis may be the first manifestation of temporal arteritis and can be the cause of sudden death from catastrophic cardiovascular complications. Follow-up of treated patients suggests that adequate treatment may prevent fatal coronary and cerebral complications. Such treatment, however, does not appear to prevent rupture of an aortic aneurysm, aortic dissection or manifestations of peripheral vascular disease. When elderly patients present with atypical atherosclerosis a diagnosis of giant cell arteritis should be considered.

TAKAYASU'S DISEASE

Takayasu's arteritis is an inflammatory disease of large vessels, particularly the aorta and its larger branches, causing luminal stenoses and aneurysm formation. Inflammatory granulomatous changes develop in the adventitia and the outer layers of the media with severe fibrous thickening of the intima in the late stages. The aetiology of Takayasu's arteritis still remains obscure and an autoimmune reaction to aortic tissue has been proposed as the cause. The disease is prevalent throughout the world and appears to affect all races but has a high incidence in the Orient.

The first case of Takayasu's arteritis was reported in 1905 by Dr Mikota Takayasu, Professor of Ophthalmology in Kanaza University in Japan.[7] The patient was a 21-year-old woman who exhibited a peculiar wreath-like arteriovenous anastomosis around the papillae. Since then the disease has been frequently observed in Japan and a research committee sponsored by the Japanese Government's Ministry of Health and Welfare studied the disease and gave it the name of Takayasu's arteritis.[8] Between 1973 and 1975, 2148 new cases were recorded, of whom 89% were female. The aetiology of the disease remains unknown but a relationship with tuberculosis has been speculated because of the pathology looking rather like that of tuberculosis. However, Takayasu's arteritis is prevalent among those who have no evidence of tuberculosis and few of these patients go on to develop obvious signs of tuberculosis. The most important aetiological agent in the disease is the autoimmune mechanism. In 1964 Ueda's research group detected an anti-aortic antibody among patients with this disease using a compliment fixation reaction.[9] The disease is reported to be more prevalent in India, Thailand, China, Korea and Israel and also amongst the black population in South Africa. A hereditary factor seems to be important in the development of the disease and HLA, AW24-BW52-DW12 haplotype patients are prone to develop rapid progression of the disease and also show resistance to steroid therapy.[10]

The disease is most prevalent in the aortic arch area but may affect any of the large vessels.[11] Histologically the inflammatory process is seen in the media of the arteries but may extend to include the adventitia and intima. The cell infiltration is characteristically composed of lymphocytes and epithelioid cells and there is usually destruction of the elastic fibres of the media with replacement by fibrous tissue and smooth muscle cells. Calcification within the media may also occur and when the arteritis develops rapidly then aneurysm formation may also be present.

Types of Takayasu's disease

The disease is classified according to site and pattern. Currently four types have been described,[12] which are shown pictorially in Fig. 5. Type IV was added as a type of arteritis of similar distribution with aneurysmal involvement.

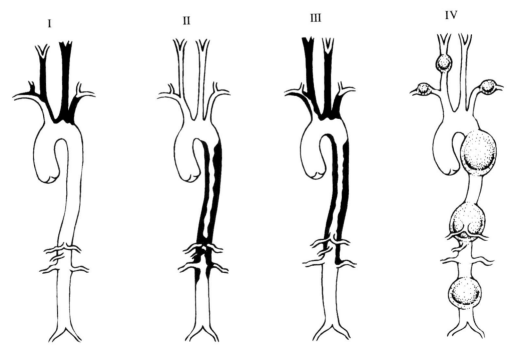

Fig. 5.   Four types of Takayasu's disease. Type IV has been added as a type of arteritis of similar distribution with aneurysmal involvement.

A fifth type has also been described, characterized by isolated medium sized artery involvement, e.g. axillary or subclavian arteries, with no evidence of aortic involvement.

Diagnosis

Classically the patients are young and female and the disease has been described from the age of 3 years to the age of 45 years with a median age at presentation of 30 years. Patients may present with a variety of rather vague clinical symptoms such as fatigue, vertigo and cold extremities. Clinically the diagnosis can be made by the absence of peripheral pulses, particularly the radial pulse, which may be absent at initial clinical examination. The patient may have an unexplained cardiac murmur suggestive of aortic regurgitation or severe unexplained hypertension. The patients frequently have a raised sedimentation rate or a raised C-reactive protein.

Table 1.   Typical presentation of Takayasu's disease

Symptoms
1. Early middle-aged female
2. Patients may describe cerebral ischaemia or fainting, visual disturbance.
3. Ischaemia of the extremities, claudication or cold fingers.
4. Headache, vertigo, shortness of breath, symptoms of hypertension.
5. General malaise and fever.

Important findings
6. Absent pulses in the upper extremities or the lower extremities
7. Murmurs in the arteries of the neck, back or abdomen.
8. Ophthalmic abnormalities.

Laboratory tests
1. Raised erythrocyte sedimentation rate.
2. Raised C-reactive protein.
3. Increase in gamma globlin levels.

Confirmatory findings
Typical abnormalities on angiography or MRI.

Diagnosis is typically made on angiography or MRI scan. The pattern of the disease on angiography will depend on the type and is usually localized to segments of disease. There may be areas of stenosis associated with areas of aneurysmal dilatation in the typical distribution of Takayasu's arteritis. Takayasu's disease has also been described in children and can occur at any time from the age of 3 years to 16 years but is very uncommon under the age of 5 years.[13] The distribution of the disease in children is similar to that in adults although renal artery stenosis appears to be more common than aortic arch disease.

Treatment

In children when the tuberculosis skin test is positive then isoniazid should be given with steroids. Even in adults if there is any suspicion of tuberculosis then anti-tuberculous treatment should be given, particularly if intervention is contemplated. Angioplasty may be effective in both children and adults with short lesions proving better than long lesions. The dilatation may be repeated if required when re-stenosis occurs, but there is little long-term data on large series.

Good reports of surgical treatment are reported by Robbs *et al.*[14] and Tarda *et al.*[12] In principle, reconstruction is done by bypass grafting from a normal artery above to normal artery below the lesion where possible. Carotid reconstruction is done by taking a graft off the normal part of the arch of aorta up to the carotid bifurcation and the thoracic aneurysm is usually bypassed from the arch of the aorta down to normal aorta below the renals. If there is associated narrowing or aneurysm or dilatation of branch vessels then these can be treated by branch reconstructions as illustrated below.

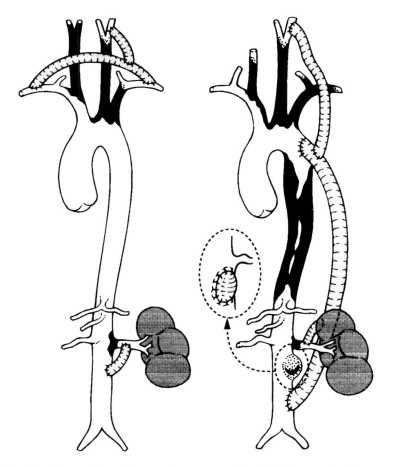

Fig. 6. Examples of types of reconstruction in Takayasu's disease.

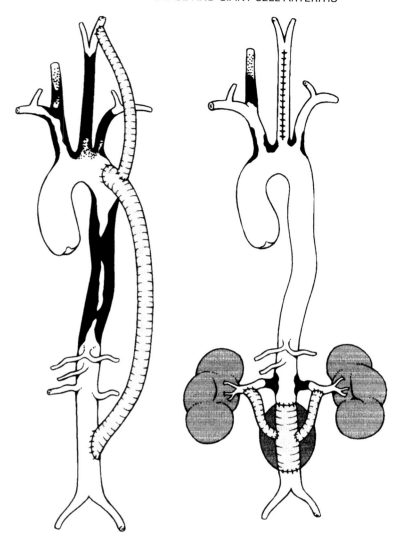

Fig. 7.   Examples of types of reconstruction in Takayasu's disease.

In the series by Robbs *et al.*[14] those with a higher sedimentation rate were treated with steroids for several weeks before surgery was contemplated in order to control the acute phase of the disease. However, in the emergency situation such as aneurysm rupture or acute ischaemia, surgery was performed on an emergency basis. Of those with type I disease (n=28) 14 were treated with interpostion graft, 12 with aortic arch reconstruction, one with a subclavian bypass and one by ligation of the internal carotid artery. In the other types (n=49) 26 were treated by thorocoabdominal aortic replacement or bypass, 18 by aorta iliac aneurysm replacement, two by nephrectomy, one by aortobifemoral bypass, one by ileorenal bypass. All four patients who had type V were treated by interposition graft.

Mortality was low (4%) and both patients who died presented with aortic rupture. There were no deaths from elective procedures. Long-term results were good although 11 developed evidence of recurrent disease with an average follow-up period of 1.2 years after operation. The high incidence of aneurysm disease in this series was discussed and appears to be at variance with other series from Japan where mainly occlusive disease is reported.

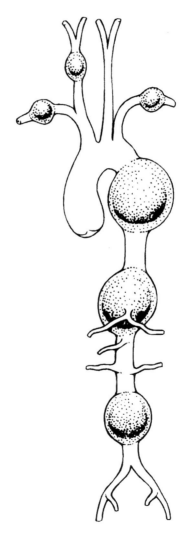

Fig. 8. Distribution of aneurysmal disease in Takayasu's disease.

The results of angioplasty in this disease are equally good early on although recurrence rates appear to be somewhat higher.[15] In a review article on the subject Bongard *et al.* reported four restenoses out of 12 renal arteries dilated.[16] Focal disease appears to do well but signs of acute inflammation at the time of the procedure appear to predict a poor outcome. Long areas of stenosis tend to do better with bypass than angioplasty. In one series from China, nine patients with stable Takayasu's arteritis suffering from lower limb insufficiency and hypertension due to aortic stenosis were treated by percutaneous transluminal angioplasty. Immediate success was obtained in all but one patient, but there was one recurrence amongst the seven patients who were followed up. However, the criteria for defining re-stenosis was not clear and the results may need to be interpreted with some caution.

CONCLUSION

Giant cell arteritis appears to be an underdiagnosed condition in the UK leading to unexplained, sudden cardiovascular death particularly in elderly females. A high index of suspicion is needed and temporal artery biopsy is required to make the definitive diagnosis. Patients with atypical upper limb arterial stenoses or occlusions should have this diagnosis considered and treatment in the first place is by steroids with angioplasty or surgery reserved for life or limb-threatening disease.

Takayasu's disease is a rare condition in the UK being much more common in Africa and the Orient. The most common presentation is hypertension in young females and typical diagnostic features are revealed on angiography or MRI. Aggressive treatment of stenotic or aneurysmal lesions by angioplasty or surgery appears to be rewarded with good short- and long-term results.

REFERENCES

1. Horton BT, Magath TB, Browne GE: An undescribed form of arteritis of the temporal vessels. *Proc Staff Meet Mayo Clinic* 7: 700–701, 1932
2. Jennings GH: Arteritis of temporal arteries. *Lancet* **i**: 323–329, 1938
3. Lie JT: Aortic and extracranial large vessel giant cell arteritis. *Semin Arth Rheum* **24**: 422–431, 1995
4. Aburahma AF, Witsberger TA: Diagnosing giant cell temporal arteritis. *West Virgina Med J* **88**: 188–193, 1992
5. Kyle V: Giant cell arteritis. *Br Med J* **305**: 524, 1992
6. Evans JM, Bowles CA, Bjornsson J, *et al.*: Thoracic aortic aneurysm and rupture in giant cell arteritis. *Arth Rheum* **37**: 1539–1547, 1994
7. Takayasu M: A case of peculiar changes in the central retinal vessels. *Arch Soc Ophth Japan* **12**: 554–555, 1908
8. Shimizu K, Saimo K: Pulseless disease. *Clin Surg (Tokyo)* **3**: 377–396, 1948
9. Ueda H, Saito Y, Ito I *et al.*: Imnological studies of aortits syndrome. *Jap Heart J* **8**: 4–18, 1967
10. Numano F, Isohisa I, Maezawa H *et al.*: HLA antigens in Takayasu's disease. *Am Heart J* **88**: 153–159, 1979
11. Procter CD, Hollier LH: Takayasu's arteritis and temporal arteritis. *Ann Vasc Surg* **6**: 195–197, 1992

12. Tarda Y, Sato, O, Oshima A *et al.*: Surgical treatment of Takayasu's disease. *Heart Vessel* **7**(Suppl): 159–167, 1992
13. Hong CY, Yun YS, Choi JY *et al.*: Takayasu's arteritis in Korean children. *Heart Vessel* **7**(Suppl): 91–96, 1992
14. Robbs JV, Abdool-Carrim ATO, Kadwa AM: Arterial reconstructions for non-specific arteritis (Takayasu's disease). Medium to long term results. *Eur J Vasc Surg* **8**: 401–407, 1994
15. Khalilullah M, Tyagi S: Percutaneous transluminal angioplasty in Takayasu's arteritis. *Heart Vessel* **7**(Suppl): 146-153, 1992
16. Bongard O, Schneider, P, Krahenbuhl *et al.*: Transluminal angioplasty of the aorta, renal and mesenteric arteries in Takayasu's arteritis. *Eur J Vasc Surg* **6**: 507–571, 1992

Raynaud's Phenomenon

C. B. Bunker

INTRODUCTION

Raynaud's phenomenon is an important clinical syndrome tightly associated with many inflammatory and thrombotic diseases of the vasculature. An understanding of its pathogenesis, aetiology, diagnosis and management is crucial to vascular surgical practice.

DEFINITION AND CLINICAL FEATURES

Raynaud's phenomenon is defined as episodic digital ischaemia in response to cold or emotional stimuli and is characterized by sequential colour changes (white, blue and red) in the affected parts. Pallor is essential for the diagnosis (Fig. 1) but attacks in patients where pallor does not occur can be called *atypical* Raynaud's phenomenon. The classical clinical features of 25 cases were first described in 1862 by the Parisian physician Maurice Raynaud in his MD thesis.[1]

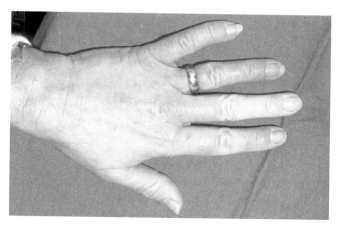

Fig. 1.   The classical pallor of Raynaud's phenomenon affecting the left middle finger of a patient with systemic sclerosis.

Raynaud's phenomenon may be primary or secondary to other causes. Historically a controversy has surrounded the terminology, definition and pathophysiology of Raynaud's phenomenon and this has affected the selection of subjects for clinical reports and research and influenced attitudes to treatment.

The concept of 'Raynaud's disease' emerged largely through the publication of many case reports. But this concept became too broad to be useful because of the reporting of cases which did not marry with Raynaud's original description and/or where the clinical signs were secondary to an overt disease process such as trauma, arterial disease, systemic sclerosis and paroxysmal haemoglobinuria. Idiopathic Raynaud's disease is now also termed primary Raynaud's phenomenon. The differential diagnosis of secondary Raynaud's phenomenon (i.e. occurring in association with a recognizable underlying pathology) is an important excercise for the vascular surgeon, general physician and dermatologist.

Raynaud was precise in delineating his criteria of intermittent attacks of pallor, cyanosis and then rubor complicated by 'symmetrical gangrene' limited to the skin of the finger tips but was not so careful in applying them to the cases he described. He did recognize that some of his cases had underlying causes for their clinical signs but, as stated above, subsequent authors have been less rigorous.

The prevalence of Raynaud's phenomenon is variously quoted as 5–30%. Most studies suggest that it is more common in women but the differences are due to the sizes and origins of the populations studied and the diagnostic criteria used by the researchers particularly with regard to colour changes.[2,3]

As many as 13% of patients with Raynaud's phenomenon in one hospital based study had systemic sclerosis (Figs 2–5). But, by contrast, far fewer (about 3%) of the patients in another family practice based survey had even the suspicion of underlying disease. Rigorous investigation may not therefore be fruitful in general

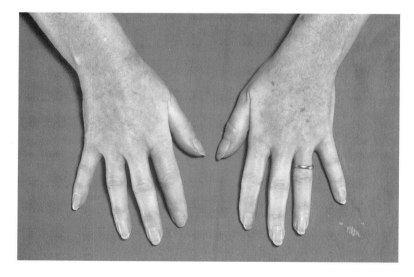

Fig. 2.   Sclerodactyly in systemic sclerosis.

practice. However, it has been suggested that all patients with Raynaud's phenomenon should be regarded as being at high risk of developing a connective tissue disease and this may well be good advice regarding the selected population of patients who present to hospital specialists, usually dermatologists, rheumatologists or vascular surgeons.[2,3]

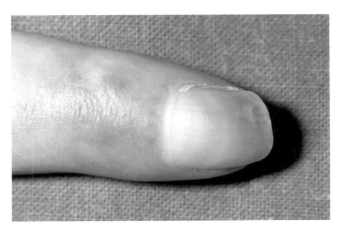

Fig. 3. Nailfold changes (erythema, telangectasia, cuticular abnormalities) in systemic sclerosis.

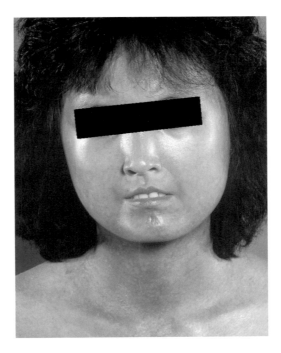

Fig. 4. Facies of systemic sclerosis (tight, waxy, shiny skin extending onto the neck).

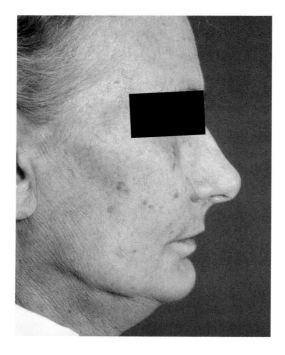

Fig. 5.   Facies of systemic sclerosis (telangectasia).

PATHOLOGY AND PATHOGENESIS

Pathological changes can be found in the digits of nearly all patients with Raynaud's phenomenon secondary to other causes. Cutaneous vessels may be abnormal clinically and on nailfold microscopy (as in systemic sclerosis), and vascular lesions amounting to narrowing and obstruction may be demonstrated by angiography. However, the consensus has been that the presence of abnormal capillaries on nailfold microscopy or structural defects on angiography is incompatible with primary Raynaud's phenomenon and should lead to a search for an underlying cause.[2,3]

Sir Thomas Lewis found atherosclerotic changes in the digital arteries of patients who probably had underlying disease but not in patients with primary Raynaud's phenomenon. Another investigator studied the digital artery pathology from 16 patients who had died with systemic sclerosis and reported severe intimal hyperplasia consisting predominantly of collagen. Some also had severe luminal narrowing and some had thrombosis. Other workers have shown diminuition of blood vessels, glomus body fibrosis and replacement of the dermis with collagen in patients with systemic sclerosis. Digital glomus body pathology has also been demonstrated in secondary Raynaud's phenomenon. Digital vasculitis has also been reported in some patients with connective tissue disease.[2,3]

Vadja et al.[4] took finger pulp biopsies from 31 patients with a large variety of underlying causes for their Raynaud's phenomenon. On electron microscopy they found endothelial cell swelling in the dermal capillaries resulting in a narrowed lumen and thickened basement membranes. The basement membranes of the unmyelinated nerves were similarly affected and there was marked degeneration of myelinated nerves.[4] Thompson et al. studied nailfold biopsies and showed a decreased number of cutaneous nerve bundles, deposition of a globular, eosinophilic, periodic acid-Schiff (PAS)-positive material in systemic sclerosis and mixed connective tissue disease.[5]

In *primary* Raynaud's phenomenon there is scanty pathological data. Video capillary microscopy has shown that the capillary morphology in patients with primary Raynaud's phenomenon does not differ from controls. The findings that some patients with primary Raynaud's phenomenon have reduced capillary numbers and increased luminal diameters can be interpreted as characterizing those patients with Raynaud's phenomenon predicted on the basis of abnormal nailfold microscopy to develop connective tissue disease.[2]

The pathophysiology of Raynaud's phenomenon has eluded definition despite much conjecture and investigation. Early work has to be interpreted carefully in view of confusion over definitions and terminology. For example, most commentators have accepted that pallor and cyanosis in the skin have different pathophysiological explanations but many investigators have not separated patients for investigative purposes according to these criteria.

Raynaud himself first suggested that Raynaud's phenomenon may result from faulty neurovascular control and envisaged a 'local syncope', due to 'increased irritability of the central parts of the cord presiding over vascular innervation'. The classic experiments of Sir Thomas Lewis led him to propose a 'local fault' in the digital arteries leading to vasoconstriction in the cold but the nature of the local fault has not hitherto been satisfactorily characterized.[8,9] Lewis also recognized that skin pallor, which occurs in the digits in Raynaud's phenomenon, can only be achieved if the capillaries are emptied and considered that cutaneous capillaries are capable of independent vasoconstriction.[10] He pointed out that simple closure of the arterioles would not be sufficient to account for the 'dead whiteness' seen in Raynaud's phenomenon and said that 'there must be in addition an active and strong spasm of the minute vessels themselves'. It is therefore contended that the microvasculature of digital skin must be primarily involved in the pathophysiology of Raynaud's phenomenon.

In parallel with progressive understanding of the complexity of the control of blood flow a large literature has appeared concerned with the respective roles which might be played in Raynaud's phenomenon by derangement of or defect in the physical properties of blood vessels, blood itself or their cellular constituents as well as pharmacological mediators and neurological influences which might have a bearing on vascular behaviour. Although abnormalities have been reported in most of these areas their direct relationship to the cause of Raynaud's phenomenon remains questionable.[2,3]

There has been much recent interest in the peptidergic nervous system and its participation in the innervation of blood vessels both in the normal control of the cutaneous microvasculature and in the pathogenesis of Raynaud's phenomenon. The properties of the potent endogenous vasodilator neuropeptide calcitonin gene-related peptide (CGRP) suggest that it may play a major role in neurovascular control in many organs including the skin. That a selective dysfunction in a CGRP neurovascular axis might be implicated in the pathophysiology of Raynaud's phenomenon and that such a deficit is consistent with a 'local fault' in the digital cutaneous vasculature is born out by the finding of a deficiency of such nerves in digital skin in Raynaud's phenomenon and vibration white finger. These structural abnormalities have also been corroborated pharmacologically.[3,6,7,11,12]

The potent endogenous vasoconstrictor peptide endothelin-1(ET-1) has also been implicated in the pathogenesis of Raynaud's phenomenon. In normal skin ET-1 is present and can influence microvascular endothelial cells: ET-1, acting unopposed, could be the mediator of capillary constriction thought by Lewis to be responsible for the pallor characteristic of Raynaud's phenomenon and its presence in skin provides a mechanism for the independent contractillity of cutaneous microvessels proposed by Lewis.[11,13] Raised concentrations of von Willebrand factor/factor VIII are also found in some patients with Raynaud's phenomenon pointing to the 'stress' effect of cold on the endothelium. Therefore, cold-stress induced endothelial release of ET-1 might be behind the digital pallor in Raynaud's phenomenon.

The deficiency of CGRP in digital nerves in Raynaud's phenomenon suggests the possibility that it is the action of the cold stress-induced release of physiological amounts of ET-1, unopposed in the pathological state by a deficient CGRP vasodilating axis, that results in the classical pallor.

One of the physiological roles of the cutaneous neurovascular network could be the modulation of blood flow in response to environmental temperature. The widespread localization of CGRP-immunoreactive fibres in skin suggests that epidermal fibres may be concerned with cold nociception controlling both reflex local (through antidromic release of peptides from perivascular fibres) and systemic (through their central sensory connections and projections) neurovascular responses. Peripheral cutaneous vasoconstriction in response to cold may be physiologically balanced or dampened by reflex antidromic CGRP release from dermal nerve fibres in intimate apposition to the cutaneous blood vessels including the papillary capillary loops.

The purpose of cold-stimulated cutaneous vasoconstriction is probably the interest preservation of core temperature and the ET-1 response may be part of a more complex mechanism involving other influences such as the sympathetic nervous system. It is conceivable that a protective cold-nociceptive reflex vasodilator response has evolved in finger skin for the preservation of tactile sensation in the cold. This might account for the alleged richness of the CGRP innervation in the digital extremities.

In Raynaud's phenomenon the CGRP axis may be dysfunctional in the fingers, so that in the presence of an intact cutaneous vasoconstrictor mechanism provided by ET-1 the classical series of events of RP is initiated.

In some people Raynaud's phenomenon may represent the cutaneous manifestation of a generalized vasospastic disorder. It has been long observed that some patients have hypertension and migraine. There is a high prevalence of

Raynaud's phenomenon and migraine in patients with variant (Prinzmetal) angina where altered adrenergic activity and high circulating thromboxane levels have been two of the explanations advanced for the coronary artery spasm.[2]

In connective tissue diseases cold-related paroxysmal alterations in the vasculature of the lung and the kidney analogous to Raynaud's phenomenon have been proposed to contribute to the pathology. Yamauchi *et al.*[14] have shown alterations in the glomerular filtration rate after cold exposure in systemic sclerosis and in systemic lupus erythematosus. Changes in pulmonary capillary blood volume during cold exposure of the hands in patients with Raynaud's phenomenon have been recorded. These are tantalising phenomena to investigators because the identification of the cause of the vasospasm may shed needed light upon the pathogenesis of these ill-understood conditions.[2,3,14]

DIAGNOSIS AND DIFFERENTIAL DIAGNOSIS

Since the time of Raynaud many causes of Raynaud's phenomenon have been established. The most important are structural or traumatic factors such as cervical rib (Figs 6, 7) and vibration white finger, organic vascular disease and associated connective tissue disease. For the clinician the principal challenge is to exclude an

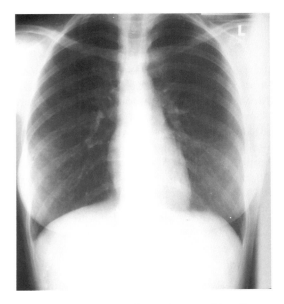

Fig. 6. Chest X-ray of patient with Raynaud's phenomenon. Cervical rib cannot be diagnosed or excluded because the radiographer has not included C7 in the study. A common pitfall.

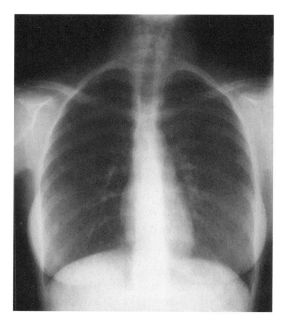

Fig. 7. Chest X-ray of the same patient with Raynaud's phenomenon as Fig. 6 but with the final cervical vertebra identifiable (downward facing costal processes) and cervical rib can now be diagnosed.

underlying cause such as a connective tissue disease, although Maricq *et al.* have recently suggested that connective tissue disease may not be as important as classically stated and have pointed to a correlation with cardiovascular disease.[15] Careful history taking and complete physical examination are mandatory. Investigations are indicated if primary Raynaud's phenomenon cannot be diagnosed with confidence and are directed by the clinical context.

The causes of Raynaud's phenomenon are given in Table 1.

Primary Raynaud's phenomenon is diagnosed according to the modified criteria of Allen and Brown (1932).[16]

1. Intermittent attacks of discolouration of extremities
   (which precede trophic changes, if present, by many years).
2. Absence of evidence of organic peripheral arterial occlusion.
3. Symmetrical or bilateral distribution.
4. Trophic changes
   (if present, limited only to the skin, never consisting of gross gangrene).
5. Exclusion of any disease that could give rise to vasospastic symptoms.

Secondary criteria are a) female sex and b) absence of severe pain during attacks

The prognosis of Raynaud's phenomenon depends upon the presence or absence of an associated disease at the time of initial assessment and the later progression to systemic disease in initially apparently uncomplicated patients. Poor prognostic features of Raynaud's phenomenon are severity, age, male sex, unilaterality, skin changes (scleroderma, vasculitis) and abnormal investigations (antinuclear antibodies, nailfold capillary microscopy).

Table 1. Causes of Raynaud's phenomenon[3]

Primary (or idiopathic) Raynaud's phenomenon

Trauma or vibration
  reflex sympathetic dystrophy
  occupational/vibration white finger
  arteriovenous fistula (for haemodialysis)
  hypothenar hammer syndrome (ulnar artery thrombosis)
  intra-arterial drug administration

Connective tissue disease and vasculitis
  systemic sclerosis
  systemic lupus erythematosus
  rheumatoid arthritis
  Sjogren's syndrome
  mixed connective tissue disease (Fig. 9)
  dermatomyosistis
  temporal arteritis[20]
  hepatitis B antigen vasculitis

Obstructive arterial disease
  arteriosclerosis
  thromboangiitis obliterans (Buerger's disease)
  thoracic outlet syndrome (cervical rib)
  carpal tunnel syndrome
  hypothenar hammer syndrome (ulnar artery thrombosis)

Neurological disease
  thoracic outlet syndrome (cervical rib)
  carpal tunnel syndrome
  reflex sympathetic dystrophy

Haematological disease
  cryoglobulinaemia
  cold agglutinins
  paroxysmal haemoglobinuria
  Waldenstrom's macroglobulinaemia

Drugs and toxins
  ergot, β-blockers, methysergide, vinblastine, bleomycin, amphetamines
  imipramine, bromocriptine, clonidine, cyclosporin-A, oral contraceptives
  vinyl chloride, nitroglycerine, heavy metals

Miscellaneous
  paraneoplastic syndrome
  chronic renal failure
  primary pulmonary hypertension
  hypothyroidism
  anorexia nervosa[21]

After Coffman.[2] Extra references are given if not discussed by these authors.

The features of sclerodactyly may not predict a poor prognosis. In one study 48% of patients worsened, 40% remained in status quo and 12% regressed. In another report sclerodactyly disappeared in 19 of 27 patients, but developed in 3-4%. Interestingly, tobacco habits did not appear to affect the prognosis and none of the patients with onset of symptoms before the age of 10 years or after the age of 55 years had, or developed, a serious underlying diagnosis.

In another follow-up of 71 patients, only three were said to have developed scleroderma with sclerodactyly at follow-up. Another author has said that three of his 39 patients developed a connective tissue disease. In a review of 87 patients: 17 had antinuclear antibodies and four of these eventually progressed to CREST (Calcinosis, Raynaud's, Eosophagitis, Sclerodactyly,Telangectasia).[2,3]

These studies comprised variable periods of follow-up, most of which were short. They represent reports both from general and hospital practice. One worker looked at systemic involvement and antibody results in patients presenting with Raynaud's phenomenon. Of 91 patients presenting to a hospital clinic with Raynaud's phenomenon, 32 had no evidence of organ involvement whereas impaired lung function was found in 23%, oesophageal hypomotility in 14%, renal involvement in 5%, arthralgia or arthritis in 27%, skin involvement in 33% the majority (26) of whom had systemic sclerosis. Twenty patients had organ involvement at presentation but with no unifying diagnosis. Most importantly, the severity of the Raynaud's phenomenon correlated with organ involvement and the presence and the titre of auto-antibodies.[2,3]

It is has been asserted that Raynaud's phenomenon occurs in 10–45% of patients with systemic lupus erythematosus (Fig. 8) and symptomatically precedes the disease in approximately 10%. In a report of 137 hospitalized patients 20% allegedly

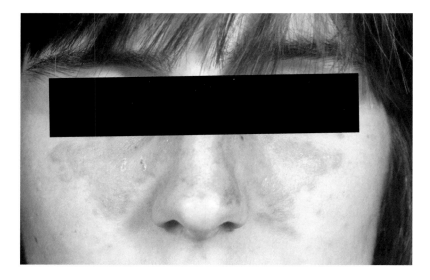

Fig. 8.   Butterfly malar erythema of systemic lupus erythematosus.

had primary disease and 42% had connective tissue disease (36 had systemic sclerosis and ten lupus erythematosus); 38% had other disease related to trauma, occupation, atherosclerosis, thrombosis or hypertension. However, the majority of the primary Raynaud's phenomenon patients also had other disease to judge from the clinical features and results of investigations reported.[2,3]

A study of capillary microscopy included 73 patients. None of the 49 patients who had a history, examination, hand radiology or nailfold capillary microscopy which suggested primary Raynaud's phenomenon subsequently developed secondary Raynaud's phenomenon over 5 years but 14 of 24 thought to be secondary because of their nailfold capillary morphology subsequently did get secondary disease. However, patients with normal capillary patterns have developed secondary diseases and patients with abnormal patterns do not always develop connective tissue disease.[2,3]

There is reason to suppose that unilaterality signifies secondary arterial pathology, cervical rib or vibration injury and should therefore be specially investigated and treated.[2,3] Moreover, according to the criteria of Raynaud and Allen and Brown this should not strictly speaking be called Raynaud's phenomenon.

TREATMENT

Treatments that have been used in the management of Raynaud's phenomenon are listed in Table 2. The specific significant advances provided by nifedipine and prostacyclin are discussed: despite these drugs some patients still suffer gross morbidity and there is a need for additional vasoactive drugs such as CGRP which may also have indications in other diseases where the peripheral vasculature is impaired.

Raynaud's phenomenon represents a therapeutic challenge because despite the use over the years of many therapies and drugs a significant number of patients remain grossly symptomatic, especially in the winter. Some patients suffer pain and disability from digital ulceration and infection with the risk of gangrene and amputation despite the important advances provided by the oral calcium channel blocking agent, nifedipine and the intravenous vasodilator, prostacyclin.

Nifedipine was introduced as a treatment for Raynaud's phenomenon 20 years ago. Subsequent controlled and double-blind studies have established its efficacy including specifically in systemic sclerosis. Other calcium channel blocking drugs have also proved useful such as diltiazem and nicardipine, but verapamil was disappointing.[2,3,17]

The calcium channel blocker, nifedipine is the drug of first choice in the management of Raynaud's phenomenon. Treatment can be initiated at initial doses of 10mg three times daily or 20mg twice daily of the sustained release preparation. The dose can be increased steadily to control symptoms but to avoid side-effects such as dizziness, headache and leg swelling. Doses of 100mg daily are sometimes usefully achieved and tolerated. The dosage can be varied during the year or the drug discontinued in the summer.

The use of prostaglandins in the treatment of vasospastic disease began with

Table 2.   Treatments for Raynaud's phenomenon[3]

Surgery
   cervical sympathectomy
   local resection
   local vascular reconstruction
   local sympathetic blockade
   (*e.g.* Bier's block, stellate ganglion block)

Vasoactive substances
   fibrinolytic agents
      (*e.g.* stanazolol)
   plasma expanders
      (*e.g.* dextran)
   sympatholytic agents
   (*e.g.* reserpine, guanethidine, methyl dopa, prazosin, phenoxybenzamine,
   phentolamine, indoramine, thymoxamine)
   β-adrenergic stimulation
      (*e.g.* terbutaline)
   directly acting vasodilators
      (*e.g.* calcitonin gene-related peptide, inositol nicotinate, hexyl nicotinate,[22] glyceryl
      trinitrate, griseofulvin,[23] hydrallazine, alcohol)
   prostanoids (e.g. prostacyclin)
   calcium channel blockers
      (*e.g.* nifedipine, diltiazem, nicardipine)
   angiotensin-converting enzyme inhibitors
      (*e.g.* captopril)
   serotonin receptor blockers
      (e.g. ketanserin)
   behavioural treatment
      (*e.g.* biofeedback and conditioning)[24]
   miscellaneous
      hyperbaric oxgen,[25] transcutaneous nerve stimulation, plasmaphaeresis, hand
      warming,[26] tri-iodothyronine[27]

Modified from Coffman[2] and Dowd.[17] Extra references given if not discussed by these authors.

promising studies of prostaglandin E_1. Prostacyclin (prostaglandin I_2) was subsequently investigated and found to be efficacious including in a double-blind controlled study. Treatment with prostaglandins evolved with the introduction of a prostacyclin analogue, iloprost. Controlled studies demonstrated the benefit of this agent as a vasodilator and there has been speculation about the contribution made by red blood cells, platelets and the endothelium. It has been suggested that intermittent iloprost infusions may have benefits over continuous nifedipine.[2,3,17,18]

   Guidelines from clinical studies as to regimens for dose, frequency and duration of iloprost infusions are largely empirical although a consensus has emerged. The drug that is available to clinicians, epoprostenol (Flolan, Wellcome) does not have a licence for use in Raynaud's phenomenon or any peripheral vascular disease. It is licensed as an inhibitor of platelet aggregation in haemodialysis. In this author's experience 5- to 10-day infusions of 1–5ng/kg/min for 4–8 hours a day can be used to good effect but the infusion rate is often limited by side-effects such as flushing, headache, nausea and bradycardia.

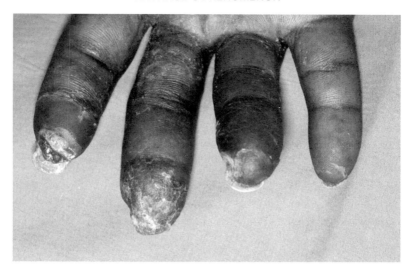

Fig. 9. Digital vasculitic ulcers in a patient with mixed connective tissue disease.

Studies of prostaglandins have been undertaken in patients with systemic sclerosis who represent those patients with the most morbidity from Raynaud's phenomenon. They are nonetheless a clinically heterogenous group which presents problems in evaluation. Furthermore, measurement of improvement of parameters such as platelet aggregation or blood flow measured by thermography or laser Doppler flowmetry may not correlate with clinical objectives such as relief of symptoms and healing of ulcers, especially in the long term, although such claims have been made.

Although nifedipine and intravenous prostanoids have a useful role in the management of Raynaud's phenomenon, neither is a panacea nor free from side-effects.

Recently, intravenous infusions of CGRP have been shown to increase the acral cutaneous blood flow and promote healing of digital ulceration but CGRP is not yet commercially available.[19]

REFERENCES

1. Barlow T: On local asphyxia and symmetrical gangrene of the extremities (Raynaud M) In: Barlow T (trans.) Selected Monographs Vol 121: London: New Sydenham Society, 1888
2. Coffman JD: *Raynaud's Phenomenon*. New York, Oxford: Oxford University Press, 1989
3. Bunker CB: The role of calcitonin gene-related peptide in the pathophsiology and treatment of Raynaud's phenomenon. MD Dissertation, University of Cambridge, 1992
4. Vajda K, Kadar A., Kali A, Urai L: Ultrastructural investigations of finger pulp biopsies: a study of 31 patients with Raynaud's syndrome. *Ultrastruct Pathol* **3:** 175–186, 1982

5. Thompson RP, Harper FE, Maize JC et al.: Nailfold biopsy in scleroderma and related disorders. Correlation of histologic, capillaroscopic and clinical data. *Arthritis Rheum* **27:** 97–103, 1984
6. Bunker CB, Terenghi G, Springall DR et al.: Deficiency of calcitonin gene-related peptide in Raynaud's phenomenon. *Lancet* **336:** 1530–1533, 1990
7. Goldsmith PC, Molina FA, Bunker CB et al.: Cutaneous nerve fibre depletion in vibration white finger. *J Roy Soc Med* **87:** 377–381, 1994
8. Lewis T: Experiments relating to the peripheral mechanism involved in spasmodic arrest of the circulation in the fingers, a variety of Raynaud's disease. *Heart* **15:** 7–101, 1929
9. Lewis T: Supplemenary notes on on the reactions of the human skin to cold. *Heart* **15:** 351–358, 1931
10. Lewis T: *The blood vessels of the human skin and their responses.* London: Shaw and Sons, 1927
11. Bunker CB: Neuropeptides and Raynaud's phenomenon. *Rheumatology* 1997 (in press)
12. Bunker CB, Foreman J, Dowd PM: Digital cutaneous vascular responses to histamine, compound 48/80 and neuropeptides in normal subjects and Raynaud's phenomenon. *J Invest Dermatol* **96:** 314–317, 1991
13. Dowd PM, Bunker CB, Bull HA et al.: Raynaud's phenomenon, calcitonin gene-related peptide, endothelin and cutaneous vasculature. *Lancet* **336:** 1014, 1990
14. Yamauchi K, Arimori S: Alterations of glomerular filtration rate during cold exposure in progressive systemic scleriosis: measurement with Technetium-99m DTPA. *Jap J Med* **29:** 208–211, 1990
15. Maricq HR, McGregor AR, Diat F et al.: Major clinical diagnoses found among patients with Raynaud phenomenon from the general population. *J Rheumatol* **17:** 1171–1176, 1990
16. Allen EV, Brown GE: Raynaud's disease: a critical review of the minimum requisites for diagnosis. *Am J Med Sci* **183:** 187–200, 1932
17. Dowd PM: The treatment of Raynaud's phenomenon. *Br J Dermatol* **114:** 527–533, 1986
18. Dowd PM, Martin MFR, Cooke ED et al.: Treatment of Raynaud's phenomenon by intravenous infusion of prostacyclin (PGI$_2$). *Br J Dermatol* **106:** 81–89, 1982
19. Bunker CB, Reavley C, O'Shaughnessey D, Dowd PM: Calcitonin gene-related peptide in treatment of severe peripheral vascular insufficiency in Raynaud's phenomenon. *Lancet* **342:** 80–84, 1993
20 Klein RG, Hunder GG, Stanson AW, Sheps SG: Large artery involvement in giant cell (temporal) arteritis. *Ann Intern Med* **83:** 806–812, 1975
21. Rustin MHA, Foreman JC, Dowd PM: Anorexia nervosa associated with acromegaloid features, onset of acrocyanosis and Raynaud's phenomenon and worsening of chilblains. *J R Soc Med* **83:** 495–496, 1990
22. Bunker CB, Cooper F, Dowd PM: A double-blind placebo controlled trial of topical hexyl nicotinate in primary Raynaud's phenomenon. *Br J Dermatol* **121** (Suppl 34): 51–52, 1989
23. Allen BR: Griseofulvin in Raynaud's phenomenon. *Lancet* **ii:** 840–841, 1971
24. Jobe JB, Sampson JB, Roberts DE, Beetham WP: Induced vasodilatation as treatment for Raynaud's disease. *Ann Intern Med* **97:** 706–709, 1982
25. Copeman PWM, Ashfield R: Raynaud's phenomenon in scleroderma treated with hyperbaric oygen. *Proc R Soc Med* **60:** 1268–1269, 1967
26. Goodfield MJD, Rowell NR: Hand warming as a treatment for Raynaud's phenomenon in systemic sclerosis. *Br J Dermatol* **119:** 643–646, 1988
27. Dessein PH, Morrison RC, Lamparelli RD, Van der Merwe CA: Triiodothyronine treatment for Raynaud's phenomenon: a controlled trial. *J Rheumatol* **17:** 1025–1028, 1990

Smoking and Vasospasm

D. J. Higman and J. T. Powell

EFFECTS OF SMOKING ON THE CIRCULATION

Cigarette smoking is the single most important risk factor for the development of peripheral atherosclerosis. For the majority of smokers, atherosclerosis only becomes apparent after several decades of smoking. However, even in the absence of gross structural changes in the arterial wall, smoking has effects on the circulation. First, smoking induces vasospasm, resulting in anoxia of the vessel wall to stimulate an influx of inflammatory cells.[1] Second, smoking modulates the concentration and activities of the clotting factors. The smoking-induced increase in fibrinogen concentration will increase plasma viscosity, the exudation of fibrinogen into the arterial wall as well as the tendency to thrombosis. These prothrombotic mechanisms are thought to account for a large part of the increased risk of cardiovascular disease in smokers.[2] Third, smoking impairs the activity of platelets, provoking their tendency to aggregate and release vasoconstrictors.[3] Therefore, in smokers vasospasm has the potential to initiate a severe inflammatory thrombotic reaction, as is most clearly seen in Buerger's disease. We will discuss here how smoking can cause such intense vasospasm that the inflammatory thrombotic reaction is initiated.

SMOKING AND VASOSPASM

The inhalation of cigarette smoke causes vasospasm. This can be demonstrated as an acute event in the microvascular circulation, by a rapid decrease in cutaneous blood flow. There is digital blanching in smokers, due to acute vasoconstriction of the digital arteries in response to the circulating products of cigarette smoke.[4] Acute vasospasm of penile arteries has also been demonstrated in response to smoking.[5]

Digital artery vasospasm in smokers is more than just a physiological observation; it is important in a number of clinical situations. Smokers appear to have greater sensitivity to other environmental vasoconstrictors. For example, cold-induced digital vasoconstriction is more intense in smokers than non-smokers.[6] This is relevant in conditions in which vasospasm is a prominent feature, particularly Raynaud's syndrome, where cold-induced vasospasm with characteristic colour changes of the digits, is the prominent feature. Patients suffering from Raynaud's syndrome who also smoke, will exacerbate the cold response, and the avoidance of these two factors are the mainstays of conservative management.

Vasospasm is the normal acute response in small arteries to smoking. In situations where the flow in these vessels is already compromised, this superimposed vasospasm may make a difference to the survival of the extremity. Heavy smoking following digital reimplantation surgery has been implicated as a cause of failure of digit revascularization.[7] It is likely in this situation that vasospasm critically compromises the flow throughout the microvascular anastomoses. The most severe form of vascular pathology, that seen in Buerger's, disease, occurs almost exclusively in young male smokers, with a dramatic regression of disease following cessation of smoking.[8] In the acute stages of the disease the small vessels of the limb are inflamed and have a tendency to thrombosis. Occlusion becomes more likely when there is a superimposed vasospasm from continued smoking, and immediate cessation is required to reduce the risk of distal tissue ischaemia.

Another condition which is exacerbated by smoking is reflex sympathetic dystrophy (RSD). The precise aetiology of RSD is not known but the condition occasionally follows trauma or ischaemia to a limb, and hyperactivity of the sympathetic nerves and secondary vasospasm are thought to be important in the pathophysiology. Studies of patients with this condition have found that smoking is the most important associated factor.[9]

Coronary artery spasm plays an important role in acute ischaemic events. It is now recognized that spasm can occur in angiographically normal vessels, producing angina in young people. Several studies have shown that symptomatic coronary artery spasm is more common in smokers, and is clearly implicated in its aetiology although the reason why this occurs in some smokers and not others is not known.[10]

THE CONTROL OF VASCULAR TONE

Vascular tone is controlled both centrally by the release of catecholamines which circulate to induce vasoconstriction in distant vessels, and peripherally by the release of local mediators. These local mediators include the endothelium-derived vasodilators, endothelium dependent relaxing factor (EDRF) and prostacyclin, and vasoconstrictors which include endothelin and thromboxane A_2 produced by platelets.[11] The balance of these factors in the normal subject regulates smooth muscle contactility in the vessel wall in response to a variety of physiological stimuli. The endothelium produces EDRF (nitric oxide) and endothelin, and normal endothelial function is important in the regulation of vascular tone. For instance, in response to increased blood flow the endothelium increases the production of both EDRF and prostacyclin, permitting the vessel to dilate to accommodate the increased flow without deleterious changes in pressure and wall shear stress. The increased production of these vasodilators following release of temporary limb occlusion is critical for the normal hyperaemic response.

THE INFLUENCE OF SMOKING ON VASOMOTOR CONTROL

Smoking affects both the central and peripheral mechanisms of vasomotor control. Nicotine in cigarette smoke activates the sympathetic nervous system. This causes an increase in heart rate and blood pressure, and peripheral vasoconstriction. These effects are associated with an increase in the plasma levels of adrenaline and noradrenaline.[12,13]

The principal vasoactive eicoisanoids are thromboxane A_2 and prostacylin, both of which are metabolites of arachidonic acid. Thromboxane A_2 is the principal arachidonic acid metabolite in platelets and in addition to promoting platelet aggregation, is a powerful vasoconstrictor. In contrast, prostacyclin, which is synthesized in the the endothelial cell, inhibits platelet aggregation and is a vasodilator.[11] In a study of monozygotic twins discordant for smoking, metabolites of both thromboxane A_2 and prostacyclin were significantly higher in the smokers, with a relatively greater increase in thromboxane metabolites, thereby favouring vasoconstriction in the smoking subjects.[14] Further evidence for alteration in prostacylin metabolism in smokers is provided by work showing that cutaneous vascular reactivity, in response to inflammatory stimuli such as ultraviolet B radiation and topical hexyl nicotinate, is depressed in smokers.[15] The inflammatory response to both of these agents is mediated by locally synthesized prostaglandins. Smoking impairs the synthesis of prostacyclin by cultured endothelial cells and this may be a direct response to nicotine, since nicotine inhibits the production of prostacyclin from human vein rings.[16]

Cumulatively, this evidence indicates that smoking alters the balance of synthesis of eicoinasoids, from prostacyclin to thromboxanes, to promote vasoconstriction.

THE INFLUENCE OF SMOKING ON NITRIC OXIDE METABOLISM

The most important modulator of vasomotor tone is endothelium-dependent relaxing factor, a diffusible compound with a short half-life which is now known to be nitric oxide (NO). The arterial endothelium constantly synthesizes NO to maintain vascular tone but synthesis and release can be increased in response to a variety of physiological stimuli such as shear stress and substances released from aggregating platelets. Nitric oxide controls vascular tone by stimulating guanylate cyclase and increasing the levels of cyclic guanosine monophosphate (GMP) in underlying vascular smooth muscle cells, causing vasodilatation.[17]

Reduction in the release of NO from the endothelium, evidenced by impaired endothelium-dependent relaxation appears to be a sensitive indicator of endothelial dysfunction, and evidence for endothelial dysfunction has been identified in the vasculature of smokers. Celermajer et al. devised a non-invasive method of measuring the vasodilatation of the superficial femoral artery and brachial artery in vivo, in response to both reactive hyperaemia (endothelium-dependent vasodilatation) and oral glyceryl trinitrate (endothelium-independent relaxation) in young volunteers without clinical evidence of atherosclerotic disease.[18] It was found that in young heavy smokers, the vasodilatation of these major arteries in response to hyperaemic blood flow was significantly lower than that observed in non-smokers. This suggests that smoking causes endothelial dysfunction long before any atherosclerotic lesions can be discerned. Evidence of endothelial dysfunction has also been demonstrated in the coronary circulation of young heavy smokers with angiographically normal arteries. In these subjects, infusion of acetylcholine-induced paradoxical vasoconstriction rather than endothelium-dependent relaxation, suggesting that in these vessels, there is an abnormal response to acetylcholine.[19]

Our own research has centred on the endothelial function of the saphenous vein, as this vessel is used widely in vascular surgery as a bypass conduit. The patency of such bypass grafts is known to be adversely affected by continued smoking.[20,21] Veins appear to release less NO than arteries, which may account, in part, for the superiority of internal mammary artery as a coronary bypass graft compared with saphenous vein.[22] However, in peripheral vascular bypass surgery, saphenous vein is the bypass of choice. Our *in vitro* studies have shown that production of NO is impaired significantly in the endothelium of saphenous vein excised from heavy smokers.[23] First, saphenous vein rings excised from smokers show a reduction in endothelium-dependent relaxation, by about 50%, compared with vein rings from non-smokers, when stimulated with either bradykinin or calcium ionophore A23187, both of which are known to stimulate the release of NO. Second, vein strips from smokers, maintained in culture stimulated with A23187, have a marked reduction in the accumulation of nitrite (a spontaneous oxidation product of NO) in the culture medium.

Our most recent experimental work has shown that, in the saphenous vein, there is a slow recovery of endothelial function, over several months, in patients who have stopped smoking.[24] This is demonstrated by both an improvement in endothelium-dependent relaxation of vein rings and an improvement in the production of nitrite (Fig. 1). Both these indicators of the NO pathway suggest that a period of

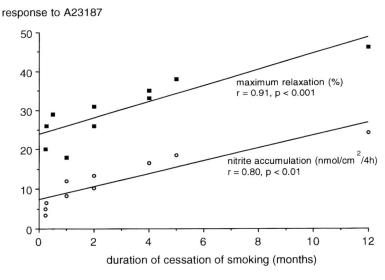

Fig. 1. Improvement of endothelial function in saphenous vein rings following cessation of smoking. The filled squares show the maximum relaxation of a saphenous vein ring in response to increasing doses of A23187, plotted against the period of abstinence from smoking. The open circles show the accumulation of the spontaneous oxidation product of NO, nitrite, from vein strips stimulated with 1μM A23187 over the same time period. The length of smoking is from patient history and cannot be evaluated objectively. After 12 months both endothelium-dependent relaxation and nitrite production have been normalized.

approximately 9–12 months smoking cessation is required before endothelial function in ex-smokers approaches the normal range of endothelial function observed in non-smokers.

There has been considerable discussion as to the mechanism underlying the impaired endothelial production of nitric oxide in smokers. Again we have investigated this using saphenous vein; nicotine was not the culprit (Fig. 2).[25] The concentration of the enzyme synthesizing nitric oxide, nitric oxide synthase, appears very similar in non-smokers and smokers but the activity of the enzyme appears to be reduced in smokers.[25] Supplementation with L-arginine, the substrate required for nitric oxide synthase to yield NO, has been considered in many clinical situations. However, supplementation of saphenous vein rings from smokers with L-arginine did not appear to improve the endothelial synthesis of NO. One of the co-factors required for optimal nitric oxide synthase activity is tetrahydrobiopterin, which usually is synthesized *de novo* in endothelium. Supplementation of vein rings from

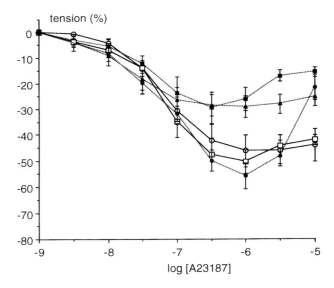

Fig. 2. The impaired vasorelaxation of saphenous vein rings from smokers: correction by tetrahydrobiopterin. The cumulative concentration response curve to calcium ionophore A23187 is shown for rings from smokers (filled squares, n=8) and non-smokers (open circles, n=8): the impaired function of vein rings from smokers is evident. Preincubation of vein rings from non-smokers with nicotine, 30ng/ml, did not impair the vasorelaxation (open squares, n=6). Similarly pre-incubation of vein rings from smokers with 3mmol L-arginine did not alter the vasomotor response to A23187 (filled triangles, n=4). In contrast, preincubation of vein rings with 20μmmol tetrahydrobiopterin (filled circles, n=5) improved the vasomotor responses of vein rings from smokers, without similar effect on vein rings from non-smokers (data not shown).

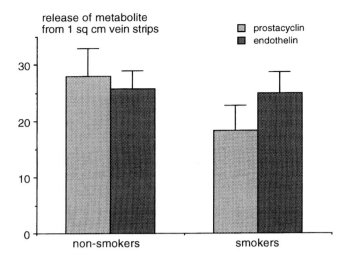

Fig. 3. Comparison of the production of prostacyclin and endothelin by saphenous vein strips from non-smokers and smokers. Prostacyclin was determined as its metabolite PGF$_{1\alpha}$ and results are given as pg/15 min. Endothelin was determined by radioimmunoassay and results are given as fmol/h.

smokers with tetrahydrobiopterin improved the production of NO and vasorelaxation (Fig. 2).[25] Therefore, a critical smoking-induced lesion in endothelium may be the inhibition of tetrahydrobiopterin synthesis by metabolites resulting from the absorption of tobacco combustion products. The wider use of tetrahydrobiopterin supplementation is being considered.[26]

Although NO is the principal endogenous vasodilator produced by endothelium under circumstances where the production of NO is compromised, prostacyclin becomes more important. However, our own work confirms that of others to show that smoking also is associated with a decreased production of prostacyclin (Fig. 3).[25,27] In contrast, the production of the vasoconstrictor endothelin is not affected by smoking (Fig. 3).[25]

MANAGEMENT OF VASOSPASM IN THE SMOKING PATIENT

Clearly the imperative in the management of any patient in whom smoking is associated with vasospasm, is to get the patient to stop smoking. In assessing smoking as a contributary factor in vasospasm, it is important to be aware that the history can be unreliable. Of patients who continue smoking after vascular surgery, approximately 40% will claim to have stopped.[20] This may be the explanation behind a lack of improvement in vasospastic symptoms following apparent smoking cessation. The lack of long-term success in cessation programmes, including the use of nicotine gum and patches, is discouraging but every effort must be made to

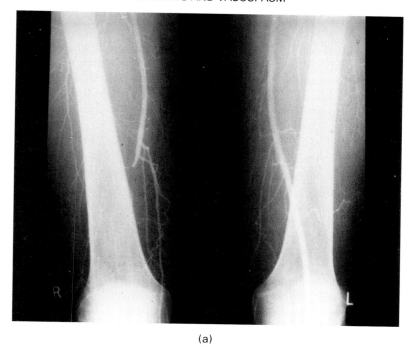

(a)

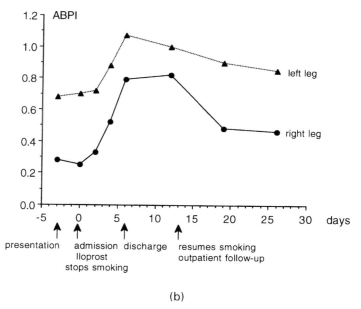

(b)

Fig. 4. Resolution of acute occlusion of the superficial femoral artery following cessation of smoking and prostacyclin infusion. The patient was a 28-year-old woman who smoked 30–40 cigarettes/day and presented with rest pain (a) admission angiogram (b) change in ankle/brachial pressure index from presentation through admission and treatment to discharge and resumption of smoking.

convince patients that the first essential stage in their management is to quit the smoking habit.

Prostaglandin infusions have a role in the acute management of arterial vasospasm. The compound commercially available is an analogue of prostacyclin, and is given as an intravenous infusion over a 72 hour period. Its use is limited by adverse reactions such as vomiting and hypotension, but may be effective in situations where vasospasm, including that induced by smoking, is threatening distal tissue viability.

The combination of smoking cessation and prostaglandin infusions occasionally can produce dramatic improvement in patients with smoking-related vasospasm. This approach requires hospitalization of the patients, hence removing them from a social environment where smoking is the norm to one where smoking is actively discouraged. The angiogram (Fig. 4a) shows occlusion of the superficial femoral artery in a 28-year-old female patient, a persistent heavy smoker who presented with ipsilateral critical ischaemia. Admission to a hospital bed for prostaglandin infusions and monitored smoking cessation produced rapid resolution of the vasospasm, with restoration of blood flow in the superficial femoral artery and marked clinical improvement in ankle/brachial pressure index (Fig. 4b).

Our very recent work indicates that there may be a vasospastic component in vein graft stenoses. The local application of glyceryl trinitrate (GTN) patches to the skin overlying a vein graft stenosis causes local dilatation of the graft, evidenced by a reduction in the velocity ratio at the point of stenosis, detected by duplex ultrasonography.[28] Glyceryl trinitrate is a nitric oxide donor, and acts on the smooth muscle cells of the vein graft to cause vasodilation, in the same way as endogenous NO released from the endothelium. If the vasospasm associated with smoking is due, in part, to endothelial dysfunction and a lack of endogenous NO, then the use of nitrates and NO donors may represent a novel therapy in the future management of vasospastic ischaemia.

SUMMARY

The vasospasm associated with smoking is an important component in a variety of clinical situations and may exacerbate distal ischaemia. It is caused by a combination of hyperactivity of the adrenergic system and an alteration in the balance of local vasoactive mediators. The production of the vasodilators, synthesized locally by endothelium, NO and prostacyclin is impaired by smoking. Cessation of smoking is the mainstay of therapy, but the infusion of prostaglandin vasodilators and possibly the use of nitrate vasodilators have a role in overcoming vasospasm in the acute stage. In addition, the very mechanisms by which smoking impairs the production of NO and prostacyclin by endothelium are likely to operate in parallel in platelets, where the diminished production of NO and prostacyclin will promote platelet activation and aggregation. The importance of vasospasm in initiating inflammatory-thrombotic events at the vessel wall has been neglected and requires emphasis.

ACKNOWLEDGEMENTS

Important contributions to this research were made by Rachid Mir-Hasseine, Alex Strachan, Robert Hicks, Lee Buttery and Jon Golledge. Research support came from the Tobacco Products Research Trust and the A.F.G. Research Foundation.

REFERENCES

1. Gerlis LM: The significance of adventitial infiltrations in coronary atherosclerosis. *Br Heart J* **18**: 166–172, 1955
2. Meade TW, Iveson J, Stirling Y *et al.*: Effects of changes in smoking and other characteristics on clotting factors and the risk of ischaemic heart disease. *Lancet* **ii**: 986–988, 1987
3. Nowak J, Murray JJ, Oates JA, Fitzgerald GA: Biochemical evidence of a chronic abnormality in platelet and vascular function in healthy individuals who smoke cigarettes. *Circulation* **76**: 6–14, 1987
4. Bornmyr S, Svensson H: Thermography and laser-Doppler flowmetry for monitoring changes in finger skin blood flow upon cigarette smoking. *Clin Physiol* **11**: 135–141, 1991
5. Levine LA, Gerber GS: Acute vasospasm of penile arteries in response to cigarette smoking. *Urology* **36**: 99–100, 1990
6. Bovenzi M: Finger systolic pressure during local cooling in normal subjects aged 20–60 years. *Int Arch Occup Environ Hlth* **61**: 179–181, 1988
7. Harris JD, Finseth F, Buncke HJ: The hazard of cigarette smoking following digital replantation. *J Microsurg* **1**: 403–404, 1980
8. Mills JL, Porter JM: Buerger's disease: a review and update. *Semin Vasc Surg* **6**: 14–23, 1993.
9. An HS, Hawthorne KB, Jackson WT: Reflex sympathetic dystrophy and cigarette smoking. *J Hand Surg Am* **13**: 458–460, 1988
10. Sugiishi M, Takatsu F: Cigarette smoking is a major risk factor for coronary spasm. *Circulation* **87**: 76–79, 1993
11. Oates JA, Fitzgerald GA, Branch RA: Clinical implications of prostaglandin and thromboxane A2 formation. *N Engl J Med* **319**: 689–697, 1988
12. Benowitz NL: Nicotine and coronary heart disease. *Trends Cardiovasc Med* **1**: 315–321, 1991
13. Ward KD, Garvey AJ, Bliss RE: Changes in urinary catecholamine excretion after smoking cessation. *Pharmacol Biochem Behav* **40**: 937–940, 1991
14. Lassila R, Seyberth HW, Haapanen A: Vasoactive and atherogenic effects of cigarette smoking: a study of monozygotic twins discordant for smoking. *Br Med J* **297**: 955–957, 1988
15. Mills CM, Hill SA, Marks R: Altered inflammatory responses in smokers. *Br Med J* **307**: 911, 1993
16. Sonnenfeld T, Wennmalm A: Inhibition by nicotine of the formation of prostacyclin-like activity in rabbit and human vascular tissue. *Br J Pharmacol* **71**: 609–613, 1980
17. Komori K, Okadome K, Sugimachi K: Endothelium-derived relaxing factor and vein grafts. *Br J Surg* **78**: 1020–1022, 1991
18. Celermajer DS, Sorensen KE, Gooch VM: Non-invasive detection of endothelial dysfunction in children and adults at risk of atherosclerosis. *Lancet* **340**: 1111–1115, 1992
19. Nitenberg A, Antony I, Foult JM: Acetylcholine-induced coronary vasoconstriction in young heavy smokers with normal coronary arteriographic findings. *Am J Med* **95**: 71–77, 1993
20. Wiseman S, Kenchington G, Dain R *et al.*: Influence of smoking and plasma factors on patency of femoropopliteal vein grafts. *Br Med J* **299**: 643–646, 1989

21. Hicks RCJ, Ellis M, Mir-Hasseine R *et al.*: The influence of fibrinogen concentration on the development of vein graft stenoses. *Eur J Vasc Endovasc Surg* **9:** 415–420, 1995

22. Barner HB, Swartz MT, Mudd JG, Tyras DH: Late patency of the internal mammary artery as a coronary bypass conduit. *Ann Thorac Surg* **34:** 408–411, 1982

23. Higman DJ, Greenhalgh RM, Powell JT: Smoking impairs endothelium-dependent relaxation of saphenous vein. *Br J Surg* **80:** 1242–1245, 1993

24. Higman DJ, Strachan AMJ, Powell JT: Reversibility of smoking-induced endothelial dysfunction. *Br J Surg* **81:** 977–978, 1994

25. Higman DJ, Strachan, AMJ, Buttery L *et al.*: Smoking impairs the activity of endothelial nitric oxide synthase in saphenous vein. *Arterioscler Thromb Vasc Biol* **16:** 546–552, 1996

26. Cosentino F, Katusic ZS: Tetrahydrobiopterin and dysfunction of endothelial nitric oxide synthase in coronary arteries. *Circulation* **91:** 139–144, 1995

27. Reinders JH, Brinkman HJM, van Mourik JA, de Groot PG: Cigarette smoking impairs endothelial prostacyclin production. *Arteriosclerosis* **6:** 15–23, 1986

28. Golledge J, Hicks RCJ, Ellis M, Greenhalgh RM, Powell JT: Dilatation of saphenous vein grafts by nitric oxide. *Eur J Vasc Endovasc Surg* 1997 (in press)

Mechanisms of Carotid Restenosis

Paolo Fiorani, Francesco Speziale, Maurizio Taurino, Enrico Sbarigia
and Alessandro Mauriello

INTRODUCTION

Recurrent carotid artery stenosis is the most frequent late complication after carotid endarterectomy (CEA). The reported incidence ranges from 0.6% to 20%[1-3] according to the diagnostic procedures used, surveillance protocol and length of follow-up. The term recurrent stenosis usually excludes residual stenoses due to technical faults because improved surgical techniques and intraoperative, perioperative and postoperative monitoring have gradually reduced their frequency.[3,4] It now customarily refers to the lesion described in 1976 by Stoney,[5] which usually becomes manifest within 1 or 2 years of surgery. The morphologic features, clinical appearances and course unmistakably distinguish recurrent stenoses from primary arteriosclerotic lesions. A recurrent stenosis appears as a whitish, shiny, mother of pearl-like fibrous wall thickening generally without surface ulcerations or thrombi (Fig. 1). These anatomic and pathologic features explain why recurrent stenoses rarely occasion overt clinical symptoms. The typical histological finding is myointimal hyperplasia that may stabilize in time, regress or progress to occlusion.

AIM OF THE STUDY

In this study we sought to verify whether the latest research findings on the morphology and pathophysiological features of recurrent stenoses would provide new information on factors likely to influence the onset and development of this lesion, with the purpose of reappraising its management.

MATERIAL AND METHODS

From 1985 to 1995, 892 consecutive patients admitted to our department underwent 1020 CEAs. The group of 892 patients comprised 714 men (80%) and 178 women (20%) with a mean age of 63 years (range 33–80 years). General risk factors for atherosclerosis included cigarette smoking in 550 patients (61%), hypertension in 530 (59%), diabetes in 153 (17%), hypercholesterolaemia in 134 (15%).

Clinical and morphological data were considered for each carotid axis operated on;

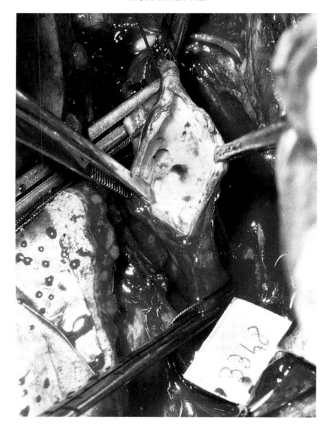

Fig. 1. Macroscopic appearance of a carotid restenosis at operation.

933 CEAs (91.4%) were performed because of symptomatic lesions and 87 (8.6%) because of asymptomatic lesions.

All patients underwent preoperative morphological and haemodynamical assessment by duplex scanning (Spectra, Diasonic Inc.). Preoperative diagnostic studies included conventional or digital angiography in 745 carotid axes (73%) and non-invasive imaging alone in 275 (27%).

Overall results of imaging demonstrated 367 (36%) monolateral stenoses: 286 (78%) haemodynamic (i.e. >50% diameter reduction) and remaining ulcerated lesions in 22%; 459 (45%) bilateral stenoses (381 haemodynamic (81%) and 19% ulcerated lesions). In 194 (19%) stenoses with contralateral occlusion, the operated lesion was haemodinamically significant in 89% of the cases. Specifically in the 275 cases in which operation was performed without angiography, duplex identified 212 (77%) haemodynamic stenosis (v2/v1 ratio greater than 2.5) and 63 ulcerated non-haemodynamic lesions (33%). Cerebral computed tomographic (CT) or magnetic resonance imaging (MRI) scans were obtained in 806 cases (79%): scans in 290 cases (36%) disclosed an ischaemic lesion, and in 516 (64%) no lesions.

In 337 (33%) CEAs patients received general anaesthesia and in 683 (33%) locoregional anaesthesia by C_2–C_4 cervical block. Up to December 1992, in 443 CEAs (43%) cerebral function was monitored by stump pressure measurement at clamping and all patients underwent continuous monitoring by quantitative electroencephalography (QEEG). Before clamping, all patients received heparin in a single 50 mg bolus dose intravenously (5000 IU). The mean clamping time was 17 minutes (range 11–37 min). In 330 CEAs (32%) arteriotomies were closed with a Dacron patch and in 690 (68%) by primary closure. All patients received postoperative heparin–calcium therapy followed by platelet antiaggregation therapy (aspirin 300 mg/day or ticlopidine (250 mg/day).

Postoperative surveillance included clinical assessment and non-invasive diagnostic imaging procedures at 1 month, 3, 6 and 12 months after surgery, thereafter yearly. Patients underwent angiography only if they had rapidly progressive or high-grade stenosis (Fig. 2), regardless of accompanying neurological symptoms, even non-focal symptoms. Morphological and haemodynamic data from duplex scanning identified 45 cases of recurrent stenosis (4.6%). Recurrent stenosis was defined as a lesion occupying more than 50% of the lumen, on the basis of echo-duplex criteria.

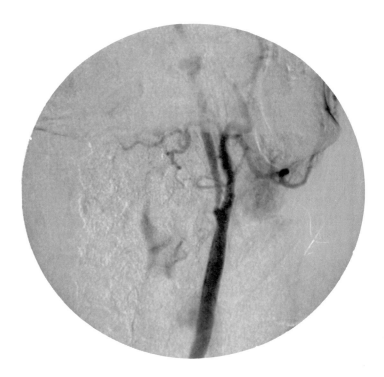

Fig. 2. Angiographic finding of a carotid restenosis.

RESULTS

Follow-up in 827 patients lasted a mean 46 months; 65 patients were lost to follow-up. In 43 of the 827 patients recurrent stenosis developed early after surgery (within 24 months); in two cases (4.6%), both atherosclerotic recurrences, it developed later. The 43 patients (35 men and 8 women, mean age 62 years) with early recurrences had the following risk factors: cigarette smoking (58%), diabetes (27%), and hypercholesterolaemia (14%). During follow-up only 20% of the initially hypertensive patients effectively controlled their pressures, whereas 57% stopped smoking, and 63% of patients who had diabetes and 35% of those with hypercholesterolaemia normalized their glucohaemia and cholesterol values. In 14 patients the indications for angiography were restenosis >70%. Four patients had asymptomatic lesions and five had symptoms of vertigo. In 31 (4.5%) of the recurrences the arteriotomy had been closed with a primary suture, in 12 (3.3%) with Dacron patching. Of the two late recurrent stenoses, both in men, one was treated surgically. Eight recurrences (18.5%) were repaired surgically; five (12%) regressed spontaneously (within 1 year); 25 (58%) remained stable, as documented by repeated 2-monthly assessments; and five (12%) were internal carotid artery occlusions. Four patients had asymptomatic occlusions; one patient had amaurosis fugax. The initial surgical indication in eight repaired recurrent stenoses was severe or progressive stenosis and in five the concurrent onset of vertigo. None of the surgical repair procedures led either to mortality or to neurological or cranial nerve deficits during the immediate postoperative follow-up. In 19 patients follow-up lasted a mean 36 months (range 2 months to 7 years).

DISCUSSION

Although the indications for carotid CEA seem clear, even for haemodynamic stenoses in asymptomatic patients,[6-8] the indications for treatment of its most frequent complication, recurrent stenosis, still need defining. Because the causes of carotid artery restenosis remain doubtful debate continues on its course and treatment. Especially controversial is the aetiology. The genesis of recurrent carotid stenosis encompasses matters of surgical technique as well as an array of variables pertaining to the patient. Technical points centre first on the presence of residual stenoses (proximal or distal);[9-13] and second on whether to close the arteriotomy with a patch.[4,14-17]

The increasingly frequent introduction of intraoperative quality control with various procedures (angiography, duplex scanning, and more recently angioscopy) has reduced the incidence of residual stenoses or other defects from the 26% reported in 1978 by Anderson *et al.*[18] to the currently reported figure ranging from 2 to 12%.[3,4,18,19]

Many vascular surgeons recommend patch angioplasty as an effective means of reducing acute internal carotid artery thrombosis after CEA and of reducing myointimal hyperplasia in the operated vessel thereby also reducing recurrent stenosis and late recurrent atherosclerotic lesions. In practice, conclusively determining the effectiveness of patch angioplasty remains arduous, not least because the multitude of studies defy comparison owing to their non-homogeneous designs, methods for patient selection and surveillance protocols. In retrospective[12,20,21] and prospective studies[16] some investigators report a lower incidence of recurrent stenosis after patch angioplasty using either prosthetic or autologous materials. Supporting these opinions, Zeirler and Deriu[22,23] showed that angioplasty-induced changes in vascular geometry, with a consequent increase in calibre, act as factors able to delay arterial repair mechanisms thus preventing the development of intimal lesions. Others[17,24,25] who disagreed with this view found no significant difference in outcome between patients treated with patch angioplasty or primary closure.

Far more numerous are the variables pertaining not to surgical techniques but to the specific characteristics of the lesion. Some evidence suggests that early recurrent stenosis should be considered as an overexuberant reaction to injury rather than a new atherosclerotic lesion.[1] Recurrent stenoses indeed exhibit neither macroscopic nor histopathological features typical of an atheroma.[26-27]

Morphology

Macroscopically, recurrent stenoses are seen as a whitish, smooth, fibrous wall thickening, generally without ulcerations or surface thrombi. Many investigators have studied the histological appearances of these lesions.[1,5,14,26,27] Electron microscopy has disclosed a series of morphological patterns originating from a cascade of events that Stemmerman and Ross[28] have reproduced experimentally. After platelet deposition and thrombus formation on the subendothelial layer, activated platelets secrete platelet derived growth factor, a protein that exerts a positive chemotactic action on polymorphonuclear neutrophils, monocytes, smooth muscle cells and fibroblasts, thus causing these cells to proliferate. Activated monocytes, macrophages, endothelial cells and smooth muscle cells secrete platelet-derived growth factor-like substances.

Endothelial cells also secrete factors that inhibit smooth muscle cell proliferation.[29,30] During the normal healing process all these cell types act in equilibrium, but factors as yet unknown can alter the balance. Especially in areas of high flow or turbulent flow, among them the carotid bifurcation, the mechanical stimulus acts even on the outer medial layers, breaking up the lamina elastica and disrupting its elastic fibres. At this stage platelets seem not to have a key role. Within 6 months of injury the blood vessel regains its elasticity and the regenerated intima begins to undergo fibrous thickening. Yet it undergoes no atherosclerotic changes even in the presence of high atherogenic risk factors.[31] Later on, the elastic structures surrounding the smooth muscle cells become even more disrupted and disorganized and realign in relation to the lumen. Immunocytologic staining shows that most cells in intimal hyperplasia originate from smooth muscle cells although many seem to be derived from circulating leukocytes.[32]

Recent studies attribute increasing importance to the potential role of immunological mechanisms in chronic degenerative arterial lesions. Noteworthy is the role of T lymphocytes in fatty streaks, the earliest lesion of atherosclerosis and in advanced lesions.[33-35] As well as T lymphocytes diseased intimal tissue frequently contains monocytes and macrophages. Although how these two cell types intervene remains unclear, T lymphocytes have a well-established role in favouring adhesion and migration of circulating monocytes, so that release of lymphokines or interleukin by activated T lymphocytes regulates macrophage recruitment thereby increasing the formation of foam cells. The role of these cytokines against growth factor receptors or smooth muscle cell growth indicates that T lymphocytes probably have a key role in atherogenesis or in blood vessel repair.[33,34] Interactions between these cells indicate numerous mechanisms that might mediate the inflammatory, repair and proliferative processes observed both in stable atherosclerotic lesions and accelerated atherosclerosis typical of recurrences.[34-37]

As our knowledge clarifies the various interacting mechanisms it should be possible to identify a pharmacological agent able to prevent recurrent stenosis. The ideal drug would be one that exerts antithrombotic and antiproliferative effects without inducing bleeding complications. Recent research has proposed the use of omega-3 fatty acids and low molecular-weight heparin. Although clinical studies report encouraging evidence that these substances reduce recurrent coronary artery stenoses after percutaneous transluminal coronary angioplasty they have are not yet widely used in clinical practice.[38]

Course of disease

The course of post-carotid endarterectomy recurrent stenoses varies according to the numerous variables that intervene either to disturb the equilibrium or to correct the dysequilibrium in arterial wall repair processes. Hence the occasional observations of restenosis that regress spontaneously. Although the mechanisms remain conjectural, an action able to block the disease or cause it to regress acts on platelet-derived growth factor, by blocking the arachidonic acid cascade.

Apart from the pharmacological effects exerted by numerous substances commonly prescribed in clinical practice (antiplatelet drugs, calcium-antagonists, cortisone, prostaglandins, colchicine, ACE-inhibitors, heparin, warfarin, dextran, hirudin and lovastatin) much interest centres on the efficacy of gene transfer in promoting specific functions capable of reducing cell responses to arterial wall damage, thereby diminishing intimal hyperplasia.

Even though the mechanisms underlying the anatomic course, especially those responsible for regression, still need clarifying experimentally, several clinical studies report imaging evidence of regression in 30% of recurrent stenoses.[39-42] Five (16%) of the demonstrable restenoses in our series regressed spontaneously.

Principles of treatment

In the rare patients with recurrent stenoses in whom a severe clinical evolution (neurological disorders of recent onset) or evidence of rapid progression to occlusion indicate surgical treatment, reoperation is the procedure widely used. The surgical indications for treatment of carotid artery recurrent stenoses depend closely on how these lesions evolve anatomically and clinically. As our review underlines, these lesions rarely produce clinically important effects; focal neurologic deficits, which none of our patients had, have a reported frequency of 1% per year, equal to the rate in the general age-matched population.[25,43-45] The most frequent symptom of restenosis is vertigo. Yet some lesions progress anatomically to haemodynamic stenosis and therefore ultimately to occlusion. This rare event (16% of our series) is reported in 8–16% of cases.[39–42]

Hence the indications for surgical treatment should be reserved for symptomatic patients with disease progressing to occlusion in whom stroke seems foreseeable. In assessing the likelihood of stroke, transcranial Doppler seems a useful technique for identifying patients without cerebral functional reserve. As we showed in an earlier study,[46] by identifying subjects in whom administration of acetazolamide (Diamox) causes the medium cerebral artery flow rate to fall by about 6 cm ± 3.0 cm, it provides evidence of a loss of functional cerebral reserve. During the postoperative period this loss becomes evident as a hyperperfusion syndrome.

The operation initially proposed and most frequently performed is a re-do carotid endarterectomy or patching without endarterectomy. The decision to do patching alone arose from the difficulty in identifying the proper cleavage plane for CEA.[20] Partly owing to these drawbacks, and also because the diseased artery remains, many vascular surgeons prefer to remove the stenotic tract en bloc and replace it with a prosthetic graft. Owing to the presence of scar tissue, grafting is technically simpler and less risky than a repeat CEA.[47] Yet it has the undoubted disadvantage of a higher rate of neurological and cranial nerve complications.[48–50] None of the patients in our re-do CEA series had perioperative strokes or cranial nerve deficits. Despite this satisfactory result a sample of only eight patients does not allow us to draw definitive conclusions.

Recently some have proposed an endovascular treatment, the rationale being that because of their morphological characteristics recurrent stenoses might respond to treatment with percutaneous transluminal angioplasty. The risks seemed reasonable, considering that restenoses rarely give rise to emboli. But the first reports[51] actually showed otherwise, complications being no less frequent than those after the primary operation. Nonetheless, later reports identified certain typical lesions (distal internal carotid artery) possibly more amenable to endovascular treatment. Primary stenting also proved far more reliable than percutaneous transluminal angioplasty plus stent both for treating recurrent stenoses and more recently for primary carotid artery stenosis.[52] Yet not all reports agree on the results of primary stenting; Dietrich et al.[53] reported neurological complications in 10.9% of the cases, one-third being in patients with recurrent stenoses. Nonetheless, the indications for the treatment of recurrent stenosis now seem oriented towards endovascular procedures because they are undoubtedly more simple than conventional surgery. If the surgical risks are similar, or better still, lower than those for the conventional operation, then an endovascular procedure could be the treatment of choice.

REFERENCES

1. Callow A, J. O'Donnell: Recurrent carotid stenosis. In: Bergan JJ, Yao JST (Eds) *Reoperative Arterial Surgery* pp. 523–535. London: Grune and Stratton
2. Kieny R, Mantxz F, Kurtz TH, Kretz JC: Les restenoses carotidiennes après endartrectomie. In: *Indication et resultats de la chirurgie carotidienne* pp. 77–100. Paris: AERCV, 1988

3. Courbier R, Jausseran JM, Reggi M *et al.*: Routine intraoperative carotid angiography: its impact on operative morbidity and carotid restenosis. *J Vasc Surg* **135**: 221, 1986
4. Flanigann DP, Schuler JJ, Vogel M *et al.*: The role of carotid duplex scanning in surgical decision making *J Vasc Surg* **2**: 15, 1985
5. Stoney RJ, String ST: Recurrent carotid stenosis. *Surgery* **80**: 705–710, 1976
6. North American Symptomatic Carotid Endarterectomy Trial Collaboration: Beneficial effect of carotid endarterectomy in symptomatic patients with high grade stenosis. *N Engl J Med* **325**: 445–453, 1991
7. MRC European Carotid Surgery Trial: Interim results for symptomatic patients with severe (70–99%) or with mild (0–29%) carotid stenosis. *Lancet* **337**: 1235–1243, 1991
8. Asymptomatic Carotid Atherosclerotic Study Participants: Endarterectomy for asymptomatic carotid artery stenosis. *JAMA* **273**: 1421–1428, 1995
9. Barnes RW, Nix ML, Nichols BT: Recurrent versus residual carotid stenosis:incidence detected by Doppler ultrasound. *Ann Surg* **203**: 652–660, 1986
10. Keagy BA, Edrington RD, Poole MA, Johnson G: Incidence of recurrent or residual stenosis after carotid endarterectomy. *Am J Surg* **149**: 722–725, 1985
11. Pierce JE, Iliopulos JI, Holcomb MA: Incidence of recurrent stenosis after carotid endarterectomy determined by digital subtraction angiography. *Am J Surg* **148**: 848–854, 1984
12. Ouriel K, Green RM: Clinical and technical factors influencing recurrent carotid stenosis and occlusion after endarterectomy. *J Vasc Surg* **5**: 702–706, 1987
13. Clagett GP, Robinowitz M, Youkey JR *et al.*: Morphogenesis and clinico-pathologic characteristics of recurrent carotid disease. *J Vasc Surg* **3**: 10–23, 1986
14. Hertzer NR, Beven EG, O'Hara PJ, Lrajewski LP: A prospective study of vein patch angioplasty during carotid endarterectomy: three years results for 801 patients and 917 operations. *Ann Surg* **206**: 628–638, 1987
15. Archie JP: Prevention of early restenosis and thrombosis occlusion after carotid endarterectomy by saphenous vein patch angioplasty. *Stroke* **17**: 901–905, 1986
16. Eikelboom BC, Ackerstaff RGA, Ludwig JW *et al.*: Interet du patch en chirurgie carotidienne. In: Kieffer E, Natali J (Eds) *Aspects techniques de la chirurgie carotidienne* pp. 171–181. Paris: AERCV, 1987
17. Katz MM, Jones GT, Degenhardt J *et al.*: The use of patch angioplasty to alter the incidence of carotid restenosis following thromboendarterectomy. *J Cardiovasc Surg* **28**: 2–8, 1987
18. Anderson CA, Collins GJ, Rich NM: Routine operative arteriography during carotid endarterectomy: a reassesment. *Surgery* **83**: 67, 1978
19. Jernigan WR, Fulton RL, Hamman JL *et al.*: The efficacy of routine completien operative angiography in reducing the incidence of perioperative stroke associated with carotid endarterectomy. *Surgery* **5**: 831, 1984
20. Gagne PJ, Riles RS, Imparato AM *et al.*: Redo endarterectomy for recurent carotid stenosis. *Eur J Vasc Surg* **5**: 135–140, 1991
21. Hertzer NB, Beven EG, Modic MT *et al.*: Early patency of the carotid artery after endarterectomy: digital substraction angiography after two hundred and sixty-two operations. *Surgery* **92**: 1049, 1982
22. Zierler RE, Bandik DF, Thiele BL, Strandness DE: Carotid artery stenosis following carotid endarterctomy. *Arch Surg* **117**: 1408–1412, 1982
23. Deriu GP, Ballotta E, Bonavina L *et al.*: The rationale for patch graft angioplasty after carotid endarterectomyearly and long-term follow-up. *Stroke* **15**: 972–979, 1984
24. Rosenthal D, Archie JP, Garcia-Rinaldi R *et al.*: Carotid patch angioplasty: immediate and long term results. *J Vasc Surg* **12**: 326–333, 1990
25. Fiorani P, Sbarigia E, Speziale F *et al.*: Risultati a distanza della chirurgia della carotide. *Minerva Angiologica* **17**: 143–147, 1992
26. Schwarcz TH, Yates GN, Ghobria LM, Baker WH: Pathologic characteristics of recurrent carotid artery stenosis *J Vasc Surg* **5**: 280–288, 1987
27. O'Donnel TF, Callow A: Ultrasound characteristics of recurrent carotid disease: Hypothesis explaining the low incidence of asymptomatic recurrence. *J Vasc Surg* **3**: 26–41, 1985

28. Stemmerman MB, Ross R: Experimental atherosclerosis. Fibrous plaque formation in primates, an electron microscopic study. *J Exp Med* **136**: 767–789, 1972

29. Ross R, Raines EW, Bowen-Pope DF: The biology of platelet-derived growth factor. *Cell* 115–169, 1986

30. Limanni A, Fleming T, Molina R, Hufnagel H *et al.*: Expression of genes for platelet derived growth factor in adult human venous endothelium. A possible non platelet dependent cause of intimal hyperplasia in vein graft and perianastomotic areas of vascular protheses. *J Vasc Surg* **7**: 10–20, 1988

31. Imparato AM, Baumann GF: Electromicroscopic studies of fibromuscular lesions experimentally produced. *Surg Gynec Obst* **139**: 497–504, 1974

32. Clowes AW, Clowes MM, Reidy MA: Kinetics of cellular proliferation after arterial injury. *Lab Invest* **54**; 295–303, 1986

33. Hansson GK, Jonasson L, Lojsted B, Stemme S *et al.*: Localization of T lymphocytes and macrophages in fibrous and complicated human atherosclerotic plaques. *Atherosclerosis* **72**: 135–141, 1988

34. Hansson GK, Jonasson L, Selfert PS, Stemme S *et al.*: Immune mechanisms in atherosclerosis. *Arteriosclerosis* **9**: 567–578, 1989

35. van der Wal AC, Das PK, van der Berg DB *et al.*: Atherosclerotic lesions in humans: *in situ* immunophenotypic analysis suggesting an immune-mediated response. *Lab Invest* **61**: 166–170, 1989

36. Hansson GK, Holm J, Kral JG, Cristea A: Accumulation of IgG and complement factor C3 in human arterial endothelium and atherosclerotic lesions. *Acta Pathol Microbiol Immunol Scand* **92A**: 429–435, 1989

37. Vlaicu R, Niculescu F, Rus HG, Cristea A: Immunohistochemical localization of the terminal C5b-9 complement complex in human aortic fibrous plaque. *Atherosclerosis* **57**: 163–177, 1985

38. Ip JH, Fuster V, Badimon L *et al.*: Syndromes of accelerated atherosclerosis: Role of vascular injury and smooth muscle cells proliferation. *J Am Coll Cardiol* **15**: 1667–1687, 1990

39. Schwarcz TH, Yates GN, Ghobrial M, Baker WH: Patholoigc characteristics of recurrent carotid artery stenosis. *J Vasc Surg* **5**: 280–288, 1987

40. Mattos MA, Van Bemelen PS, Barkmeir LD *et al.*: Routine surveillance after carotid endarterectomy. Does it affect clinical management? *J Vasc Surg* **17**: 819–831, 1993

41. Bertin VJ, Plecha FB, Roger J *et al.*: Recurrent stenosis by duplex scan following carotid endarterectomy. *Arch Surg* **125**: 866–869, 1989

42. Healy DA, Zierler RE, Nicholls SC *et al.*: Long-term follow-up and clinical outcome of carotid restenosis. *J Vasc Surg* **10**: 662–669, 1989

43. Sumner DS, Mattos MA, Hodgson KJ: Surveillance program for vascular reconstructive procedures. In: Yao TJS, Pearce W (Eds) *Long-term Results in Vascular Surgery* No.33, p. 59, 1993

44. Washburn WK, Mackey WC, Belkin M, O'Donner TF: Late stoke after carotid endarterectomy: the role of recurrent stenosis. *J Vasc Surg* **15**: 1032–1037, 1992

45. Fiorani P, Sbarigia E, Giannoni MF *et al.*: For how long should carotid endarterectomy surveillance be contunued? *Int Angiol* **13**: 190–195, 1994

46. Sbarigia E, Speziale F, Giannoni MF *et al.*: Post carotid endadrterectomy hyperperfusion syndrome: preliminary observations for identifying at risk by transcranial Doppler sonography and acetazolamide test. *Eur J Vasc Surg* **7**: 252–256, 1993

47. Treiman GS, Jenkins JM, Edwards WH *et al.*: The evolving surgical management of recurrent carotid stenosis. *J Vasc Surg* **16**: 354–363, 1992

48. Callow AD: Recurrent stenosis after carotid endarterectomy *Arch Surg* **117**: 1082–1085, 1982

49. Bernstein EF, Torem S, Dilley RB: Does carotid restenosis predict an increased risk of late symptoms, stroke or death? *Ann Surg* **212**: 629–636, 1990

50. Das MB, Hertzer NR, Ratcliff NB *et al*: Recurrent carotid stenosis: a 5-year series of 65 reoperation. *Ann Surg* **202**: 28–35, 1985

51. Bergeron P, Rudondy P, Benichou H *et al.*: Transluminal angioplasty for recurrent stenosis after carotid endarterectomy *Int Angiol* **12**: 256–259, 1993

52. Bergeron P, Chambran P, Benichou H, Alessandri C: Recurrent carotid disease: will stents be an alternative to surgery? *J Endovasc Surg* **3:** 76–79, 1996

53. Dietrich EB, Ndiaye M, Reid DB: Stenting in the carotid artery: initial experience in 110 patients. *J Endovasc Surg* **3:** 42–62, 1996

VEIN GRAFT STENOSIS

Structural Predictors of Vein Graft Stenosis

David K. Beattie and Alun H. Davies

INTRODUCTION

Autogenous vein is the preferred conduit for infrainguinal arterial reconstruction.[1,2] Despite this, up to 30% of vein grafts fail, often within 12 months of surgery[3] and this may affect both limb salvage and level of amputation.[4] Graft failure is conventionally described as occurring in one of three postoperative periods[5] and preoperative graft morphology has been shown to correlate with graft patency in each of these.

GRAFT FAILURE

Early graft failure occurs within 30 days of surgery and accounts for 5–30% of failures. Technical problems may occur in 15% of femorodistal bypasses. Twisting and kinking of the graft causes malalignment, the former being more common in reversed and fully mobilized grafts, though the latter is less common than in synthetic grafts.[6–8] Insertion of the graft under tension may jeopardize flow. Persistent valves and tributaries may not always be immediately detectable, even with on-table arteriography[9] and failure to identify these correlates with occlusion. Non-division of saphenous tributaries leads to arteriovenous fistulae[10] and may occur in 20% of *in situ* grafts.[11] Anastomoses are particularly prone to technical error, especially distally, the more common problems being intimal dissection and luminal narrowing. Early graft patency is also dependent on graft inflow, and hence upon cardiac output and proximal atherosclerotic disease.[12,13] However, a runoff deficiency is the most common cause of early graft failure;[5] it has been demonstrated that graft outcome correlates to tibial vessel patency[14] and that an intact pedal arch is vital.[15]

Intermediate graft failure occurs between 1 and 12 months. Up to 75% of failures occur during this period,[16] by far the most common cause being the development of neointimal hyperplasia with resultant, usually single, discrete stenoses,[17] though valve cusp fibrosis and aneurysmal dilatation may also be responsible. Neointimal hyperplasia is a uniform vascular response to vessel injury, which can range from mild endothelial denudation to severe medial disruption. Histologically, medial smooth muscle cells alter phenotype, proliferate and migrate to the intima. In the intima a second phase of proliferation occurs and the cells become embedded in an extracellular matrix comprising mainly collagen.[18] Lesions develop quickly, often within 2 weeks of surgery.[19]

Late graft failure is significantly rarer than intermediate and early failure. The primary cause is disease progression in the native inflow, or more commonly runoff, vessel compromising graft flow and leading to thrombosis.[20] It has been suggested that the act of grafting itself increases the rate of progression of native vessel disease,[21] though failure may also be due to the development of atheroma in the vein graft itself.[22]

FACTORS ASSOCIATED WITH VEIN GRAFT STENOSIS AND THEIR IDENTIFICATION

There are many techniques available for optimizing patient selection and defining the most appropriate vascular procedure to be performed. Full use of these can minimize the risk of many of the causes of graft failure discussed above. Clinical examination,[23] biplanar arteriography,[24] subtraction techniques,[25] ultrasound,[26] and magnetic resonance imaging all have a place. However, the recognition that the majority of graft attrition is due to neointimal hyperplasia and subsequent vein graft stenosis has led to strenuous efforts to identify and correct this problem before the 'at risk' graft becomes an occluded graft, though the former may not necessarily result in the latter.

VEIN GRAFT SURVEILLANCE

The precise aetiology of the lesion of vein graft stenosis is much debated, but the importance of identification and subsequent intervention has been extensively reviewed. Despite the paucity of randomized trials, there is evidence that vein graft stenosis is a structural predictor of a failing graft, with at least a three-fold increase in the risk of occlusion for uncorrected lesions.[27-30] One small randomized trial supports this.[31] For this reason many units now consider it mandatory to enter all vein graft patients into duplex-based graft surveillance programmes. Doubt still exists, however, as to the validity of these reports[32] and a recent large literature review of duplex surveillance reported that, whilst surveillance led to superior graft patency rates, there was no concomitant improvement in limb salvage.[33] Despite this, the presence of postoperative intimal hyperplasia as a potential structural predictor of graft failure can not be ignored.

PRE-EXISTING VEIN MORPHOLOGY – THE CONCEPT OF VEIN QUALITY

Only relatively recently has it been recognized that the changes of intimal hyperplasia, sclerosis and muscle hypertrophy, as shown in Fig. 1, may pre-exist the insertion of vein into the arterial system.[34-37] More recently still, these changes have been positively correlated with vein graft stenosis. Marin *et al.* concluded that veins with thick and calcified walls or hypercellular intima at the time of grafting are at increased risk of developing intragraft lesions that may lead to graft failure.[38] Our own unpublished data yielded statistical significance for a sample size as small as 24 patients when looking at graft outcome in veins showing preoperative intimal

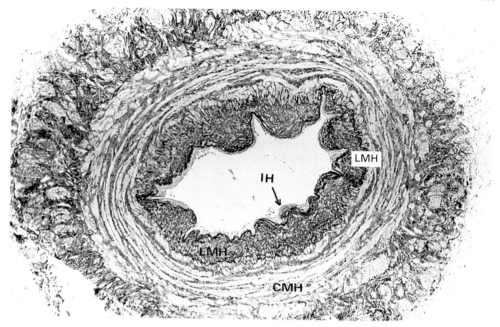

Fig. 1. Histology of an abnormal vein showing classical features of pre-existing intimal hyperplasia (IH), longitudinal (LMH) and circular muscle hypertrophy (CMH) with a magnification of x320. Haematoxylin and eosin staining were used.

hyperplasia compared with those showing no such change. However, one recently published series of 53 patients undergoing infrainguinal bypass surgery failed to show a correlation between either preoperative intimal or medial thickness and graft stenosis after 12 months postoperative surveillance.[39] The presence of a macrophage infiltrate, a lymphocytic infiltrate or of subendothelial smooth muscle cells have also been shown to be associated with the development of a stenosis, though the presence of vein incompetence, the site of valves or tributaries, and the degree of endothelial loss are not.[40] Furthermore, despite early reports to the contrary, there appears to be no difference in either patency or stenosis rates between *in situ* and reversed vein techniques.[41,42] Similarly, although the initial reports on the use of arm vein were disappointing, early interpretation failed to take into account the fact that such vein is often used in secondary intervention where outcome is expected to be poorer. A number of reports now confirm the acceptability of arm vein in infrainguinal reconstruction.[43,44]

The use of the pre-bypass vein morphology as a predictor of graft outcome has been further advanced by the demonstration that the internal diameter of vein correlates with graft patency, as shown in Fig. 2, and that mean vein compliance is lower in patients who go on to develop graft stenosis, as demonstrated in Fig. 3. Furthermore, the vein diameter, and hence the likelihood of graft stenosis, may vary as the donor vein becomes more distal, as shown in Table 1.[40,45] The results of comparing a preoperative internal diameter of less than 3mm with a compliance of

0.15 or less as being predictive of the development of graft stenosis are shown in Table 2.[40]

These findings introduce the important concept of vein quality and demonstrate that the outcome of bypass grafting may be primarily dependent upon the quality of the intended conduit, although the importance of patient selection and the avoidance of technical errors is recognized. For this reason a method for the assessment of bypass vein is mandatory either pre- or intraoperatively, or preferably both.

Table 1. The distribution of internal vein diameter for 53 long saphenous veins and the numbers within each group that developed a stenosis

	<3mm	3–5mm	>5mm
Groin	4(2)	35(4)	14(1)
Mid thigh	14(2)	31(4)	8(1)
Knee	16(3)	32(3)	5(1)
Mid calf	32(3)	20(4)	1(0)

Values in parentheses are numbers of stenoses.

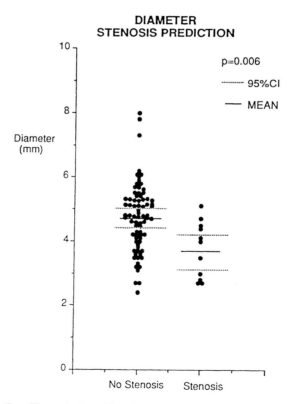

Fig. 2. The relationship of preoperative graft diameter to the subsequent development of vein graft stenosis.

Table 2. The diameter of 3mm as a predictor of graft stenosis or a compliance value of 0.15 or less as a predictor of graft stenosis

	Compliance (%)	Diameter (mm)
Sensitivity	91	57
Specificity	94	91
Positive predictive value	67	36
Negative predictive value	99	96
Accuracy	93	87

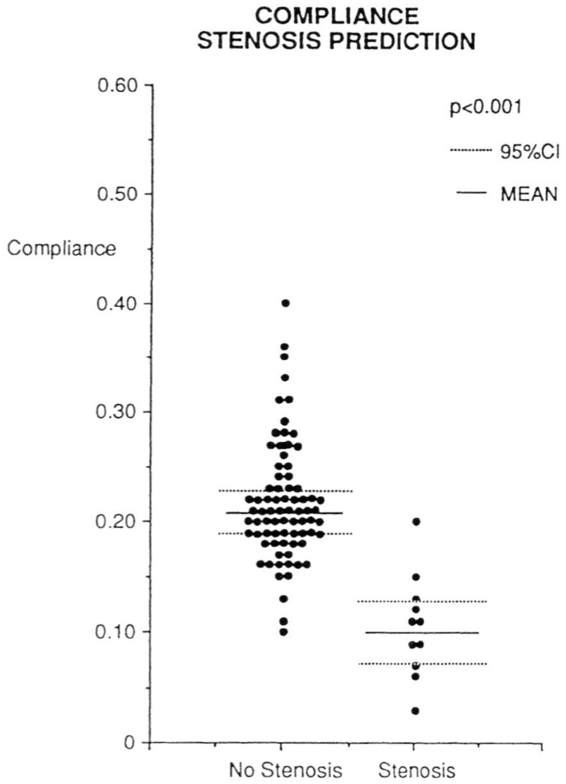

Fig. 3. The lowest compliance value found in the vein as a predictor of subsequent vein graft stenosis (compliance shown in percentage per mmHg)

PRE-BYPASS ASSESSMENT

Preoperatively, an assessment of vein anatomy, compliance and internal diameter are all feasible. Previously, venography was the gold standard as it can accurately replicate the operative findings,[46] though it is not reliable in defining vein calibre, and perforators may lead to poor filling of the proximal system.[47] Inability to assess depth means that vein mapping, and hence the aiding of placement of incisions, may not be possible.[48] In many units, duplex Doppler is now the mainstay for preoperative venous assessment. Information on vein wall morphology,[49] blood flow, calibre, varicosities and tributaries, as well as cusps, is given.[50] Duplex accurately predicts vein location, size and quality[51] and is better than venography in assessing calf vein diameter.[48] In one series, duplex directly diagnosed pre-existing venous disease, with respect to wall thickness, calcification and occlusion, in 62% of cases.[52]

An extension of the use of duplex in the structural assessment of vein has been proposed.[45] Compliance measurements, made using a duplex scanner with venous occlusion for distension, have been compared with vein histology and found to be significantly smaller in veins with moderate or severe pre-existing intimal hyperplasia. As noted earlier, there is also a positive correlation with vein graft stenosis, and hence preoperative compliance measurements may be a predictor of vein graft outcome (Fig. 2).

INTRAOPERATIVE ASSESSMENT

The intraoperative assessment of vein quality, and the identification of pre-existing intimal hyperplasia, has hitherto been difficult. However, identification of hyperplastic but otherwise 'normal' vein at operation might indicate a graft requiring intensive surveillance, or even dictate that an alternative conduit be used. Visualization and palpation, whilst important, are inaccurate, though irrigation of a vein via an umbilical feeding catheter, or failure to pass a catheter, may identify graft thickening.[52] It is not always possible, particularly in very distal bypasses, to spare enough vein for histological analysis. Furthermore, results are not immediately available and can have no bearing on the intraoperative course. However, a prospective trial by Wilson et al.[53] evaluated angioscopy in this role, using a novel semiquantitative grading system for vein scoring. Lesions detected by angioscopy included haemorrhagic mural plaques, flimsy intraluminal strands, webs and mobile and adherent thrombus. There was a significant association between both angioscopy scores and semiquantitative vein histology scores, and between angioscopy scores and graft outcome, as shown in Table 3.[53]

A further role for angioscopy has been advocated. Completion arteriography has limitations; the proximal graft is not visualized, no haemodynamic information is provided and retained valves and cusps may be missed.[54] Angioscopy has been proposed as an effective and relatively atraumatic way of assessing a bypass graft; immediate identification and correction of incomplete valvulotomy, identification of persistent side branches and assessment of anastomotic integrity are all possible.[55] Some authors claim superiority for angioscopy over arteriography.[56,57] Despite these applications, angioscopy remains an underutilized tool in arterial reconstruction.

Table 3. The association between angioscopy grade and graft outcome (χ^2 test compares 'failed' grafts (stenosis + occlusion) with normal grafts)

| | Semi quantitative angioscopy grade | | | |
	0	1	2	3
Occlusion before 30 days	0	0	3	8
Occlusion/stenosis after 30 days	0	1	3	1
Patent graft	7	9	6	0
$\chi^2 = 22.00$				
$p<0.001$				

LABORATORY ASSESSMENT

Whilst not strictly identifying structural predictors of graft stenosis, a number of methods of laboratory identification of the 'at risk' graft have been suggested. Chan[58] has investigated the characteristics of human vascular smooth muscle cells in culture and found that cell growth, and heparin inhibition of that growth, is a characteristic of an individual patient which is preserved or unmasked in culture. Heparin resistance in culture was clearly associated with peripheral bypass graft restenosis. Hence cellular heparin resistance may be a risk factor for, and predictive of, restenosis. Other investigators have used organ culture, which is an established model of intimal hyperplasia.[59] Pre-bypass intimal thickness has been correlated with the development of neointimal hyperplasia after 14 days in organ culture.[60] This suggests that veins with pre-bypass changes are more likely to develop graft stenoses *in vivo*. This has been disputed however by another series where there was no such correlation and, in addition, a clinical series showed no association between the behaviour of vein in culture and the development of graft stenosis *in vivo*.[39] Systemic factors may be predictive and these are dealt with elsewhere in this book. There is no reliable method at present for predicting vein graft failure in the laboratory.

CONCLUSION

Despite evolving operative techniques, there has been little improvement in graft patency rates in peripheral bypass surgery. This represents two failings; a failure to fully understand, and hence to manipulate, the pathophysiological mechanisms implicated in graft failure, and a failure to recognize the concept of preoperative vein quality and its implications for graft patency at an earlier stage.

The technology is now becoming available to allow a detailed assessment of vein quality prior to its use as a conduit. Such assessment will ensure that each patient receives a bypass comprising the best quality vein available. Whilst it is recognized that the quality of vein eventually used may not be optimal, it may indicate a patient who requires more intensive graft surveillance and may dictate that, even in distal bypass surgery, recourse to a synthetic conduit is the better option. It is incumbent upon each surgeon to make use of these techniques if bypass patency and limb salvage rates are to be improved.

REFERENCES

1. Michaels JM: Choice of materials for above-knee femoro-popliteal bypass graft. *Br J Surg* **76:** 7–14, 1989
2. Tilanus HW, Obertop H, Van Urk H: Saphenous vein or PTFE for femoropopliteal bypass – A prospective randomised trial. *Ann Surg* **202:** 780–782, 1985
3. Szilagyi DE, Elliot JP, Hageman JH *et al.*: Biologic fate of autogenous vein implants as arterial sustitutes – Clinical, angiographic and histologic observations in femoro-popliteal operations for atherosclerosis. *Ann Surg* **178:** 232–246, 1973
4. Evans WG, Hayes JP, Vermilion BD: Effect of a failed distal reconstruction on the level of amputation. *Am J Surg* **160:** 217–220, 1990
5. LiCalzi LK, Stansel HC: Failure of reversed autogenous saphenous vein femoropoliteal grafting: Pathophysiology and prevention. *Surgery* **91:** 352–358, 1982
6. Taylor RS, McFarland RJ, Cox MI: An investigation into the causes of failure of PTFE grafts. *Eur J Vasc Surg* **1:** 335–343, 1987
7. Stept LL, Flinn WR, McCarthy WJ *et al.*: Technical defects as a cause of early graft failure after femorodistal bypass surgery. *Arch Surg* **122:** 599–604, 1987
8. Kehler M, Albrechtsson U, Alwmark A *et al.*: Intra-operative digital angiography as a control of the *in-situ* saphenous vein bypass graft. *Acta Radiol* **29:** 645–648, 1988
9. Bush HL, Corey CA, Nabseth DC: Distal *in situ* saphenous vein grafts for limb salvage – Increased operative blood flow and post-operative patency. *Am J Surg* **145:** 542–548, 1983
10. Gannon MX, Goldman MD, Simms MH *et al.*: Peri-operative complications of *in situ* vein bypass. *Ann Roy Coll Surg Eng* **74:** 252–255, 1987
11. Shearman CP, Gannon MX, Gwynn BR, Simms MH: A clinical method for the detection of arteriovenous fistulas during *in situ* great saphenous vein bypass. *J Vasc Surg* **4:** 578–581, 1986
12. Hollier LH: Cardiac evaluation in patients with vascular disease – Overview: A practical approach. *J Vasc Surg* **15:** 726–729, 1992
13. Charlesworth D, Harris PL, Cave FD, Taylor L: Undetected aortoiliac insufficiency: A reason for early failure of saphenous vein bypass grafts for obstruction of the superficial femoral artery. *Br J Surg* **62:** 567–570, 1975
14. Szilagyi DE, Hageman JH, Smith RF *et al.*: Autogenous vein grafting in femoropopliteal atheroclerosis: The limit of its effectiveness. *Surgery* **86:** 836–51, 1979
15. Cutler BS, Thompson JE, Keinasser LJ, Hempel GK: Autogenous saphenous vein femoro-popliteal bypass analysis of 298 cases. *Surgery* **79:** 325–331, 1976
16. Brewster DC, Lasalle AJ, Robison JG *et al.*: Femoropoliteal graft failures: Clinical consequences of success of secondary reconstructions. *Arch Surg* **118:** 1043–1047, 1983
17. Moody P, Gould DA, Harris PL: Vein graft surveillance improves patency in femoropopliteal bypass. *Eur J Vasc Surg* **4:** 117–121, 1990
18. Davies MG, Hagen PO: Pathobiology of intimal hyperplasia. *Br J Surg* **81:** 1254–1269, 1994
19. Brody WR, Angell WW, Kosek JC: Histologic fate of the venous coronary artery bypass in dogs. *Am J Path* **66:** 111–130, 1972
20. Whittlemore AD, Clowes AW, Couch NP, Mannick JA: Secondary femoropopliteal reconstruction. *Ann Surgery* **193:** 35–42, 1981
21. Morris PE, Hessel SJ, Couch NP, Adams DF: Surgery and the progression of the occlusive process in patients with peripheral vascular disease. *Radiology* **124:** 343–348, 1977

22. DePalma RG: Atherosclerosis in vascular grafts. *Atheroscler Rev* **6:** 147–176, 1979
23. Brewster DC, Waltman AC, O'Hara PJ, Darling RC: Femoral artery pressure during aortography. *Circulation* **60:** 120–124, 1979
24. Currie JC, Wilson YG, Davies AH *et al.*: Pulse generated run-off versus dependent doppler ultrasonography for assessment of calf vessel patency. *Br J Surg* **81:** 1448–1456, 1994
25. Sumner DS, Porter DJ, Moore DJ, Winders RE: Digital subtraction angiography: Intravenous and intra-arterial techniques *J Vasc Surg* **2:** 344–353, 1985
26. Beattie D, Golledge J, Hicks RCJ *et al.*: Duplex alone as a diagnostic test for management of lower limb ischaemia *Br J Surg* **83** (Suppl 1): 47, 1996
27. Mills JL, Fujitani RM, Taylor SM: The characteristics and anatomic distribution of lesions that cause reversed vein graft failure: A five-year prospective study *Vasc Surg* **17:** 382–398, 1993
28. Idu MM, Blankenstein JD, De Gier P *et al.*: Impact of a color-flow duplex surveillance programme on infrainguinal vein graft patency: A five-year experience. *J Vasc Surg* **17:** 42–53, 1993
29. Mattos MA, Van Bremmelen PS, Hodgson KJ *et al.*: Does detection of stenoses identified with colour duplex scanning improve infrainguinal graft patency? *J Vasc Surg* **17:** 54–66, 1993
30. Griff MJ, Nicolaides AN, Wolfe JHN: Detection and grading of femorodistal vein graft stenoses: duplex velocity measurements compared with angiography. *J Vasc Surg* **8:** 661–666, 1988
31. Lundell A, Lindblad B, Bergqvist D, Hansen F: Femoropopliteal-crural graft patency is improved by an intensive graft surveillance programme: A prospective randomised study. *J Vasc Surg* **21:** 26–34, 1995
32. Beattie DK, Greenhalgh RM, Davies AH: Vein graft surveillance; Is the case proven? *Ann Roy Coll Surg Eng* **79:** 1–2, 1997
33. Golledge J, Beattie DK, Greenhalgh RM, Davies AH: Have the results of infrainguinal bypass improved with the widespread utilisation of postoperative surveillance? *Eur J Vasc Endovasc Surg* **11:** 388–392, 1996
34. Waller BF, Roberts WC: Remnant saphenous veins after aortocoronary bypass grafting: Analysis of 3394 centimeters of unused vein from 402 patients. *Am J Cardiol* **55:** 65–71, 1985
35. Scott DJA, McMahon JN, Beard JD *et al.*: Histology of the long saphenous vein: a cause of femorodistal bypass failure. *J Cardiovasc Surg* **29:** 84, 1988
36. Davies AH, Magee TR, Baird RN *et al.*: Pre-bypass morphological changes in vein grafts. *Eur J Vasc Surg* **7:** 642–647, 1993
37. Marin ML, Gordon RE, Veith FJ *et al.*: Human greater saphenous vein: histologic and ultrastructural variation. *Cardiovasc Surg* **2:** 56–62, 1994
38. Marin ML, Veith FJ, Panetta TF *et al.*: Saphenous vein biopsy: A predictor of vein graft failure. *J Vasc Surg* **18:** 407–415, 1993
39. Varty K, Porter K, Bell PRF, London NJM: Vein morphology and bypass graft stenosis. *Br J Surg* **83:** 1375–1379, 1996
40. Davies AH, Magee TR, Sheffield E *et al.*: The aetiology of vein graft stenoses. *Eur J Vasc Surg* **8:** 389–394, 1994
41. Taylor LM, Phinney ES, Porter JM *et al.*: The present status of reversed vein bypass for lower extremity revacularisation. *J Vasc Surg* **3:** 288–297, 1986
42. Harris PL, Veith FJ, Shanik GD *et al.*: Prospective randomised comparison of *in situ* and reversed infrapopliteal vein grafts. *Br J Surg* **80:** 173–176, 1993
43. Grigg MJ, Wolfe JHN: Combined reversed and non-reversed upper arm vein for femoro-distal grafting. *Eur J Vasc Surg* **2:** 49–52, 1988
44. Harward TRS, Coe E, Flynn TC, Seeger JM: The use of arm vein conduits during infra geniculate arterial bypass. *J Vasc Surg* **16:** 420–427, 1992
45. Davies AH, Magee TR, Baird RN *et al.*: Vein compliance: A preoperative indicator of vein morphology and of veins at risk of vascular graft stenosis. *Br J Surg* **79:** 1019–1021, 1992
46. Veith FJ, Moss CM, Sprayregen S, Montefusco C: Preoperative saphenous venography in arterial reconstructive surgery of the lower extremity. *Surgery* **85:** 253–256, 1979

47. Harris PL, Nott DM: Venous evaluation for *in situ* bypass surgery. *Ann Chirurg Gynaecol* **81:** 137–140, 1992
48. Leopold PW, Strandall AA, Corson JD *et al.*: Initial experience comparing B-mode imaging and venography of the saphenous vein before *in situ* bypass. *Am J Surg* **152:** 206–210, 1986
49. Kupinsky AM, Evans JM, Khan AM *et al.*: Ultrasonic characteristics of the saphenous vein. *Cardiovasc Surg* **1:** 513–517, 1993
50. Katz ML, Pilla TS, Comerota AJ: Technical aspects of venous duplex imaging. *J Vasc Technol* **12:** 100–102, 1988
51. Seeger JM, Schmidt JH, Flynn TC: Pre-operative saphenous and cephalic vein mapping as an adjunct to reconstructive arterial surgery. *Ann Surg* **205:** 733–739, 1987
52. Panetta TF, Marin ML, Veith FJ *et al.*: Unsuspected pre-existing saphenous vein disease: an unrecognised cause of vein bypass failure. *J Vasc Surg* **15:** 102–112, 1992
53. Wilson YG, Davies AH, Currie IC *et al.*: Angioscopy for quality control of saphenous vein during bypass grafting. *Eur J Vasc Endovasc Surg* **11:** 12–18, 1996
54. Thiele BL, Strandness DE: Accuracy of angioscopic quantification of peripheral atherosclerosis. *Prog Cardiovasc Dis* **26:** 223–236, 1983
55. Fleisher HL, Thompson BW, McCowan TC *et al.*: Angioscopically monitored saphenous vein valvulotomy. *J Vasc Surg* **4:** 360–364, 1986
56. Ritchie JL, Hansen DD, Johnson C *et al.*: Combined mechanical and chemical thrombolysis in an experimental animal model: evaluation by angiography and angioscopy. *Am Heart J* **1:** 64–72, 1990
57. Miller A, Marcaccio EJ, Tannenbaum GA *et al.*: Comparison of angioscopy and angiography for monitoring infra-inguinal bypass vein grafts: Results of a prospective randomised trial. *J Vasc Surg* **17:** 382–398, 1993
58. Chan P: Cell biology of human vascular smooth muscle. *Ann Roy Coll Surg Eng* **76:** 298–303, 1994
59. Soyombo AA, Angelini GD, Bryan AJ: Intimal proliferation in an organ culture of human saphenous vein. *Am J Path* **137:** 1401–1410, 1990
60. Wilson YG, Davies AH, Southgate K *et al.*: The influence of angioscopic vein graft preparation on development of neointimal hyperplasia in an organ culture of human saphenous vein. *Eur J Vasc Endovasc Surg* 1997 (in press)

Fibrinogen as an Inflammatory Mediator in the Development of Vein Graft Pathology

Jonathan Golledge and Janet T. Powell

INTRODUCTION

Saphenous vein has been demonstrated to be the best conduit for femorodistal bypass; however, 20–30% of vein grafts occlude or require revision within 1 year of surgery.[1,2] The reported 5–10% perioperative (30-day) occlusion rate is attributed to technical problems at the time of operation, such as twisting of the bypass conduit, poor distal runoff and hypercoaguable states.[3,4] The principal cause of vein graft failure between 1 and 12 months is the development of focal stenosis within the body of the graft or at the arteriovenous anastomosis.[5,6] Studies in which duplex surveillance is performed report graft stenosis in between 10 and 25% of vein bypasses, with an average being 19% from a recent review of 17 series.[7] Tight stenosis has been shown to be associated with an increased risk of thrombotic graft occlusion; however, not all stenoses are progressive. Duplex surveillance allows identification of graft stenosis but does not necessarily identify the grafts likely to go on to occlude.[8] The patency of revised stenotic grafts is better than that of revised occluded grafts.[1] However, since intensive surveillance probably means revising some grafts which may never have occluded, some vascular surgeons do not feel duplex surveillance is justified. Therapy which prevented the development of graft stenosis would therefore be of great importance.

Present understanding of the mechanisms leading to graft stenosis have come from a number of different types of study including experimental studies in animal models, *in vitro* studies of human tissue or cultured cells and clinical studies of predictors of graft stenosis. These studies have highlighted a number of potential factors associated with the development of graft stenosis, including the characteristics of vein used (see chapter by AH Davies), injury to the vein at the time of graft preparation and anastomosis, the response of the vein to its new haemodynamic environment and the interaction between the vein and blood elements.[9–11] These factors should not be considered in isolation since it is likely that graft stenosis has a multifactorial aetiology.

CLINICAL STUDIES IDENTIFYING PREDICTORS OF GRAFT FAILURE AND STENOSIS

Factors associated with graft failure

A number of studies have demonstrated high plasma fibrinogen concentration to be significantly associated with infrainguinal vein graft occlusion.[12,13] Both Harris *et al.*[13]

and Wiseman *et al.*[12] demonstrated plasma fibrinogen concentration to be the most significant biochemical predictor of vein graft occlusion. Wiseman and colleagues studied 157 patients following infrainguinal vein bypass.[12] One-year patency for patients with below median fibrinogen concentration was 90% compared with 57% for patients with above median fibrinogen concentration (p<0.0002).[12] Smoking was also associated with vein graft occlusion, but at a less significant level: the 1-year patency was 84% for non-smokers (serum thiocyanate <70 μmol/l) and 63% for smokers (serum thiocyanate >70 μmol/l), p=0.02. These two factors of plasma fibrinogen and smoking are not unrelated, since smoking is associated with raised plasma fibrinogen levels.[14] Other factors which influence plasma fibrinogen concentration include age, obesity, the acute phase response, diabetes and genetic status.[15]

Factors associated with graft stenosis

Relatively few studies have investigated predictors of graft stenosis. Hicks *et al.* studied 75 patients following infrainguinal vein bypass with duplex surveillance to identify factors associated with graft stenosis.[16] From a range of patient and biochemical factors assessed by multiple regression analysis, high plasma fibrinogen was identified as the single factor associated with graft stenosis (p=0.003). By life table analysis, at 1-year only 46% of grafts remained free of stenosis in patients with above median fibrinogen concentrations compared with 84% of grafts in patients with below median fibrinogen concentrations.[16] Cheshire *et al.* also found an association between plasma fibrinogen concentration and vein graft stenosis.[17] These authors studied the factors associated with occlusion or stenosis of 79 infrainguinal bypass grafts; this was a mixed series and 56 were vein grafts and 23 prosthetic grafts. Smoking, plasma fibrinogen, and plasma 5-hydroxy-tryptamine were associated with graft stenosis on univariate analysis; at a similar level, p=0.001, no multivariate analysis was performed.[17]

VIRCHOWS TRIAD

The factors predicting thrombosis have been traditionally defined by Virchow's triad: comprising circulatory stasis, damage to the lumen of the vessel and hypercoagulable states (Fig. 1). High plasma fibrinogen by providing further substrate for the formation of fibrin would be expected to be a risk factor for thrombosis. Indeed plasma fibrinogen concentration has been demonstrated as a risk factor for thromboembolism at sites other than infrainguinal vein grafts, including the coronary and carotid arteries.[14] Thus patients with high plasma fibrinogen would be expected to be at increased risk of thrombosis. This rational would explain the association between vein graft occlusion and plasma fibrinogen concentration. However, other theories are required to explain the association between vein graft stenosis and plama fibrinogen concentration.

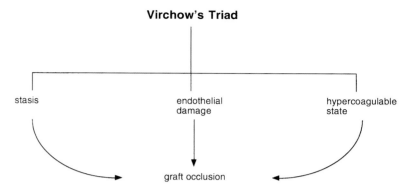

Fig. 1. Virchow's triad.

EXPERIMENTAL STUDIES

The clinical studies discussed above suggested an important role for fibrinogen in the aetiology of vein graft stenosis, the mechanisms which may be involved are beginning to be unravelled by *in vitro* studies.

Fibrinogen and leukocytes

In the experimental situation in animal models of vein bypass, leukocyte accumulation is an early event, with a dense collection of platelets, blood factors and leukocytes developing at the site of endothelial injury within 24 hours of graft implantation. Inhibiting leukocyte accumulation with antibodies to leukocyte markers, such as anti-CD 18, has been shown to decrease the development of intimal hyperplasia in rabbits.[18] Studies in cultured cells have demonstrated that leukocytes are able to stimulate the release of smooth muscle cell mitogens from endothelial cells.[19] Accumulated leukocytes may also be of importance by releasing oxygen-derived free radicals and lysosomal proteinases which by direct effects on smooth muscle cells and also modulation of endothelial products, e.g. inactivation of nitric oxide, may influence smooth muscle cell proliferation and migration.[20] The role of leukocytes in the development of vein graft stenoses is further suggested by their demonstration at the site of stenoses explanted from failing grafts.[21]

Studies on cultured cells, both human venous umbilical cells (HUVEC) and human saphenous endothelial cells, have demonstrated that fibrinogen facilitates leukocyte adhesion and transmigration across endothelial monolayers.[22,23] The specific endothelial-fibrinogen and leukocyte-fibrinogen receptors involved have been identified. A site on the γ-chain of fibrinogen, termed γ-3 (sequence 117-133 of the γ-chain) binds to the endothelial receptor ICAM-1.[22,24] Whereas, a site on the D fragment of fibrinogen termed P1 (sequence 190-202 of the γ-chain) binds to the leukocyte receptor CD11b/CD18 (MAC-1).[25] Fibrinogen appears to be able to act as a bridging molecule between leukocytes and vascular endothelium to facilitate both leukocyte adhesion and transmigration (Fig. 2).

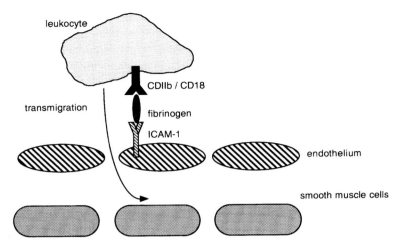

Fig. 2. Fibrinogen acts as a bridging molecule to facilitate leukocyte adhesion and transmigration.

Thus, soon after vein grafting, fibrinogen has the potential to facilitate leukocyte adhesion to the lumen of the graft. This possibility is made more likely by the demonstration that the endothelial fibrinogen receptor ICAM-1 is shear stress responsive, and in an *in vitro* model of vein bypass the endothelial concentration of this adhesin is increased two-fold as early as 45 minutes in response to arterial flow.[26,27] In addition to ICAM-1, leukocyte adhesion and transmigration is also dependent on a number of other leukocyte adhesins, including the selectins, and soluble factors, such as monocyte chemotactic factor and nitric oxide.[28] Thus the overall effect of this increase in ICAM-1 concentration soon after vein grafting requires further investigation.

Fibrinogen and platelets

The endothelial loss and injury that results from saphenous vein preparation and anastomosis would be expected to encourage platelet adhesion soon after vein grafting, and this has been demonstrated in animal vein grafts.[29] Platelet adhesion takes place at the site of endothelial loss where collagen is exposed to interact with plasma von Willebrand factor (VIII:vWF) and platelet glycoprotein Ib (Fig. 3). Following adhesion, platelets release the contents of their cytoplasmic granules, including platelet-derived growth factor (PDGF), and expose a fibrinogen receptor, the glycoprotein IIb-IIIa complex on their surface. Fibrinogen bridges between IIb-IIIa complexes to bind platelets into activated aggregates (Fig. 3).[30] Subsequent activation of the coagulation pathway results in the formation of a vessel wall thrombus.

This sequence of events, resulting in a localized collection of blood cells and constituents on the vessel wall, has long been suspected of playing an important role

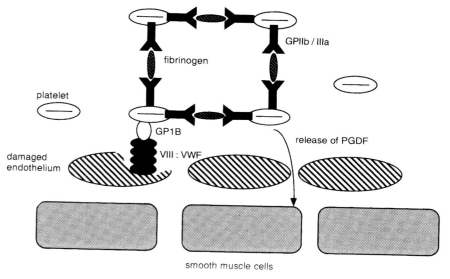

Fig. 3. Role of fibrinogen in platelet aggregation at the site of vessel wall injury.

in subsequent vessel wall pathology. In the 1970s Ross and colleagues proposed that platelet accumulation at the vessel wall was involved in the subsequent development of atherosclerosis.[31] More recently, the accumulating platelets with release of smooth muscle cell mitogens and chemoattractants, such as PDGF, have been suggested to play a role in the development of intimal hyperplasia. However, the use of antiplatelet aggregants, such as aspirin has been unsuccessful in improving the patency of vein bypass or the restenosis rate following angioplasty.[32,33] This appears to reflect the ineffectiveness of such drugs in inhibiting platelet aggregation.[34] Recently studies using a more powerful means of inhibiting platelet aggregation have reported more promising results in reducing the development of restenosis following coronary angioplasty;[35] c7E3, a monoclonal antibody against the fibrinogen receptor platelet glycoprotein (GP) IIb-IIIa inhibits platelet aggregation in man by 80%.[36] The Evaluation of c7E3 Fab in Preventing Ischaemic Complications of High-Risk Angioplasty (EPIC) has recently reported reduced 30-day postangioplasty ischaemic events[35] and clinical restenosis rates at 6 months in a large study randomizing over 2000 patients.[37] Whether GP IIb-IIIa plays a similarly important role in the development of vein graft stenosis is unknown. However, it is possible that part of the association between fibrinogen and graft stenosis may be explained by encouragement of platelet aggregation at the site of endothelial injury with resultant release of smooth muscle cell mitogens (Fig. 3).

Fibrinogen and endothelial-smooth muscle cell signalling

Recent work has demonstrated that fibrinogen has vasomotor effects on saphenous vein, involving cell signalling via ATP-dependent potassium channels.[27] Addition of fibrinogen to human saphenous vein segments placed in an organ bath produces a dose-dependent relaxation. The effect is endothelium-dependent, partially inhibited by antibodies to ICAM-1 and abolished by potassium channel blockers, such as glibenclamide and tetraethylammonium. Thus it appears that fibrinogen binding to ICAM-1 induces the release of an endothelial vasorelaxant.[27] This vasorelaxant does not appear to be nitric oxide or a prostanoid since the relaxation is not significantly inhibited by the nitric oxide synthase inhibitor L-NAME or indomethacin, and is most probably endothelium-derived hyperpolarizing factor.[27] Subsequent studies have demonstrated that this fibrinogen mediated vasorelaxation is linked to the tyrosine phosphorylation of endothelial proteins. It is possible that the association between plasma fibrinogen concentration and vein graft stenosis, and the vasomotor effects exerted by fibrinogen may be related in that the pathway leading to the release of vasoactive mediators may be coupled to the synthesis of smooth muscle mitogens (Fig. 4). This pathway appears to be even more active in saphenous vein when it is placed in the arterial circulation. Segments of saphenous vein exposed to arterial flow *in vitro* demonstrate a significant increase in fibrinogen mediated endothelium-dependent relaxation.[27]

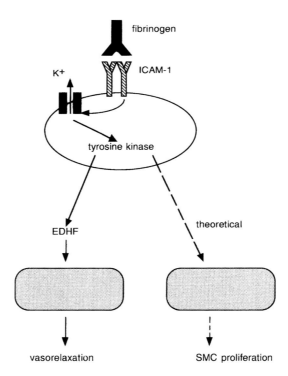

Fig. 4. The pathway of fibrinogen mediated vaso-relaxation in saphenous vein.

Fibrin and fibrinopeptides

The products of enzymic action on fibrinogen may also have a role in vein graft failure (Fig. 5). Early in the process of fibrinolysis the carboxyl terminus of the α-chain as well as β15-42 are cleaved from fibrin, followed by more complete enzymic release of fragments E and D;[38] β15-42 is chemotactic for neutrophils and β1-42 induces endothelial cell retraction and fibroblast migration.[39] Products arising from the conversion of fibrinogen to fibrin may have additional effects on cellular proliferation in the vessel wall. There is evidence from animal studies that local implantation of fibrinopeptide B into animal vessels stimulates smooth muscle proliferation.[40] Fibrinogen degradation products have been demonstrated to release growth factors from endothelial cells,[41] and may have mitogenic effects in the vessel wall.[41,42] Fibrin also may interact with specific receptors on the endothelium to release inflammatory mediators, such as interleukin-8.[43] Moreover, both fibrin and its degradation products impair the release of nitric oxide from cultured endothelial cells.[44]

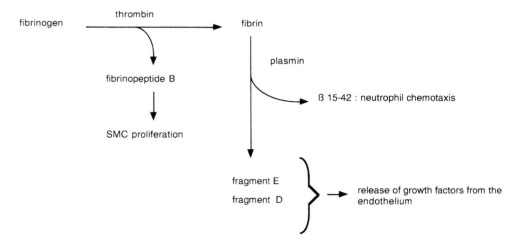

Fig. 5. Effects of fibrinogen breakdown products. SMC: Smooth muscle cell.

SUMMARY

Raised plasma fibrinogen is a powerful predictor of the development of vein graft stenosis. Fibrinogen appears to have an important influence on the interaction at and within the vessel wall of the vein graft. Fibrinogen has been demonstrated to enhance leukocyte accumulation, platelet aggregation and signalling from endothelial to medial smooth muscle cells (Figs 2–4). These effects are likely to have detrimental effects and appear to be exaggerated in the newly implanted vein graft. It is hoped that further understanding of these fibrinogen-saphenous vein interactions will lead to therapeutic interventions which will inhibit the development of vein graft stenosis.

REFERENCES

1. Bandyk DF, Bergamini TM, Towne JB *et al*.: Durability of vein graft revision: The outcome of secondary procedures. *J Vasc Surg* **13**: 200–210, 1991
2. Harris PL, Veith FJ, Shanik GD *et al*.: Prospective randomized comparison of *in situ* and reversed infrapopliteal vein grafts. *Br J Surg* **80**: 173–176, 1993
3. Donaldson MC, Mannick JA, Whittemore AD: Causes of primary graft failure after *in situ* vein bypass grafting. *J Vasc Surg* **15**: 113–120, 1992
4. Stept LL, Flinn WR, McCarthy WJ *et al*.: Technical defects as a cause of early graft failure after femorodistal bypass. *Arch Surg* **122**: 599–604, 1987
5. Berkowitz HD, Greenstein S, Barker CF, Perloff LJ: Late failure of reversed vein bypass grafts. *Ann Surg* **210**: 782–786, 1989
6. Mills JL: Mechanisms of vein graft failure: the location, distribution, and characteristics of lesions that predispose to graft failure. *Semin Vasc Surg* **6**: 78–91, 1993
7. Golledge J, Beattie DK, Greenhalgh RM, Davies AH: Have the results of infrainguinal bypass improved with the widespread utilisation of postoperative surveillance? *Eur J Vasc Endovasc Surg* **11**: 388–393, 1996
8. Brennan JA, Walsh AKM, Beard JD *et al*.: The role of simple non-invasive testing in infrainguinal vein graft surveillance. *Eur J Vasc Endovasc Surg* **5**: 13–17, 1991
9. Panetta TF, Marin MI, Veith FJ *et al*.: Unsuspected pre-existing saphenous vein disease: An unrecognised cause of vein bypass failure. *J Vasc Surg* **15**: 102–112, 1992
10. Soyombo AA, Angelini GD, Newby AC: Neointimal formation is promoted by surgical preparation and inhibited by cyclic nucleotides in human saphenous vein organ cultures. *J Cardiovasc Surg* **109**: 2–12, 1995
11. Dobrin PD, Littooy FN, Endean ED: Mechanical factors predisposing to intimal hyperplasia and medial thickening in autogenous vein grafts. *Surgery* **105**: 393–400, 1989
12. Wiseman SA, Kenchington GF, Dain R *et al*.: The influence of smoking and plasma factors on femoropopliteal vein graft patency. *Br Med J* **299**: 643–646, 1989
13. Harris PL, Harvey DR, Bliss BP: The importance of plasma lipid, glucose, insulin and fibrinogen in femoropopliteal surgery. *Br J Surg* **65**: 197–200, 1978
14. Meade TW, Iveson J, Stirling J: Effects of changes in smoking and other characteristics on clotting factors and the risk of ischaemic heart disease. *Lancet* **ii**: 986–988, 1987
15. Humphries SE, Dubowitz M, Cook M *et al*.: Role of genetic variation at the fibrinogen locus in determination of plasma fibrinogen concentrations. *Lancet* **i**: 1452–1454, 1987
16. Hicks RCJ, Ellis M, Mir-Hasseine R *et al*.: The influence of fibrinogen concentration on the development of vein graft stenosis. *Eur J Vasc Endovasc Surg* **9**: 415–420, 1995
17. Cheshire N, Barradas M, Chambler A *et al*.: Systemic factors in early graft failure and stenosis. *Br J Surg* **81**: 617, 1994
18. Kling D, Fingerle J, Harlan JM: Inhibition of leukocyte extravasation with a monclonal antibody to CD18 during formation of experimental intimal thickening in rabbit carotid arteries. *Arterioscler Thromb* **12**: 997–1007, 1992
19. Totani L, Piccoli A, Pellegrini G *et al*.: Polymorphonuclear leukocytes enhance release of growth factors by cultured endothelial cells. *Arterioscler Thromb* **14**: 125–132, 1994
20. Weiss SJ: Tissue destruction by neutrophils. *N Engl J Med* **320**: 365–376, 1989
21. Kockx MM, Cambier BA, Bortier HE *et al*.: Foam cell replication and smooth muscle cell apoptosis in human saphenous vein grafts. *Histopathology* **25**: 365–371, 1994
22. Languino LR, Plescia J, Duperray A *et al*.: Fibrinogen mediates leukocyte adhesion to vascular endothelium through an ICAM-1 dependent pathway. *Cell* **73**: 1423–1434, 1993
23. Languino LR, Duperry A, Joganic KJ *et al*.: Regulation of leukocyte-endothelium interaction: transendothelial migration by intercellular adhesion molecule-1 fibrinogen recognition. *Proc Natl Acad Sci USA* **92**: 1505–1509, 1995
24. Altieri DC, Duperray A, Plescia J *et al*.: Structural recognition of a novel fibrinogen γ chain sequence (117-133) by intercellular adhesion molecule-1 mediates leukocye-endothelium interaction. *J Biol Chem* **270**: 696–699, 1995
25. Altieri DC, Plescia J, Plow EF: The structural motif glycine 190-valine 202 of the

fibrinogen γ chain interacts with CD11b/CD18 integrin and promotes leukocyte adhesion. *J Biol Chem* **268:** 1847–1853, 1993

26. Golledge J, Turner RJ, Harley SL *et al.*: Response of saphenous vein endothelium to pulsatile arterial flow and circumferential deformation. Presented at The ESVS, Venice, 1996

27. Hicks RCJ, Golledge J, Mir-Hasseine R, Powell JT: Vasoactive effects of fibrinogen on saphenous vein. *Nature* **379:** 818–820, 1996

28. Tedder TF, Steeber DA, Chen A, Engel P: The selectins: vascular adhesion molecules. *FASEB* **9:** 866–873, 1995

29. Clowes AW, Reidy MA: Prevention of stenosis after vascular reconstruction: Pharmacologic control of intimal hyperplasia: A review. *J Vasc Surg* **13:** 885–891, 1991

30. Houdijk WP, Sakariassen KS, Nievelstein PF, Sixma JJ: Role of factor VII-von Willebrand factor and fibronectin in the interaction of platelets in flowing blood with monomeric and fibrillar human collagen types I and III. *J Clin Invest* **75:** 531–540, 1985

31. Ross R, Raines E, Bowen-Pope D: Growth factors from platelets, monocytes, and endothelium: their role in cell proliferation. *Ann N Y Acad Sci* **397:** 18–24, 1982

32. McCollum C, Alexander C, Kenchington G *et al.*: Antiplatelet drugs in femoropopliteal vein bypasses: a multicentre trial. *J Vasc Surg* **13:** 150–162, 1991

33. Schwartz L, Bourassa MG, Lesperance J *et al.*: Aspirin and dipyridamole in the prevention of restenosis after percutaneous transluminal coronary angioplasty. *N Engl J Med* **318:** 1714–1719, 1988

34. Kiss RG, Lu HR, Roskams T *et al.*: Time course of the effects of a single bolus injection of F(ab')2 fragments of the antiplatelet GPIIb/IIIa antibody 7E3 on arterial graft occlusion, platelet aggregation, and bleeding time in dogs. *Arterioscler Thromb* **14:** 367–374, 1994

35. The EPIC investigators. Use of a monoclonal antibody directed against the platelet glycoprotein IIb/IIIa receptor in high risk coronary angioplasty. *N Engl J Med* **330:** 956–961, 1994

36. Turner NA, Moake JL, Kamat SG *et al.*: Comparative real time effects on platelet adhesion and aggregation under flowing conditions of *in vivo* aspirin, heparin, and monoclonal antibody fragment against glycoprotein IIb/IIIa. *Circulation* **91:** 1354–1362, 1995

37. Topol EJ, Califf RM, Weisman HF *et al.*: Randomised trial of coronary intervention with antibody against platelet IIb/IIIa integrin for reduction of clinical restenosis: results at six months. The EPIC Investigators. *Lancet* **34:** 1434–1435, 1994

38. Rowland F, Donovan M, Picciano P *et al.*: Fibrin-mediated vascular injury. Identification of fibrin peptides that mediate endothelial cell retraction. *Am J Pathol* **117:** 418–428, 1984

39. Skogen W, Senior R, Griffin G, Wilner G: Fibrinogen-derived peptide B beta 1-42 is a multidomained neutrophil chemoattractant. *Blood* **71:** 1475–1479, 1988

40. Kadowaki MH, Singh TM, Zarins TM *et al.*: Role of fibrinopeptide B in early atherosclerotic lesion formation. *Am J Surg* **160:** 156–159, 1990

41. Lorenzet R, Sobel JH, Bini A, Witte LD: Low molecular weight fibrinogen degradation products stimulate the release of growth factors from endothelial cells. *Thromb Haemost* **68:** 357–363, 1992

42. Stirk CM, Kochhar A, Smith EB, Thompson WD: Presence of growth-stimulating fibrin degradation products containing fragment E in human atherosclerotic plaques. *Atherosclerosis* **103:** 159–169, 1993

43. Qi J, Kreutzer DL: Fibrin activation of vascular endothelial cells. *J Immunol* **155:** 867–876, 1995

44. Freedman JE, Fabian A, Loscalzo J: Impaired EDRF production by endothelial cells exposed to fibrin and FDP. *Am J Physiol* **268:** C520–526, 1995

Proliferation Response After Angioplasty

Richard D. Kenagy and Alexander W. Clowes

INTRODUCTION

Successful enlargement of a stenotic artery after percutaneous transluminal angioplasty involves extensive injury to the vessel wall with increased lumen size resulting from fracture and dissection of the plaque, plaque reduction, and stretching of non-plaque areas of the vessel. The arterial response to injury has been extensively studied in various animal models. Although matrix formation, reorganization of thrombus and vasospasm are also major components of the response to arterial injury, in this brief review we will focus on proliferation and migration of smooth muscle cells (SMCs) and the role of some selected growth factors and proteinases.

CELLULAR ASPECTS OF THE RESPONSE TO INJURY

The most thoroughly understood model of arterial injury is the balloon-injured rat carotid artery. The response of the wall in this model occurs in three waves of cellular activity.[1] The first wave is medial SMC replication, which begins at about 24 hours and returns to baseline by 4 weeks.[2] The second wave is medial SMC migration into the intima starting after 3–4 days.[2,3] If a quiescent endothelial layer is regenerated within several days, SMCs do not migrate into the intima despite an initial proliferative response.[4] Some evidence suggests that mononuclear leukocytes may stimulate SMC migration.[5] The third wave is intimal SMC proliferation, which peaks at 4 days and is essentially complete by 2 weeks. These intimal SMCs are phenotypically different from medial SMC.[6] It is not clear if this results from the expansion of a subpopulation of genetically distinct medial SMCs or is caused by local regulatory factors. Finally, intimal matrix accumulates for up to 4 weeks, although the number of SCMs remains constant.[2]

Although the arteries of larger animals, such as pig and baboon, demonstrate a proliferative response to injury qualitatively similar to the rat,[7,8] there are also clear differences between rats and these animals. Examples are the response to angiotensin-converting enzyme inhibitors[9,10] and to heparin.[11,12] In human vessels proliferation is low in primary and restenotic arterial lesions, irrespective of the time after angioplasty.[13–15] Unlike the animal vessels, these diseased human arteries contain intimal lesions populated with inflammatory cells, vasa vasorum and lipids. One approach to modelling the complexity of the human atherosclerotic artery has been to perform balloon injury experiments on cholesterol-fed animals.[16–18] An additional aspect of the response to injury in arteries of these animals is macrophage proliferation.

The role of adventitial proliferation after injury has largely been ignored.[19] Although complete medial fracture allows adventitial fibroblasts to migrate into the intima and proliferate,[20] whether this occurs in the absence of complete medial rupture is not known. Also, while there is evidence for an inhibitory effect of the adventitia on SMC proliferation and migration[2,21] manipulation of the adventitia by occlusion of vasa vasorum[22] and non-restrictive cuffing[23] stimulates neointimal formation.

SOME GROWTH FACTORS IMPORTANT TO THE INJURY RESPONSE

Fibroblast growth factor (FGF)

The first wave of medial SMC proliferation in the injured rat carotid is mediated by basic fibroblast growth factor (bFGF)[24] released from damaged SMC; bFGF also stimulates endothelial cell proliferation[25] and medial SMC migration.[26] It does not play a role in intimal proliferation,[24] although large doses of bFGF give a modest stimulation of intimal SMC growth.[27]

Platelet derived growth factor (PDGF)

The major effect of PDGF is the stimulation of SMC migration from the media to the intima.[28,29] Infusion of PDGF[28] or the release of PDGF by platelets after injury[30] has little or no effect on SMC proliferation. The PDGF A and B chains and PDGF-β receptor are expressed in human coronary arteries subjected to angioplasty; these molecules might play a role in the subsequent repair.[31]

SOME PROTEINASES INVOLVED IN THE INJURY RESPONSE

Plasminogen activators and matrix metalloproteinases(MMPs)

Urokinase and MMP9 are increased within 1 day of arterial injury, while tissue plasminogen activator (tPA) and activated MMP2 are increased by day 4 or 5.[32,33] Blockade of plasminogen activators with tranexamic acid[29] or of MMPs with tissue inhibitor of metalloproteinase-1 or specific MMP inhibitors[34,35] inhibits SMC migration into the neointima; MMP2 is required for rat SMC migration through a matrix *in vitro*.[36] Of interest, the inhibitory effect of MMP inhibitors on neointimal formation is lost at late times because of increased neointimal proliferation at 7–10 days.[35,37] Mouse studies in which urokinase, plasminogen activator (uPA) inhibitor-1, and tPA are knocked out support the conclusion that urokinase is required for neointimal formation after arterial injury.[38] The uPA receptor is involved in SMC migration *in vitro*.[39,40]

Coagulation cascade

Thrombin, factors X and Xa, and protein S have been shown to be mitogens for SMC *in vitro*.[41,42] Thrombin can also stimulate SMC to secrete PDGF and bFGF.[43] A factor

VIIa inhibitor, tick anticoagulant protein (an Xa inhibitor), and tissue factor pathway inhibitor decrease intimal hyperplasia after arterial injury in rabbits and baboons.[44–47] Hirudin, an inhibitor of thrombin, is able to inhibit intimal hyperplasia in rabbits[48] and baboons.[47] Blockade of platelet aggregation with glycoprotein IIb/IIIa antagonists, such as ReoPro, is effective in preventing occlusion and restenosis after angioplasty.[49] Part of the effect of ReoPro is the result of also blocking the $\alpha_v\beta_3$ integrin, which is needed for SMC migration.[50] These results all support the conclusion that platelet and coagulation factors are probably involved in recruiting cells into the zone of injury.

RELATIONSHIPS AMONG GROWTH FACTORS AND PROTEINASES

In the vessel wall there may be a complex interplay among the plasminogen activators, MMPs and growth factors produced by the cells present. For example, PDGF and bFGF induce MMP1[51,52] and tPA[53] in SMC. In addition, the extracellular portion of a broad array of membrane spanning proteins, such as tumour necrosis factor-α (TNF-α) precursor, L-selectin and TNF receptor, is released by an enzyme, which is inhibited by MMP inhibitors.[15,54] The active ligand binding domain of the bFGF receptor 1 released by MMP2 might act as a bFGF inhibitor.[55] The transforming growth factor (TGF)-β precursor[56] and several MMPs[57] are activated by plasmin. The addition of plasminogen to SMC causes MMP2 activation[7] by an unknown mechanism possibly involving membrane-type MMP-1.[58] MMPs can degrade some serine proteinase inhibitors.[59] Finally, urokinase and MMP2 have been linked with integrin function-MMP2 with $\alpha_v\beta_3$,[60] and urokinase/urokinase receptor with $\beta2$ and $\beta1$[39] integrins. Both $\alpha_v\beta_3$[50] and the urokinase receptor[40] stimulate SMC migration.

ARTERIAL EXPLANTS AND ORGAN CULTURE AS A BRIDGE TO HUMAN DISEASE

Organ and tissue culture methods have been used to study the regulation of arterial SMC proliferation. For example, human aorta in culture develops a thickened intima,[61] which may depend on the endothelium and FGF.[62] Using rat carotids, De Mey and colleagues[63] observed that PDGF had no effect on SMC proliferation, while bFGF stimulated medial, but not extramedial, SMC proliferation. This is similar to the artery *in vivo*. A common problem in these studies is that migrating cells from the adventitia cannot be differentiated from SMC by available markers.[64] A way to avoid this pitfall when studying SMC function is to use arterial explant cultures stripped of adventitia.

We have tested in baboons the hypothesis that explants of arterial media may be a useful model of the response to injury observed *in vivo*. Baboon aortic medial explants can be made by first removing the endothelium, dissecting the inner media from the adventitia and then chopping the media into 1 mm² explants.[7] In the balloon-injured baboon saphenous artery (Fig. 1a) and in explants (Fig. 1b) SMCs enter S phase between 1 and 2 days; MMP9 and uPA are increased *in vivo* 1 day after injury and by 1 or 2 days in the explants (Fig. 2). After a lag of about 4 days SMCs begin migrating out of the explants.[7] This is similar to the lag observed in the injured rat carotid artery.[2] In the baboon artery, migrating SMCs cannot be detected since SMCs are already present in the normal arterial intima. The number of intimal SMCs increases between 4 and 14 days and could be the result of both migration and proliferation.

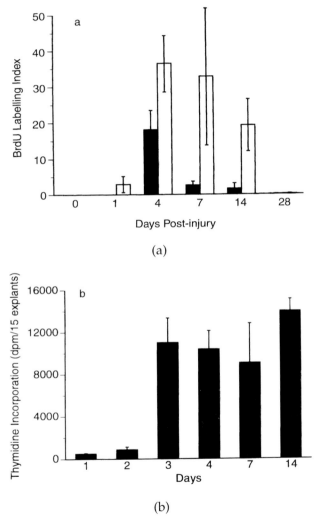

Fig. 1. (a) Time course of changes in medial (closed bars) and intimal (open bars) BrdU labelling index after injury to the saphenous artery (n=3-4). Animals received BrdU 1, 9 and 17 hours before sacrifice. (b) [³H]Thymidine incorporation into DNA by SMCs in explants. Time points represent the end of 24 hour labelling periods (n=4-7). Mean ±SEM. From ref. 7, with permission of The American Heart Association Inc.

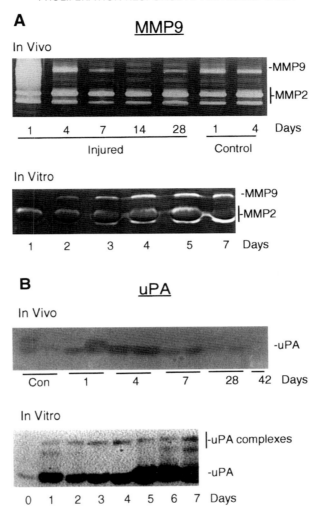

Fig. 2. (a) Gelatin zymography of extracts of saphenous artery or of medium from explants at the indicated times. Control extracts are from the uninjured contralateral artery at the indicated time after injury. Medium from explants was analysed because essentially all MMP9 is secreted and is undetectable in the explants. (b) Casein zymography for plasminogen activators (dark field photography) of extracts of saphenous artery or of explants at the indicated times after injury or explantation. Control extracts *in vivo* are from the contralateral arteries at 1 and 4 days. From ref. 7, with permission of the American Heart Association Inc.

Thus, several cellular responses to injury observed *in vivo* are replicated *in vitro* in medial explants (Fig. 3). Using this explant model we have demonstrated that primate SMC migration through the arterial matrix requires endogenous bFGF, PDGF, MMP9, uPA, tPA and plasminogen.[7,65,66] We have therefore demonstrated in a primate system the role of these growth factors and proteinases in SMC migration through arterial tissue. Having demonstrated proof of concept, we are now studying human saphenous vein and aortic medial explants and have observed MMP9, MMP2 and uPA production and a slower migration of SMC compared with baboon aortic explants.

Arterial Injury

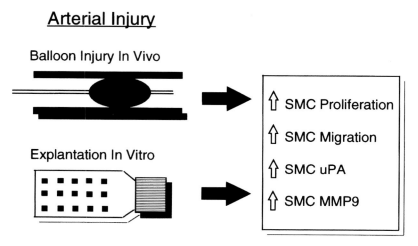

Fig. 3.   Common responses to injury of arteries *in vivo* and *in vitro*.

SUMMARY

The proliferative and migratory responses of SMC are important aspects of the arterial response to injury. Recent data suggest that arterial remodelling may be more important in restenosis after angioplasty compared with intimal hyperplasia,[1,6,67] although proliferation and migration may be more important in the restenotic process associated with stents.[68] In contrast, SMC proliferation, migration and matrix production may be beneficial in the advanced atherosclerotic plaque where the fibrous cap forms a barrier between the blood and the prothrombotic interior. The SMC response may heal and stabilize a ruptured plaque cap or injured vessel after angioplasty. Thus, pharmacological intervention should probably be designed to limit, but not eliminate, SMC growth and migration at the site of injury. Explants of human arteries and vein will be useful for studying SMC functions after injury that are difficult to study in humans. Such models may allow us to test therapeutic strategies that ultimately should prove to be useful in patients.

REFERENCES

1. O'Brien ER, Schwartz SM: Update on the biology and clinical study of restenosis. *Trends Cardiovasc Med* **4:** 169–178, 1994
2. Clowes AW, Reidy MA, Clowes MM: Kinetics of cellular proliferation after arterial injury. I. Smooth muscle growth in the absence of endothelium. *Lab Invest* **49:** 327–333, 1983
3. Clowes AW, Schwartz SM: Significance of quiescent smooth muscle migration in the injured cat carotid artery. *Circ Res* **56:** 139–145, 1985
4. Clowes AW, Clowes MM, Fingerle J, Reidy MA: Kinetics of cellular proliferation after arterial injury. V. Role of acute distension in the induction of smooth muscle proliferation. *Lab Invest* **60:** 360–364, 1989
5. Hancock WW, Adams DH, Wyner LR *et al.*: CD4+ mononuclear cells induce cytokine expression, vascular smooth muscle cell proliferation, and arterial occlusion after endothelial injury. *Am J Pathol* **145:** 1008–1014, 1994
6. Schwartz SM, DeBlois D, O'Brien ERM: The intima – Soil for atherosclerosis and restenosis. *Circ Res* **77:** 445–465, 1995
7. Kenagy RD, Vergel S, Mattsson E *et al.*: The role of plasminogen, plasminogen activators and matrix metalloproteinases in primate arterial smooth muscle cell migration. *Arterioscler Thromb Vasc Biol* **16:** 1373–1382, 1996
8. Ohno T, Gordon D, San H *et al.*: Gene therapy for vascular smooth muscle cell proliferation after arterial injury. *Science* **265:** 781–784, 1994
9. Powell JS, Clozel JP, Muller RKM *et al.*: Inhibitors of angiotensin-converting enzyme prevent myointimal proliferation after vascular injury. *Science* **245:** 186–188, 1989
10. Hanson SR, Powell JS, Dodson T *et al.*: Effects of angiotensin converting enzyme inhibition with cilazapril on intimal hyperplasia in injured arteries and vascular grafts in the baboon. *Hypertension* **18** (Suppl.) 1170–1176, 1991
11. Geary RL, Koyama N, Wang TW *et al.*: Failure of heparin to inhibit intimal hyperplasia in injured baboon arteries: the role of heparin-sensitive and insensitive pathways in the stimulation of smooth muscle cell migration and proliferation. *Circulation* **91:** 2972–2981, 1995
12. Clowes AW, Clowes MM, Kirkman TR *et al.*: Heparin inhibits the expression of tissue-type plasminogen activator by smooth muscle cells in injured rat carotid artery. *Circ Res* **70:** 1128–1136, 1992
13. Gordon D, Reidy MA, Benditt EP, Schwartz SM: Cell proliferation in human coronary arteries. *Proc Natl Acad Sci USA* **87:** 4600–4604, 1990
14. Katsuda S., Coltrera MD, Ross R, Gown AM: Human atherosclerosis: IV. Immunocytochemical analysis of cell activation and proliferation in lesions of young adults. *Am J Pathol* **142:** 1787–1793, 1993
15. Preece G, Murphy G, Ager A: Metalloproteinase-mediated regulation of L-selectin levels on leukocytes. *J Biol Chem* **271:** 11634–11640, 1996
16. Karim MA, Miller DD, Farrar MA *et al.*: Histomorphometric and biochemical correlates of arterial procollagen gene expression during vascular repair after experimental angioplasty. *Circulation* **91:** 2049–2057, 1995
17. Recchia D, Abendschein DR, Saffitz JE, Wickline SA: The biologic behavior of balloon hyperinflation-induced arterial lesions in hypercholesterolemic pigs depends on the presence of foam cells. *Arterioscler Thromb Vasc Biol* **15:** 924–929, 1995
18. Geary RL, Williams JK, Golden D *et al.*: Time course of cellular proliferation, intimal hyperplasia, and remodeling following angioplasty in monkeys with established atherosclerosis – A nonhuman primate model of restenosis. *Arterioscler Thromb Vasc Biol* **16:** 34–43, 1996
19. Doornekamp FNG, Borst C, Post MJ: Endothelial cell recoverage and intimal hyperplasia after endothelium removal with or without smooth muscle cell necrosis in the rabbit carotid artery. *J Vasc Res* **33:** 146–155, 1996
20. Scott NA, Cipolla GD, Ross CE *et al.*: Identification of a potential role for the adventitia in

vascular lesion formation after balloon overstretch injury of porcine coronary arteries. *Circulation* **93:** 2178–2187, 1996

21. Betz E, Fallier-Becker P, Wolburg-Buchholz K, Fotev Z: Proliferation of smooth muscle cells in the inner and outer layers of the tunica media of arteries: An *in vitro* study. *J Cell Physiol* **147:** 385–395, 1991

22. Barker SGE, Talbert A, Cottam S: Arterial intimal hyperplasia after occlusion of the adventitial vasa vasorum in the pig. *Arterioscler Thromb* **13:** 70–77, 1993

23. Kockx MM, De Meyer GRY, Andries LJ *et al.*: The endothelium during cuff-induced neointima formation in the rabbit carotid artery. *Arterioscler Thromb* **13:** 1874–1884, 1993

24. Lindner V, Reidy MA: Proliferation of smooth muscle cells after vascular injury is inhibited by an antibody against basic fibroblast growth factor. *Proc Natl Acad Sci USA* **88:** 3739–3743, 1991

25. Lindner V, Majack RA, Reidy MA: Basic fibroblast growth factor stimulates endothelial regrowth and proliferation in denuded arteries. *J Clin Invest* **85:** 2004–2008, 1990

26. Jackson CL, Reidy MA: Basic fibroblast growth factor: its role in the control of smooth muscle cell migration. *Am J Pathol* **143:** 1024–1031, 1993

27. Lindner V, Lappi DA, Baird A *et al.*: Role of basic fibroblast growth factor in vascular lesion formation. *Circ Res* **68:** 106–113, 1991

28. Jawien A, Bowen-Pope DF, Lindner V *et al.*: Platelet-derived growth factor promotes smooth muscle migration and intimal thickening in a rat model of balloon angioplasty. *J Clin Invest* **89:** 507–511, 1992

29. Jackson CL, Raines EW, Ross R, Reidy MA: Role of endogenous platelet-derived growth factor in arterial smooth muscle cell migration after balloon catheter injury. *Arterioscler Thromb* **13:** 1218–1226, 1993

30. Fingerle J, Johnson R, Clowes AW *et al.*: Role of platelets in smooth muscle cell proliferation and migration after vascular injury in rat carotid artery. *Proc Natl Acad Sci USA* **86:** 8412–8416, 1989

31. Ueda M, Becker AE, Kasayuki N *et al.*: *In situ* detection of platelet-derived growth factor-A and -B chain mRNA in human coronary arteries after percutaneous transluminal coronary angioplasty. *Am J Pathol* **149:** 831–843, 1996

32. Clowes AW, Clowes MM, Au YPT *et al.*: Smooth muscle cells express urokinase during mitogenesis and tissue-type plasminogen activator during migration in injured rat carotid artery. *Circ Res* **67:** 61–67, 1990

33. Zempo N, Kenagy RD, Au YPT *et al.*: Matrix metalloproteinases of vascular wall cells are increased in balloon-injured rat carotid artery. *J Vasc Surg* **20:** 209–217, 1994

34. Forough R, Koyama N, Hasenstab D *et al.*: Overexpression of tissue inhibitor of matrix metalloproteinase-1 inhibits vascular smooth muscle cell functions *in vitro* and *in vivo*. *Circ Res* **79:** 812–820, 1996

35. Bendeck MP, Irvin C, Reidy MA: Inhibition of matrix metalloproteinase activity inhibits smooth muscle cell migration but not neointimal thickening after arterial injury. *Circ Res* **78:** 38–43, 1996

36. Pauly RR, Passaniti A, Bilato C *et al.*: Migration of cultured vascular smooth muscle cells through a basement membrane barrier requires type IV collagenase activity and is inhibited by cellular differentiation. *Circ Res* **75:** 41–54, 1994

37. Zempo N, Koyama N, Kenagy RD *et al.*: Regulation of vascular smooth muscle cell migration and proliferation *in vitro* and in injured rat arteries by a synthetic matrix metalloproteinase inhibitor. *Arterioscler Thromb Vasc Biol* **16:** 28–33, 1996

38. Carmeliet P, Collen D: Gene targeting and gene transfer studies of the plasminogen/plasmin system: Implications in thrombosis, hemostasis, neointima formation, and atherosclerosis. *FASEB J* **9:** 934–938, 1995

39. Wei Y, Lukashev M, Simon DI *et al.*: Regulation of integrin function by the urokinase receptor. *Science* **273:** 1551–1555, 1996

40. Noda-Heiny H, Daugherty A, Sobel BE: Augmented urokinase receptor expression in atheroma. *Arterioscler Thromb* **15:** 37–43, 1995

41. Gasic GP, Arenas CP, Gasic TB, Gasic GJ: Coagulation factors X, Xa and protein S as

potent mitogens of cultured aortic smooth muscle cells. *Proc Natl Acad Sci USA* **89:** 2317–2320, 1992

42. Bar-Shavit R, Benezra M, Eldor A *et al.*: Thrombin immobilized to extracellular matrix is a potent mitogen for vascular smooth muscle cells: nonenzymatic mode of action. *Cell Reg* **1:** 453–463, 1990

43. Fager G: Thrombin and proliferation of vascular smooth muscle cells. *Circ Res* **77:** 645–650, 1995

44. Ragosta M, Gimple LW, Gertz SD *et al.*: Specific factor Xa inhibition reduces restenosis after balloon angioplasty of atherosclerotic femoral arteries in rabbits. *Circulation* **89:** 1262–1271, 1994

45. Jang YS, Guzman LA, Lincoff AM *et al.*: Influence of blockade at specific levels of the coagulation cascade on restenosis in a rabbit atherosclerotic femoral artery injury model. *Circulation* **92:** 3041–3050, 1995

46. Harker LA, Hanson SR, Wilcox JN, Kelly AB: Antithrombotic and antilesion benefits without hemorrhage risks by inhibiting tissue factor pathway. *Haemostasis* **26** (Suppl. 1), 76–82, 1996

47. Harker LA, Hanson SR, Runge MS: Thrombin hypothesis of thrombus generation and vascular lesion formation. *Am J Cardiol* **75:** 12B–17B, 1995

48. Sarembock IJ, Gertz SD, Gimple LW *et al.*: Effectiveness of recombinant desulphatohirudin in reducing restenosis after balloon angioplasty of atherosclerotic femoral arteries in rabbits. *Circulation* **84:** 232–243, 1991

49. Tcheng JE: Glycoprotein IIb/IIIa receptor inhibitors: putting the EPIC, IMPACT II, RESTORE, and EPILOG trials into perspective. *Am J Cardiol* **78:** 35–40, 1996

50. Choi ET, Engel L, Callow AD *et al.*: Inhibition of neointimal hyperplasia by blocking $a_v b_3$ integrin with a small peptide antagonist GpenGRGDSPCA. *J Vasc Surg* **19:** 125–134, 1994

51. Yanagi H, Sasaguri Y, Sugama K *et al.*: Production of tissue collagenase (matrix metalloproteinase 1) by human aortic smooth muscle cells in response to platelet-derived growth factor. *Atherosclerosis* **91:** 207–216, 1991

52. Kennedy SH, Qin H, Lin L, Tan EML: Basic fibroblast growth factor regulates type I collagen and collagenase gene expression in human smooth muscle cells. *Am J Pathol* **146:** 764–771, 1995

53. Kenagy RD, Clowes AW: Regulation of baboon arterial smooth muscle cell plasminogen activators by heparin and growth factors. *Thromb Res* **77:** 55–61: 1995

54. Arribas J, Coodly L, Vollmer P *et al.*: Diverse cell surface protein ectodomains are shed by a system sensitive to metalloprotease inhibitors. *J Biol Chem* **271:** 11376–11382, 1996

55. Levi E, Fridman R, Miao HQ *et al.*: Matrix metalloproteinase 2 releases active soluble ectodomain of fibroblast growth factor receptor 1. *Proc Natl Acad Sci USA* **93:** 7069–7074, 1996

56. Sato Y, Rifkin DB: Inhibition of endothelial cell movement by pericytes and smooth muscle cells: Activation of a latent transforming growth factor-like molecule by plasmin during co-culture. *J Cell Biol* **109:** 309–315, 1989

57. Murphy G, Atkinson S, Ward R *et al.*: The role of plasminogen activators in the regulation of connective tissue metalloproteinases. *Ann NY Acad Sci* **667:** 1–12, 1992

58. Sato H, Takino T, Okada Y *et al.*: A matrix metalloproteinase expressed on the surface of invasive tumour cells. *Nature* **370:** 61–65, 1994

59. Desrochers PE, Jeffrey JJ, Weiss SJ: Interstitial collagenase (matrix metalloproteinase-1) expresses serpinase activity. *J Clin Invest* **87:** 2258–2265, 1991

60. Brooks BP, Stromblad S, Sanders LC *et al.*: Localization of matrix metalloproteinase MMP-2 to the surface of invasive cells by interaction with integrin $a_v b_3$. *Cell* **85:** 683–693, 1996

61. Barrett LA, Mergner WJ, Trump BF: Long-term culture of human aortas. Development of atherosclerotic-like plaques in serum-supplemented medium. *In vitro* **15:** 957-966, 1979

62. Daley SJ, Gotlieb AI: Fibroblast growth factor receptor-1 expression is associated with neointimal formation *in vitro*. *Am J Pathol* **148:** 1193–1202, 1996

63. Schiffers PMH, Fazzi GE, Van Ingen Schenau D, De Mey JGR: Effects of candidate autocrine and paracrine mediators on growth responses in isolated rat arteries. *Arterioscler Thromb* **14:** 420–426, 1994

64. Slomp J, Gittenberger-de Groot AC, Van Munsteren JC *et al*.: Nature and origin of the neointima in whole vessel wall organ culture of the human saphenous vein. *Virchows Arch Int J Pathol* **428:** 59–67, 1996
65. Kenagy RD, Clowes AW: A Possible Role for MMP-2 and MMP-9 in the migration of primate arterial smooth muscle cells through native matrix. *Ann NY Acad Sci* **732:** 462–465, 1994
66. Kenagy RD, Clowes AW: Primate smooth muscle cell (SMC) migration is mediated by matrix metalloproteinase 9 and by urokinase. **10:** A1297(Abstract); FASEB J, 1996
67. Post MJ, Borst C, Kuntz RE: The relative importance of arterial remodeling compared with intimal hyperplasia in lumen renarrowing after balloon angioplasty: A study in the normal rabbit and the hypercholesterolemic Yucatan micropig. *Circulation* **89:** 2816–2821, 1994
68. Hoffmann R, Mintz GS, Dussaillant GR *et al*.: Patterns and mechanisms of in-stent restenosis – A serial intravascular ultrasound study. *Circulation* **94:** 1247–1254, 1996

Thrombolysis or Surgery for Vein Graft Occlusion

Anthony D. Whittemore and Michael Belkin

INTRODUCTION

Autogenous infrainguinal arterial reconstruction has become a well-established method for palliating claudication and achieving limb salvage in critically ischaemic limbs.[1-4] Primary graft patency rates are commonly reported in the 70–80% range after 5 years, with secondary patency rates 10–15% higher, and an overall limb salvage rate of nearly 90% may be anticipated. A significant minority (20–30%) of autogenous bypasses, therefore, fail during the 5-year interval following initial surgery in spite of our increased understanding of the mechanisms of failure and the initiation of current surveillance protocols designed to detect the failing graft prior to actual thrombosis. In fact, the majority of autogenous grafts requiring revision present with total occlusion despite our best efforts at diligent surveillance and patient education.[5] The occluded vein graft continues to challenge the judgment and skill of the vascular surgeon who must command a thorough knowledge of the mechanisms of graft failure, the magnitude and duration of ischaemia, the efficacy and safety of a variety of treatment options and, of increasing importance, the economic impact of each strategy.

MECHANISMS OF GRAFT FAILURE

Vein graft occlusion which occurs shortly after initial operation, usually within a few days and certainly within a month, is generally attributable to errors of operative technique or judgment.[6] Technical errors include inadequate arterial flushing resulting in thrombotic or atheroembolic complications, clamp injuries, misguided anastomotic suture technique, vein graft injuries, and retained valves, to mention just a few. Judgmental errors are characterized by the use of an inadequate venous conduit, either too small in calibre or of poor quality due to prior segmental phlebitis or sclerotic valves, or inadequate inflow or outflow. Occasionally, early graft thrombosis may result from hypercoagulability, usually superimposed upon an inadequate conduit or marginal outflow vessel.

Graft thrombosis occuring after the early postoperative period, from 3 to 18 months, is most frequently the result of fibrous intimal hyperplasia, either focal or diffuse, within the vein graft or in the perianastomotic region. With the availability of duplex surveillance, these lesions are documented in approximately one-third of all grafts and are usually evident at the first evaluation 2–3 months after surgery;[7-10] 90% of such lesions exert their maximal effect within 1 year. If such lesions become haemodynamically significant and are ignored, graft occlusion or serious deteriation occurs in 50%; if revised while the graft is still patent, however, sustained assisted patency is achieved in 80–85% of grafts for an additional 5 years.[6,11,12]

Finally, graft failure beyond the 1–2 year interval becomes increasingly the result of progressive atherosclerotic disease, usually in the outflow distribution. Once again, graft surveillance in perpetuity allows the detection of reduced flow through the conduit suggesting progressive outflow disease and provides the opportunity for revision prior to thrombosis. This appreciation of the common mechanisms of graft failure provides partial explanation for the observation that thrombectomy or thrombolysis alone does not address the underlying causative lesion and therefore assures repeated thrombosis.

MAGNITUDE AND DURATION OF ISCHAEMIA

Patients who present with limb threatening ischaemia at the time of vein graft occlusion should undergo a reasonable attempt at restoration of vein graft patency or a new bypass procedure, as most who are initially operated upon for limb salvage will develop recurrent critical ischaemia. Occasionally, a patient will experience minimal symptoms with vein graft failure due to interval development of collateral or healing of the tissue necrosis which prompted the original procedure. Subsequent development of co-morbidity may preclude persistent aggressive attempts at limb salvage. The latter consideration is particularly pertinent to the dialysis population which incurs a higher operative morbidity such that their shortened life expectancy may argue against repetitive procedures.[13] Extensive recurrent tissue necrosis in such patients may justify simple amputation.

Most patients, however, are suitable candidates for secondary intervention and the most appropriate option depends in part upon the magnitude and duration of ischaemia. It is often difficult to pinpoint the exact date of graft thrombosis since those failing from progressive fibrous intimal hyperplasia or distal atherosclerotic disease do so gradually over some ill-defined period of time. It is unlikely, however, that vein grafts occluded for more than 1 month will respond to lytic therapy; in fact, lytic therapy has proved most appropriate for those occlusions occurring within 14 days of presentation.

A second consideration in determining which treatment option to utilize is the magnitude of ischaemia. While failed grafts generally do not produce an acutely threatened limb, rapidly progressive ischaemia with neurologic deficits preclude prolonged administration of lytic agents, and might be better served with temporizing thrombectomy or immediate revision. On the other hand, provided the thrombosed graft can be traversed with a guide wire and infusion catheter, success with lytic therapy is usually evident very shortly after its initiation, and within 2–3 hours patency can be restored and subsequent correction of the underlying defect pursued.

EFFICACY OF TREATMENT OPTIONS

When Fogarty and co-workers introduced the balloon thromboembolectomy catheter in 1963, the most straightforward approach to the thrombosed vein graft consisted of surgical thrombectomy through limited incisions over the proximal and distal anastomoses. It became readily evident that simple thrombectomy alone was not durable and that sustained patency required identification and correction of the underlying defect. Initial experience with thrombectomy and simple vein patch angioplasty of focal hyperplastic lesions provided satisfactory short-term results, but the poor long-term patency rate of 20–25% was repeatedly documented.[6,11,14] The occluded vein graft was best managed, therefore, with an entirely new autogenous bypass when possible for optimal limb salvage.

With the advent of effective agents, however, vein graft occlusions were increasingly managed with thrombolysis and resulted in several evangelical reports of early technical success in the setting of multiple anecdotal experiences rendered uninterpretable due to a heterogenous patient population, to combining both acute arterial occlusion with autogenous and prosthetic bypasses, and to considerable variation in dose and delivery regimens of the three major lytic agents available. It was clear that lytic agents were effective in establishing early patency and offered several theoretical advantages over surgical thrombectomy. Endothelial damage resulting from balloon thrombectomy during surgery is minimized, the causative lesion is unmasked with the improved radiographic resolution available in an angiography suite, and outflow vessels inaccessible to surgical thrombectomy catheters might be rendered patent thereby improving outflow for a subsequent surgical correction. In fact, the technical success rate of lytic therapy led to the hope that balloon dilatation of focal lesions might obviate the necessity for surgery at all. Unfortunately this has not proven the case as balloon angioplasty of vein graft lesions provided disappointing patency rates in the range of 25–30%.[15]

Early feasibility studies with lytic therapy have been superseded by several randomized prospective trials with more clearly defined endpoints including limb salvage and death. One of the earliest of these was reported by Nilsson and co-workers in the European trial which compared surgical thrombectomy with recombitant tissue plasminogen activator in a small group of 20 patients with acute arterial occlusions of less than 7 days duration.[16] A second larger study was carried out at the University of Rochester in which 114 patients with limb threatening peripheral arterial occlusions were randomized to either surgery or interarterial catheter-directed urokinase.[17] Lytic therapy was initially successful in dissolution of the thrombus in 70% of patients, but the limb salvage rates were virtually identical in both groups (82%) after 1 year.

The Surgery vs Thrombolysis for Ischemia of the Lower Extremity (STILE) trial and was carried out in several centres throughout North America in patients randomized to surgery, intra-arterial urokinase or intra-arterial recombitant tissue plasminogen activator (rTPA).[18] This study included patients with thrombosed arteries as well as vein and prosthetic grafts with a mean length of time from onset of symptoms to treatment of 50 days. A major disadvantage of this study was the wide variety of clinical characteristics utilized to establish the occurrence of a primary endpoint. While some were obvious including death, amputation and haemorrhage, others were more subjectively defined such as ongoing ischaemia, vascular complications and perioperative complications, both major and minor. The study initially demonstrated a highly significant difference in favour of surgery in that 64% of patients achieved a positive outcome as opposed to only 38% of those undergoing thrombolysis after an early 1 month interval. The study suggested that lytic therapy resulted in a reduction in the magnitude in the planned revascularization procedure, since 56% of lytic patients were able to undergo a lesser procedure than initially planned. This reduction in magnitude, however, did not translate into a superior overall outcome compared with initial surgery.

An important observation was the significant reduction in amputation rate when thrombolytic therapy was initiated within 2 weeks of the onset of ischaemia (11%) as opposed to those with longer duration of ischaemia (30%). The amputation rate observed in those patients treated surgically after 14 days following the onset of symptoms was only 3% in the surgical group, vs 12% in the lytic group. The two major conclusions supported by data from the STILE trial established surgery as a more effective treatment option than thrombolytic therapy and, second, any benefit associated with lytic therapy is limited to patients treated within 2 weeks of the onset of symptoms.

The most recent addition to the thrombolytic literature with regard to peripheral vascular occlusion is the Thrombolysis or Peripheral Arterial Surgery (TOPAS) study.[19] This trial was designed to test the efficacy of lytic therapy utilizing recombitant urokinase (rUk) compared with surgery for the treatment of lower extremity critical ischaemia. Phase I of this trial evaluated three potential doses of rUK (2000 vs 4000 vs 6000 International Units/minute for the initial 4 hours followed by 2000 IU/min thereafter). The ongoing phase II component is designed to compare thrombolysis with the optimal dose from Phase I with surgery. Phase I established the mid-range dose of 4000 IU/min as the safest and most effective lytic treatment of occluded vein grafts. Complete lysis was achieved within 4 hours in 30% of the grafts. As reported by Oriel and associates, multivariate analysis of patients treated with intra-arterial lysis demonstrated that success is predicated upon traversing the occlusion with a guidewire and that lysis was more likely to be successful for occluded prosthetic grafts than for autogenous vein grafts.[19]

SURGICAL STRATEGIES FOR THE FAILED AUTOGENOUS VEIN GRAFT

The restoration of durable patency to thrombosed autogenous infrainguinal vein grafts has therefore proved difficult with either thrombectomy or thrombolytic therapy alone, and even when followed by appropriate surgical revision, results have proved suboptimal. This disappointing experience forms the basis underlying the general principal that the best strategy for continued limb salvage following thrombosis is an entirely new vein graft. Several reports in the past have documented 5-year primary patencies associated with such secondary autogenous recon-structions ranging from 37% to 57%.[6,12,20] We recently reviewed our experience during the past 20 years at the Brigham & Women's Hospital which consisted of 300 consecutive reoperations for infrainguinal graft occlusions.[21] The majority of secondary reconstructions (84%) were indicated for recurrent critical ischaemia and the remainder were carried out for recurrent disabling claudication. Autogenous vein was utilized in 213 (71%) reconstructions, and consisted of greater saphenous vein in 62%, with the remainder from arm or lesser saphenous sources, either single segment (27%) or composite conduits (11%). Eighty-seven prosthetic grafts (29%) were used, most of which were expanded polytetrofluoroethylene. The majority of both vein and prosthetic grafts originated from the common femoral artery. Most vein grafts (65%) terminated at the distal tibial level, while most prosthetic grafts (83%) were anastomosed to the popliteal artery.

Results were analysed with regard to primary and secondary patency, limb salvage and patient survival as primary endpoints. Primary patency refers to a continuously patent graft requiring no further intervention. Secondary patency includes grafts that have been continuously patent, those which have required revisions to sustain that patency (primary assisted patency), as well as those

Table 1. Life-table analysis of secondary infrainguinal reconstruction

Graft type or indication for surgery	No. of grafts	5-year primary patency (%)	5-year secondary patency (%)	5-year limb salvage (%)	5-year patient survival (%)
Prosthetic grafts	87	25.3 ± 5.7	27.4 ± 6.1	53.5 ± 7.5	71.5 ± 6.7
Autogenous grafts	213	43.2 ± 4.6	51.5 ± 4.6	58.7 ± 5.5	72.6 ± 4.7
p Value		0.007	<0.001	0.23	0.45
Early primary graft failure	44	27.2 ± 7.7[a]	29.8 ± 8.3[a]	43.9 ± 10[a]	81.4 ± 10.7[a]
Late primary graft failure	169	51.5 ± 4.9[a]	61.1 ± 4.7[a]	74.9 ± 4.4[a]	75.2 ± 4.6[a]
p Value		0.017	0.003	0.004	0.3
Autogenous bypass 1975–1984	59	28.8 ± 6.3	38.3 ± 6.9	40.4 ± 7.6	73.8 ± 7.6
Autogenous bypass 1985–1993	154	49.5 ± 6.3	59.1 ± 5.8	72.4 ± 6.6	74.4 ± 4.8
p Value		0.01	0.017	<0.001	0.24
Popliteal outflow	43	44.5 ± 9.7	53.8 ± 9.4	62.8 ± 12.5	NA[b]
Tibial outflow	111	51.4 ± 8.1	60.9 ± 7.4	78.2 < 5.7	NA[b]
p Value		0.295	0.281	0.174	–
GSV[b]	79	60.4 ± 7.1	68.5 ± 6.0	77.8 ± 7.4	NA[b]
Alternative vein[c]	75	35.0 ± 11.0	48.3 ± 10.5	54.2 ± 11.8	NA[b]
p Value		0.020	0.090	0.046	–
Arm veins[d]	46	46.4 ± 9.2[a]	56.5 ± 8.1[a]	65.4 ± 8.0[a]	NA[b]
LSV[e]	34	54.7 ± 9.9[a]	54.7 ± 9.9[a]	55.0 ± 14.1[a]	NA[b]
p Value		0.268	0.417	0.261	–
Claudication	35	63.8 ± 9.2	75.8 ± 8.1	87.4 ± 7.1	85.2 ± 6.9
Limb salvage	178	45.1 ± 7.7	52.3 ± 7.9	66.6 ± 9.5	72.8 ± 5.5
p Value		0.079	0.048	0.056	0.09
Primary autogenous bypass	435	65.1 ± 4.2	79.7 ± 3.3	91.3 ± 4.3	75.1 ± 4.3
Secondary autogenous bypass	154	49.5 ± 6.3	59.1 ± 5.8	72.4 ± 6.6	74.4 ± 4.8
p Value		0.020	<0.001	0.003	0.456

(From ref. 21, with permission.)
NA: Not applicable for comparison.
[a]Follow-up interval is 4 years for these groups.
[b]GSV grafts include *in situ*, non-reversed, translocated, and reversed grafts.
[c]Alternative vein grafts include arm vein grafts, LSV grafts, and composite vein grafts.
[d]Includes arm vein and arm vein composite vein grafts.
[e]Lesser saphenous vein.

disobliterated with either thrombectomy or thrombolytic therapy following occlusion and subsequently revised. The majority of grafts in the secondary patency group, however, were revised while still patent as our recent surveillance protocol allowed detection of significant lesions prior to graft thrombosis.

Follow-up was available for 284 (95%) grafts. A single operative death occurred from a myocardial infarction accounting for the 0.3% mortality rate. Overall morbidity occurred in 25% of procedures. Early graft failure was observed in 18% of the entire group resulting in a 7% overall amputation rate. As illustrated in Table 1, while the overall 5-year limb salvage and suvival rates were similar for those undergoing autogenous and prosthetic grafts, the primary and secondary patency rates achieved with autogenous grafts were significantly higher. Restoration of durable patency to grafts failing within 3 months of the original procedure was not as successful as those with delayed failure. A comparison of our recent experience since 1985 with the prior decade (Fig.1) testifies to improved surgical techniques and vigilant graft surveillance. Secondary bypasses consisting of greater saphenous vein proved superior to those using alternative sources of autogenous conduit (Fig.2). There were no differences, however, between sources of alternative conduit which included arm, lesser saphenous and composite vein grafts.

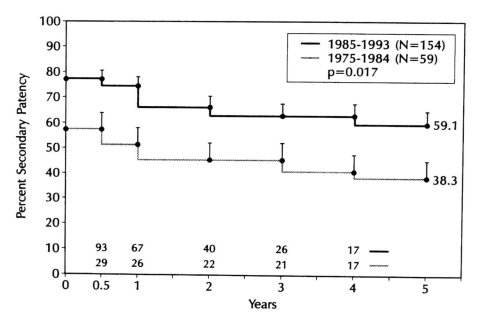

Fig. 1. Life-table analysis of secondary patency rates of autogenous vein secondary bypass grafts performed in the period 1975–1984 vs the period 1985–1993. (From ref. 21 with permission.)

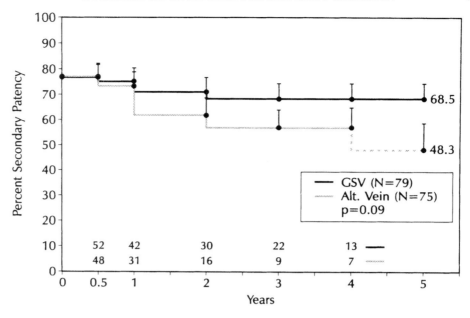

Fig. 2. Life-table analysis of secondary patency rates for secondary bypasses performed with greater saphenous vein (including *in situ*, reversed and non-reversed translocated veins with lysed valves) vs alternative vein bypasses (including composite, arm vein, and lesser saphenous vein grafts). All bypasses were performed during the period 1985–1993. (From ref. 21, with permission.)

CONCLUSIONS

Data so far available from randomized prospective thrombolytic trials fail to substantiate significant benefit over surgery either in terms of cost or efficacy at the 1-year interval. Based on our most recent experience, surgical intervention with autogenous reconstructon for thrombosed vein grafts may be expected to provide a 60–70% patency rate and a 70–80% limb salvage rate after 5 years.

REFERENCES

1. Donaldson MC, Mannick JA, Whittemore AD: Femoraldistal bypass with *in situ* greater saphenous vein: long term results using the Mills valvulatome. *Ann Surg* **213:** 457–465, 1991
2. Leather RP, Shah DJ, Chang BB *et al.*: Resurrection of the *in situ* saphenous vein bypass: 1000 cases later. *Ann Surg* **208:** 435–442, 1988
3. Taylor LM, Edwards JM, Porter JM: Present status of reversed vein bypass grafting: five year results of a modern series *J Vasc Surg* **11:** 193–206, 1990
4. Bergamini TM, Towne JB, Bandy DF *et al.*: Experience with *in situ* saphenous vein bypasses during 1981 to 1989: Determinant factors of long term patency. *J Vasc Surg* **13:** 137, 1991

5. Donaldson MC, Mannick JA, Whittemore AD: Causes of primary graft failure after *in situ* saphenous vein bypass grafting. *J Vasc Surg* **15**: 113–120, 1992

6. Whittemore AD, Clowes AW, Couch NP *et al.*: Secondary femoropopliteal reconstruction. *Ann Surg* **193**: 35–42, 1981

7. Bandyck DF, Seabrook GR, Moldhauer P *et al.*: Hemodynamics of vein graft stenosis. *J Vasc Surg* **8**: 688–695, 1988

8. Mills JL, Harris EJ, Taylor LM *et al.*: The importance of routine surveillance of distal bypass grafts with duplex scanning: a study of 379 reversed vein grafts. *J Vasc Surg* **11**: 379–389, 1990

9. Bandyck DF, Schmitt DD, Seqabrook GR *et al.*: Monitoring functonal patency of *in situ* saphenous vein bypasses: The impact of a surveillance protocol and elective revision. *J Vasc Surg* **9**: 286–296, 1989

10. Green RM, McNamara J, Ouriel K, DeWeese JA: Comparison of infrainguinal graft surveillance techniques. *J Vasc Surg* **11**: 207–215, 1990

11. Brewster DC, LaSalle AJ, Robison JG *et al.*: Femoropopliteal graft failures: clinical consequences and success of secondary reconstructions. *Arch Surg* **118**: 1043–1050, 1984

12. Bandyk DF, Bergamini TM, Towne JB *et al.*: Durability of vein graft revision: The outcome of secondary procedures. *J Vasc Surg* **13**: 200–210, 1992

13. Whittemore AD, Donaldson MC, Mannick JA: Infrainguinal reconstruction for patients with chronic renal insufficiency. *J Vasc Surg* **17**: 32–41, 1993

14. Cohen JR, Mannick JA, Couch NP *et al.*: Recognition and management of impending vein graft failure. *Arch Surg* **121**: 758–759, 1986

15. Whittemore AD, Donaldson MC, Polak JF, Mannick JA: Limitations of balloon angioplasty for vein graft stenosis. *J Vasc Surg* **4**: 340–345, 1991

16. Nilsson L, Albrechtsson U, Jonung T *et al.*: Surgical treatment versus thrombolysis in acute arterial occlusion: A randomised controlled study. *Eur J Vasc Surg* **6**: 189–193, 1992

17. Ouriel K, Shortell CK, De Weese JA *et al.*: A comparison of thrombolytic therapy with operastive revascularization in the treatment of acute peripheral arterial ischemia. *J Vasc Surg* **19**: 1021–1030, 1994

18. The STILE Investigators: Results of a prospective randomized trial evaluating surgery versus thrombolysis for ischemia of the lower extremity: The STILE trial. *Ann Surg* **220**: 251–268, 1994

19. Ouriel K, Veith FJ, Sasahara AA for the TOPAS Investigators: Thrombolysis or peripheral arterial surgery: Phase I results. *J Vasc Surg* **23**: 64–75, 1996

20. Belkin M, Conte MS, Donaldson MC *et al.*: Preferred strategies for secondary infrainguinal bypass: Lessons learned from 300 consecutive reoperations. *Soc Vasc Surg* 1995; 282–293.

21. Belkin M, Conte MS, Donaldson MC *et al.*: Preferred strategies for secondary infrainguinal bypass: Lessons learned from 300 consecutive reoperations. *J Vasc Surg* **21**: 282–295, 1995

Fluoroscopically Assisted Thromboembolectomy: An Improved Method for Performing an Old Operation

Takao Ohki, Richard E. Parsons, Michael L. Marin and Frank J. Veith

INTRODUCTION

Since 1963 when the Fogarty balloon was introduced, it has gained widespread use as a valuable tool in the management of acute limb ischaemia and has simplified and increased the effectiveness of arterial thromboembolectomy.[1] Initial reports of its use have been favourable with reduction in mortality rates and an increase in limb salvage.[2-5] However, as it gained frequent use, complications have also been encountered.[3,6-13] Foster *et al.* classified these complications into four types, all of which where due to mechanical injury caused by the blind insertion of the catheter or uncontrolled inflation of the balloon. Both of these may have been prevented if the position and the degree of the inflation of the contrast filled balloon catheter could have been visualized.[13]

Balloon thromboembolectomy may also be hampered by the inability to pass the balloon catheter through the occluded tortuous arteries, difficulties in assessing the adequacy of the clot removal or failure to identify lesions responsible for the thrombosis.

In an effort to reduce procedural complications and to increase technical success, we evaluated the efficacy of visualizing the balloon catheter with the use of a C-arm digital fluoroscope or fluoroscopically assisted thromboembolectomy (FAT-E) in the treatment of acute thrombotic arterial occlusions (Fig. 1).

MATERIAL AND METHODS

Experimental studies

A canine model was used to evaluate the degree of arterial overdistention by blind balloon embolectomy using standard techniques. Both common femoral arteries were dissected in a mongrel dog weighing 50 kg. A 5 French haemostatic introducer sheath was inserted in the left femoral artery and advanced retrograde into the distal iliac artery. A second introducer sheath was then placed into the right femoral artery and advanced antegrade into the right superficial femoral artery. The luminal diameter of both the iliac and the superficial femoral arteries were measured from the angiographic image obtained with a C-arm digital fluoroscope and were calibrated for image magnification. Vascular surgeons with various levels of clinical experience carried out

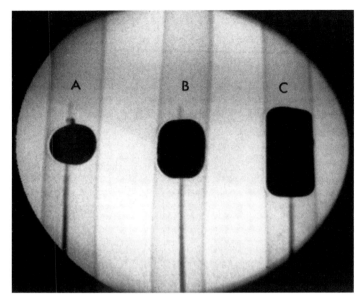

Fig. 1. Fluoroscopic *in vitro* image of a balloon thrombectomy catheter filled with radiographic contrast and distended to different balloon profiles. (a) Following minimal inflation of the balloon catheter, the balloon assumes an ovoid profile (olive shape) approximating but not directly contacting the contained vessel lumen. (b) Further inflation of the balloon catheter reveals that the ovoid appearance begins to transform into an elongated, rectangular structure which closely apposes the vessel wall. (c) Following overdistention of the balloon catheter, a rectangular profile is achieved which results in significant radial force to the underlying vessel.

standard procedures for arterial thromboembolectomy of the superficial femoral and iliac arteries using contrast filled Fogarty embolectomy balloon catheters (Baxter Healthcare Corporation, CA) (Fig. 2). The sizes of Fogarty balloon catheters used were no. 4 for the iliac artery and no. 2 for the superficial femoral artery. The operating surgeon blindly performed the embolectomy, without being able to see the fluoroscopic image (Fig. 3). Three separate catheter passes were made in each vessel, and in each instance the balloon shape and balloon dilated lumen diameter of the artery were recorded from the digital fluoroscope screen by a second observer (Table 1). The balloon dilated lumen diameters of the artery were averaged and were expressed as the percentage overdilation compared with the size of the normal artery (Table 1).

Clinical studies

In 22 patients with acute arterial occlusions FAT-E was used over a 26-month period. A standard balloon embolectomy catheter was initially inserted into each thrombosed vessel. When there were difficulties in passing the catheter through occluded or tortuous arterial segments, a haemostatic sheath was inserted in the

Table I. Experimental evaluation of vessel distention by the embolectomy balloon in a canine model

Postgraduate year	Iliac artery balloon diameter (mm) (% over-distention) n (%)	Femoral artery balloon diameter (mm) (% over-distention) n (%)
PGY-1	6 (20)	>5.5 (25)
PGY-1	6.5 (30)	3 (50)
PGY-1	6 (20)	2.5 (25)
PGY-3	6 (20)	3 (50)
PGY-3	6 (20)	3 (50)
PGY-3	6.5 (30)	2.5 (25)
PGY-5	6.5 (30)	3 (50)
PGY-7	6 (20)	3 (50)
PGY-8	6 (20)	2.5 (25)
PGY-9	6 (20)	3 (50)
PGY-14	6 (20)	2.5 (25)
PGY-40	6.5 (30)	3 (50)
Average	6.2 (23)	2.8 (40)

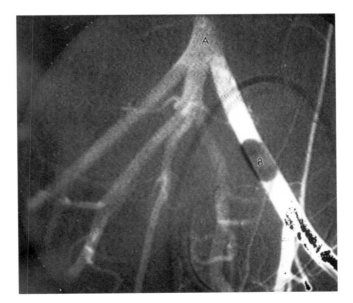

Fig. 2. Digital arteriogram of a dog during experimental FAT-E. Following contrast injection, a roadmap image is created which permits direct comparison of the size of the embolectomy balloon with the size of the underlying artery. Direct comparison of the luminal size with the balloon size can be made using this technique (A: aorta; B: contrast-filled embolectomy balloon).

common femoral artery and held in place with tensioned doubled silastic loops. A guidewire was used to cross the region and then a double lumen balloon catheter was inserted over the wire. Under fluoroscopic guidance using a digital C-arm portable fluoroscope with road mapping capability (BV 212, Philips, The Netherlands), the balloon was slowly filled with contrast media until the balloon profile approached the roadmap image of the underlying vessel lumen (Fig. 4). The

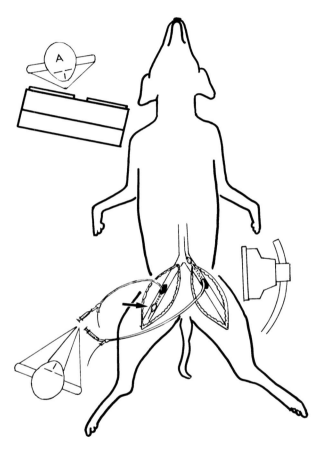

Fig. 3. The experimental technique for evaluating the efficacy of FAT-E. A 4 French balloon thrombectomy catheter is inserted into the left femoral artery and advanced through the iliac artery to the aorta. The surgeon controlling the balloon thrombectomy catheter cannot visualize the fluoroscopic image of balloon inflation and withdrawal. Under fluoroscopic guidance, a second observer (A) follows the procedure and records the diameter of the artery prior to thrombectomy as well as the diameter of the balloon as it passes through the thrombectomized vessel. A similar procedure is carried out on the superficial femoral artery of the dog (arrow), and the vessel lumen and balloon diameters of this vessel are also recorded.

balloon was then carefully withdrawn under fluoroscopic control in order to prevent overdistention of the artery. As the balloon was gently withdrawn to extract the clot, deformities of the balloon profile by underlying arterial lesions were fluoroscopically identified and their locations were marked on the skin with radiopaque metal clips (Figs 5, 6). This procedure was repeated as required to achieve optimal clot removal. At the completion of each thromboembolectomy, the existence of an underlying lesion was confirmed either by haemodynamic pull-through gradient measurements or by contrast arteriograms performed retrograde through the haemostatic sheath in the common femoral artery or prograde by a catheter inserted to a level proximal to the previous thrombosis.

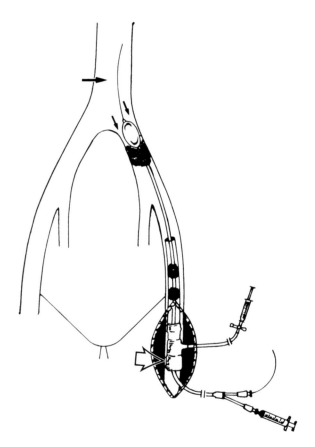

Fig. 4. Illustration of FAT-E using an over-the-wire technique. Following passage of a radiographic guidewire (closed arrow), a balloon thrombectomy catheter equipped with two lumens is passed through a haemostatic valve in a previously placed vascular sheath (open arrow). Under fluoroscopic control, the balloon is withdrawn through the vessel containing the clot and the clot is advanced into the introducer sheath. Several passages of the balloon thrombectomy catheter may be made prior to the removal of the sheath containing the thrombectomized clot.

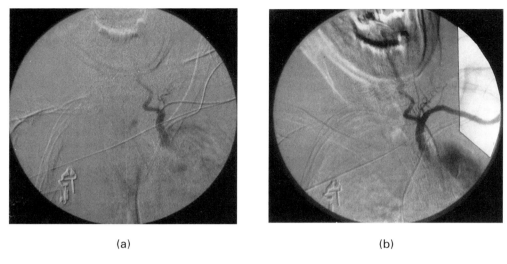

(a)   (b)

Fig. 5. FAT-E of a subclavian artery embolus. (a) An arteriogram undertaken after retrograde recanalization which was performed under fluoroscopic guidance demonstrates total occlusion of the subclavian artery distal to the take off of the left vertebral artery. In this case, gentle catheter passage through the occlusion and accurate identification of the proximal end of the occlusion were crucial, since both forceful manoeuvre or inflation of the balloon within the clot have the potential of dislodging the thrombus into the vertebral artery. (b) Following withdrawal of the subclavian artery thrombus, good flow is seen through the subclavian artery.

RESULTS

Experimental studies

The normal iliac artery and the superficial femoral artery lumen of the dog measured 5 mm and 2 mm in diameter, respectively. Twelve surgeons with various levels of clinical experience performed the balloon catheter procedures. The percentage overdistention for the entire group averaged 23 ± 5% for the iliac artery and 40 ± 13% for the superficial femoral artery (Table 1). The degree of arterial overdistention had no correlation with the duration of clinical experience. In four instances, the operator was not aware that the catheter had been placed in an aortic branch vessel which was confirmed by fluoroscopy (mesenteric and lumbar vessels). In addition, as embolectomy balloons were inflated and withdrawn from the aorta into the smaller iliac artery, marked deformation of the balloon was frequently observed indicating that a significant radial force was being applied to the iliac artery.

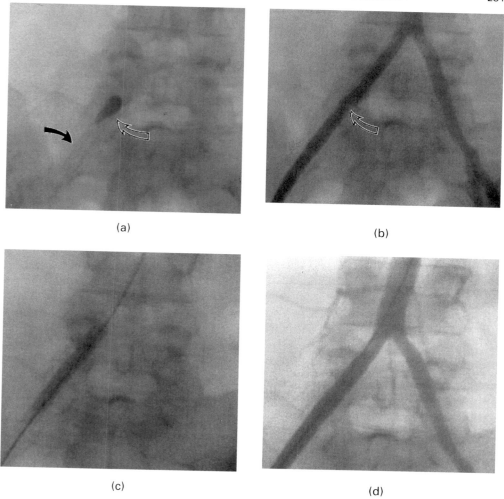

(a)

(b)

(c)

(d)

Fig. 6. FAT-E of the iliac artery. One week after the insertion of a balloon expandable Palmaz stent for an iliac artery stenosis, a thrombosis of the iliac artery occurred. (a) FAT-E was performed in this occluded iliac artery (arrow). The balloon deforms its ovoid profile conforming to an apparent lesion at the proximal portion of the iliac artery stent (double arrows). (b) A retrograde arteriogram performed from the common femoral artery demonstrates what appears to be an intimal flap just proximal to the level of the iliac stent. (c) A second stent is then deployed across the region of this intimal flap, functionally tacking the flap down to the underlying vessel wall. (d) A completion arteriogram shows good flow through the iliac artery and correction of the underlying intimal flap.

Clinical studies

After initial clot removal in the 22 patients, 15 residual lesions were fluoroscopically detected by balloon deformation at the time of its withdrawal. These were further confirmed by the existence of haemodynamic pull-through gradients or by contrast arteriograms. Repeat thrombectomy (n=8), balloon angioplasty (n=3) and placement of intravascular stents (n=4) eliminated all 15 lesions (Table 2). No arterial ruptures or intimal dissections were identified within treated vessels on completion arteriograms following FAT-E. Luminal continuity was successfully restored in all 22 of these patients, ten of whom required a distal standard arterial bypass (six vein, four polytetrafluoroethylene) to correct existing outflow occlusive disease, and two required an inflow procedure because the residual lesion could not be repaired endoluminally. One patient died from a myocardial infarction and cardiogenic shock 1 day after successful FAT-E removal of a saddle embolus. This 99-year-old individual had warm extremities and a return of all lower extremity pulses prior to

Table 2.   Results of fluoroscopically assisted thromboembolectomy

Patient no.	Sex/ age	Balloon type	Residual lesions[a]	Thrombectomy location	Supplemental procedures[b]	Patency (months)
1	M/70	SF	C	Aortoiliac	Iliofemoral	25
2	M/66	SF	A	Aortoiliac	—	23
3	M/80	SF	A	Femoropopliteal	Femoropopliteal	18[c]
4	F/76	SF	A	Tibioperoneal	Femoropopliteal	18
5	F/41	SF	C	Femoropopliteal	Femoropopliteal	16
6	F/41	SF	B	Aortoiliac	—	15
7	F/41	OW	D	Femoropopliteal	—	15[d]
8	M/70	SF	A	Aortoiliac	Femorotibial	15
9	M/63	OW	D	Femoropopliteal	Femoropopliteal	15
10	F/68	SF	A	Femoropopliteal	—	13[e]
11	M/60	SF	D	Tibioperoneal	Femoropopliteal	13
12	F/72	SF	B	Aortoiliac	—	11
13	M/70	SF	A	Tibioperoneal	Iliofemoral	10
14	M/81	OW	B	Aortoiliac	—	10
15	F/69	OW	C	Femoropopliteal	—	10
16	M/63	SF	C	Aortoiliac	Femorotibial	8[f]
17	F/70	SF	D	Aortoiliac	—	7
18	M/73	SF	A	Aortoiliac	—	6
19	M/66	SF	A	Brachial-radial-ulnar	—	2
20	F/52	SF	D	Femoropopliteal	Femoropopliteal	2
21	F/99	SF	D	Aortoiliac	—	—[g]
22	F/89	SF	D	Subclavian	—	2

SF: standard Fogarty; OW: over-the-wire.
[a]Residual lesions: A, resolved with repeat thrombectomy; B, resolved with balloon angioplasty; C, resolved with insertion of intravascular stent; D, no residual lesion after primary thrombectomy.
[b]These procedures were performed at the time of primary thrombectomy.
[c]Required tibial extension at 6 months for failing graft.
[d]Required repeat thrombectomy and femoro-above-knee popliteal bypass at 8 months.
[e]Failed at 10 months necessitating thrombectomy and extension to below-knee popliteal artery.
[f]Thrombosis with limb loss.
[g]Died in the early postoperative period from myocardial infarction.

her death. Although three patients (14%) required a subsequent late intervention (two femoropopliteal bypasses and one extension to the tibial level) to maintain arterial or bypass patency, all 21 of the remaining patients maintained patency of the arterial segment or segments originally treated by FAT-E for 2 - 25 months (mean, 14 months).

DISCUSSION

Although the balloon catheter has simplified and increased the effectiveness of arterial thromboembolectomy, it has been associated with several procedural complications which increase in frequency with and may be exacerbated by the presence of underlying occlusive disease.[3,6–13] The incidence of this underlying arteriosclerosis in patients with acute limb ischaemia has progressively increased over the last three decades, and most patients who currently present with acute lower extremity ischaemia have extensive arteriosclerosis obliterans.[14] In part because of this, Foster and his colleagues encountered 12 complications with the use of the Fogarty balloon catheter and classified these complications into four types, where type 1 is arterial perforation caused by the tip of the catheter, type 2 is arterial rupture secondary to overdilatation, type 3 is intimal dissection and type 4 is balloon rupture with distal embolization of a fragment of rubber.[13] In addition, subintimal catheter insertion and migration of the catheter into a normal critical vessel has been reported without the surgeon being aware of these potentially catastrophic events.[15–18] All these detrimental effects of standard balloon thromboembolectomy are markedly increased in arteriosclerotic patients in whom luminal irregularity is common and arteriosclerotic lesions can be disrupted by blind passage of the inflated balloon.

In order to minimize these injuries, Burdick and Williams advocated inflation of the embolectomy balloon by partial compression of a comparatively large initial volume of air in the syringe.[19] In addition, use of smaller sized catheters, minimal and variable balloon inflation and gentle catheter manipulations are also important to minimize intimal damage and enhance procedural success.[18]

Despite these precautions, however, standard balloon thromboembolectomy can cause substantial arterial damage which may promote the development of chronic arterial obstruction.[14,20–23] The atherogenic potential of balloon catheters has been documented in experimental models which have illustrated defined intimal and medial injuries and smooth muscle cell proliferative potential.[20] There is a direct correlation between the shear forces applied to the arterial wall by inflation of the balloon and the resulting degree of intimal hyperplasia, which may lead to chronic occlusion.[24–26] These observations confirm the importance of minimizing the injury applied to the arterial wall during inflation or withdrawal of the balloon embolectomy catheter.

Balloon catheters are usually inserted into affected arteries and passed without the ability to observe the degree of balloon inflation relative to the arterial lumen or catheter movement or direction within the vessel which is responsible for these mechanical injuries. Using fluoroscopic guidance, the balloon can be visualized as it approaches the limits of the arterial wall or impinges on arteriosclerotic lesions.

This eliminates the operator dependence on the sensation of friction of the balloon as it is withdrawn across the intima of the vessel. Despite great care not to overinflate the balloon while using the friction method, significant distention of the arterial wall will frequently occur by the time the surgeon feels resistance on the catheter shaft. This was well demonstrated in the experimental canine model described in this study. The techniques described in this study add direct imaging to the standard blind techniques of arterial balloon catheter passage so as to avoid many of these catheter thromboembolectomy complications and to accomplish more effective clot removal.

In addition, FAT-E facilitates the identification and accurate localization of underlying arteriosclerotic lesions. As a contrast-filled balloon is slowly withdrawn through an arterial stenosis, the balloon will deform to the shape of the underlying lesion permitting visualization and localization on fluoroscopic images. These lesions can then be immediately treated, as we have shown in the present study, by repeat thrombectomy, balloon angioplasty, the placement of intravascular stents, or the performance of an appropriate bypass.

Furthermore, intraoperative digital angiogram will permit inspection of the vessel for completeness of the thromboembolectomy procedure, technical adequacy of a bypass graft anastomosis and, finally, it will give some indication of the outflow vessel resistance as a function of the speed with which contrast flows through the target vessel.

The use of FAT-E may also provide surgeons with experience of various equipment including guidewires, directional catheters and the C-arm fluoroscope. Since these devices are essential tools in other endovascular procedures, we believe that FAT-E will be a valuable step towards developing the skills needed to perform such procedures. As greater facility is attained with imaging and catheter techniques, skills in arterial angioplasty and stenting may also be acquired.

In conclusion, FAT-E is a safer method for treating acute arterial occlusions, especially in patients with advanced arteriosclerosis. It reduces the risk of arterial damage and facilitates the accurate identification, localization and treatment of underlying arterial lesions. It can also allow vascular surgeons the opportunity to develop the necessary skills to perform other endovascular procedures.

REFERENCES

1. Fogarty T, Cranley J, Krause R *et al.*: A method for extraction of arterial emboli and thrombi. *Surg Gynecol Obstet* **116:** 241–244, 1963
2. Chassin JL: Improved management of acute embolism and thrombosis with an embolectomy catheter. *J Am Med Assoc* **194:** 845–850, 1965
3. Fogarty TJ, Cranley JJ: Catheter technique for arterial embolectomy. *Ann Surg* **161:** 325–330, 1965
4. Glotzer DJ, Glotzer P: Superior mesenteric embolectomy. *Arch Surg* **93:** 421–424, 1966
5. Krause RJ, Cranley JJ, Strasser ES *et al.*: Further experience with new embolectomy catheter. *Surgery* **59:** 81–87, 1966
6. Kendrick J, Thompson B, Read R *et al.*: Arterial embolectomy in the leg: Results in a referral hospital. *Am J Surg* **142:** 739–743, 1981
7. Panetta T, Thompson J, Talkington C *et al.*: Arterial embolectomy: A 34-year experience with 400 Cases. *Surg Clin N Am* **66:** 339–353, 1986

8. Abbott W, Maloney R, McCabe C *et al.*: Arterial embolism: A 44-year perspective. *Am J Surg* **143**: 460–464, 1982

9. Green R, DeWeese J, Rob C: Arterial embolectomy before and after the Fogarty catheter. *Surgery* **77**: 24–33, 1975

10. Haimovici H, Moss C, Veith F: Arterial embolectomy revisited. *Surgery* **78**: 409–410, 1975

11. Hogg GR, MacDougall JT: An accident of embolectomy with the use of the Fogarty catheter. *Surgery* **61**: 716–718, 1967

12. Stoney RJ, Ehrenfield WK, Wylie EJ: Arterial rupture after insertion of a Fogarty catheter. *Am J Surg* **115**: 830–831, 1968

13. Foster J, Carter J, Edwards W *et al.*: Arterial injuries secondary to the use of the Fogarty catheter. *Ann Surg* **171**: 971–978, 1970

14. Veith FJ, Panetta TF, Wengerter KR *et al.*: Femoral-popliteal-tibial occlusive disease. In: Veith FJ, Hobson RW, II, Williams RA, Wilson SE (Eds) *Vascular Surgery: Principles and Practice* 2nd edn, pp. 421–446. New York: McGraw-Hill, 1994

15. Dainko E: Complication of the use of the Fogarty balloon catheter. *Arch Surg* **105**: 79–82, 1972

16. Charlesworth PM, Brewster DC, Darling RC: Renal artery injury from a Fogarty balloon catheter. *J Vasc Surg* **1**: 573–576, 1984

17. Masuoka S, Shimomura T, Ando T *et al.*: Complications associated with the use of the Fogarty balloon catheter. *J Cardiovasc Surg* **21**: 67–74, 1980

18. Cranley JJ, Krause RJ, Strasser ES *et al.*: Catheter technique for arterial embolectomy: A seven year experience. *J Cardiovasc Surg* **11**: 44–51, 1970

19. Burdick JF, Williams GM: A study of the lateral wall pressure exerted by balloon-tipped catheters. *Surgery* **87**: 638–644, 1980

20. Chidi C, DePalma R: Atherogenic potential of the embolectomy catheter. *Surgery* **83**: 549–557, 1987

21. Hansen CP, Holtveg HM, Holstein P: Thromboembolectomy in geriatric patients from long-stay wards. *Danish Med Bull* **39**: 570–572, 1992

22. Dregelid EB, Stangeland LB, Eide GE *et al.*: Patient survival and limb prognosis after arterial embolectomy. *Eur J Vasc Surg* **1**: 263–271, 1987

23. Brgge M, Jelnes R, Aredrup H *et al.*: Arterial embolism of the legs: A follow-up study of 252 patients. *Ann Chir Gynaecol* **74**: 137–141, 1985

24. Goldberg EM, Goldberg MC, Chowdhury LN, *et al.*: The effects of balloon embolectomy-thrombectomy catheters on vascular architecture. *J Cardiovasc Surg* **24**: 74–80, 1983

25. Jorgensen RA, Drobin PB: Balloon embolectomy catheters in small arteries. IV. Correlation of shear forces with histologic injury. *Surgery* **93**: 798–808, 1983

26. Poole JCF, Cromwell SB, Benditt EP: Behavior of smooth muscle cells and formation of extracellular structures in the reaction of arterial walls to injury. *Am J Path* **62**: 391–404, 1971

VENOUS THROMBOSIS

Are Patients with Varicose Veins at Special Risk of Thromboembolism?

W. Bruce Campbell

INTRODUCTION

Patients and their doctors know that 'thrombosis' in the veins of the legs can be dangerous, leading to death as a result of 'clots to the lung'. This is the sum of most patients' knowledge of venous disease, and many people with varicose veins are worried that they are at risk of thrombosis and pulmonary embolism.

Particular concern exists for those who have suffered superficial thrombophlebitis in varicose veins, and who seldom understand clearly the difference between this condition and deep vein thrombosis (DVT). The important distinction has not been explained to them, often because doctors advising were unsure which condition they had. Even when thrombophlebitis is correctly diagnosed there is uncertainty about whether this is likely to progress to DVT.

Surgeons operating on varicose veins face a special dilemma regarding the risk of thromboembolism, and the pros and cons of prophylaxis. There is no good evidence that DVT or pulmonary embolism are special risks after varicose vein surgery, and in clinical practice their incidence seems very low. Proven mechanical methods of prophylaxis (stockings, pumps) are difficult or impossible to use during operation on the legs, while subcutaneous heparin may make bruising worse. However, varicose veins have been placed high on the list of risk factors for DVT both in national[1] and international[2] consensus statements. This means that there is a serious medicolegal threat to any surgeon who has not used 'demonstrable prophylaxis' during varicose vein surgery if thromboembolism occurs, despite inadequate evidence of the benefits and risks. This threat is enhanced by the popular belief that varicose veins are somehow associated with 'thrombosis'.

This chapter considers the available evidence on varicose veins and DVT, and includes results of a survey of vascular surgeons in Great Britain and Ireland about thromboembolism prophylaxis during varicose vein surgery.

THE EVIDENCE FOR VARICOSE VEINS AS A RISK FACTOR FOR DVT

The inclusion of varicose veins as a risk factor for DVT is based on the results of studies which examined the incidence of postoperative DVT (mostly after abdominal and pelvic surgery) by radioisotope labelling of fibrinogen to detect thrombi in the leg veins.

(i)   In 1970 Kakkar *et al.*[3] studied 203 consecutive patients aged 40 or over, having a variety of elective operations. Radioisotope evidence of thrombosis was found in 31%. Among those with varicose veins the incidence was 56% – significantly greater than in those without varicose veins. This difference was only significant in younger patients (under 60 years of age).

(ii)   Nicolaides and Irving[4] documented the results of a multivariate analysis of 624 patients screened by radioisotope scanning at the time of surgery. They observed thrombosis in 26% of 557 patients without varicose veins, but 53% of 62 patients with varicose veins ($p<0.0005$) – a relative risk of 3.39. Surprisingly, they observed no significant increase in risk for obesity, history of previous pulmonary embolism, or malignancy.

(iii)   In 1976 Clayton *et al.*[5] reported a study aimed at identifying clinical and laboratory criteria to predict a high risk of DVT, in 124 patients having major gynaecological surgery. Twenty developed detectable thrombosis, of whom 45% had varicose veins, compared with a 20% prevalence of varicose veins among those without postoperative DVT.

(iv)   Lowe *et al.*[6] detected thromboses in 33% of 63 patients after major abdominal surgery, in an initial study on predictive indices for DVT. In a second study using predictive indices derived from the first, 18 cases of thrombosis were detected after scanning 41 patients (an incidence of 44%). The percentages of patients with varicose veins among those with thrombosis were 48% in their initial study and 41% in both studies, compared with 5% and 9% respectively among those without detectable thrombosis. Although the numbers of patients were quite small, these differences were significant ($p<0.001$) for varicose veins as a risk factor.

(v)   In a study of 85 patients having abdominal operations, Sue-Ling *et al.*[7] found that the presence of varicose veins had some predictive power for the development of postoperative DVT, although the relationship between varicose veins and DVT did not reach statistical significance in this population of patients.

These studies invite a number of possible criticisms. They included only older patients (over the age of 40). The presence of varicose veins was difficult to separate from associated obesity and age in some of the studies. The severity of varicose veins was not very clear, nor was coincidence of varicose veins and postoperative DVT in the same limb (rather than in the contralateral leg). No account was taken of whether varicose veins might have been associated with prior deep venous disease. Findings in some of the trials were inconsistent for other risk factors, such as obesity and malignant disease. Finally, the technique of radioisotope scanning for detection of DVT may not differentiate clearly between thrombus in the deep and superficial veins. These comments notwithstanding, there seems clear and consistent evidence to support the belief that varicose veins are associated with DVT after major abdominal and pelvic surgery. By contrast, these studies should not automatically be extrapolated to suggest an increased risk at other times for people with varicose veins.

VARICOSE VEINS WITH A HISTORY OF PREVIOUS DVT

Obstruction to the deep veins by thrombosis can result in the appearance of large varicose veins in a few patients. There are other patients who have primary varicose veins but who also have a history of DVT associated with childbirth, operation, or illness. These patients are at increased risk of further thromboembolism, not because of their varicose veins, but on account of their damaged deep veins.

All patients presenting for treatment of varicose veins should be asked if they have had thrombosis in the past. If they have had a DVT then they must be treated as high risk. Often the history is uncertain and confused: 'I think I had a thrombosis after one of the babies', frequently turns out to indicate an attack of superficial thrombophlebitis. Questions about leg swelling, localized inflammation, hospital admission, 'special X-rays', and whether they were given warfarin for several weeks may help to elucidate the true diagnosis. Sometimes it becomes clear that the patient's medical attendants themselves were unsure about the diagnosis.

Absence of swelling or skin changes, and normal venous Doppler signals in the popliteal fossa are helpful pointers to the absence of chronic damage to larger veins by previous DVT. However, when doubt remains about possible DVT in the past, and when this is considered important in management, then venography or detailed duplex scanning should be done to look for evidence of residual signs of thrombosis.

All of the comments which follow in this chapter exclude varicose veins caused by, or associated with, prior DVT.

ARE PEOPLE WITH VARICOSE VEINS AT SPECIAL RISK IN THEIR NORMAL DAILY LIVES?

From a theoretical standpoint there is no special reason why varicose veins ought to lead to DVT. The longstanding and widespread belief that they might seems to be based largely on lack of understanding about the difference between the deep and superficial veins, and on confusion about terminology (thrombosis/thrombophlebitis).

There is no evidence, based either on trials or anecdote, to support the idea that DVT occurs more commonly in people with varicose veins and without other precipitating factors, such as a major operation. We have not observed unexpected DVT among many hundreds of duplex scans done for patients with varicose veins, and this experience is shared by others.[8]

ARE VARICOSE VEIN PATIENTS WITH SUPERFICIAL THROMBOPHLEBITIS AT SPECIAL RISK OF DVT?

A number of studies on patients with superficial thrombophlebitis (phlebitis) of the lower limbs have demonstrated associated thrombosis in deep veins, but most cases have been in circumstances of special risk. Lutter et al.[9] documented thromboembolic complications in 31% of 186 patients with phlebitis diagnosed on duplex scanning.

Predisposing factors for DVT were bilateral phlebitis, age over 60, male sex, history of DVT, bed rest, and presence of infection. Only 60% of their patients had varicose veins: in these cases DVT was more common when the long saphenous vein was involved (35% incidence) than when isolated varicosities were the site of phlebitis (8%). Skillman et al.[10] also found DVT to be more common in cases of phlebitis extending above the knee. In their study of 42 patients (93% with varicose veins) the other predisposing factor for DVT was a recent operation. By contrast, Jorgensen et al.[8] found no predictive factors in a prospective series of 57 patients with phlebitis: they made no special note of varicose veins in this study.

In a study of 56 patients with phlebitis Bergqvist et al.[11] observed a prevalence of 44% for DVT in patients without varicose veins, compared with 2.6% in those with varicose veins ($p<0.01$). The only patient in their series with varicose veins and a DVT had a history of previous DVT.

These studies suggest that DVT complicating thrombophlebitis in varicose veins below the knee is very rare. The chance of DVT is increased when other risk factors are present (for example in cases of postoperative phlebitis) and when the long saphenous vein is involved above the knee. The danger of extension of thrombus into the deep veins from phlebitis spreading proximally up the long saphenous has been recognized for a long time. Urgent saphenofemoral ligation is the best course of action, to prevent the risk of iliofemoral thrombosis.[12–14]

ARE PATIENTS HAVING OPERATIONS FOR VARICOSE VEINS AT SPECIAL RISK OF THROMBOEMBOLISM?

There is no evidence of a special risk of thromboembolism for patients having varicose vein operations. However, the association of varicose veins with thrombosis after abdominal and pelvic operations,[3–7] and their consequent inclusion high on published lists of risk factors[1–2] mean that surgeons may be sued if they have not used demonstrable prophylaxis, and if a patient then suffers a DVT or pulmonary embolus. If other risk factors exist, then there would seem to be a clear case for prophylaxis – in particular for patients with a history of thromboembolism, those taking the contraceptive pill, obese patients, and those having operations lasting more than about 30 minutes (which includes virtually all patients having bilateral varicose vein surgery). In the absence of any clinical evidence of an increased risk of DVT after varicose vein operations, the main reason for using prophylaxis in cases without other risk factors is for medicolegal protection. This requires the use of 'demonstrable prophylaxis'. The most obvious proven method is use of sub-cutaneous heparin.[15]

There seemed to be wide variation in practice with regard to thromboembolism prophylaxis for varicose vein surgery. In other areas of surgery, where good data exist on the advisability of prophylactic methods, considerable variations have been documented in their use.[16–18] A recent survey in the USA suggested that most surgeons were using prophylaxis appropriately, but this was based on a very poor response rate.[19] In order to elucidate views and practice with regard to varicose vein surgery and DVT, a questionnaire was sent to 363 members of the Vascular Surgical Society of Great Britain and Ireland, and achieved an 80% response rate.[20]

Only 29% vascular surgeons regarded varicose veins as an important risk factor for DVT, and only 12% always used subcutaneous heparin prophylaxis at the time of varicose vein surgery. Seventeen percent of surgeons never used subcutaneous heparin, while 71% did so selectively: the factors which influenced the use of heparin are shown in Table 1. A specific question was asked about why surgeons did not use heparin prophylaxis in bilateral varicose vein operations, and the responses are shown in Table 2. The most common reasons were concern about increased bleeding and bruising, and 'No evidence of DVT risk'. Concern about haematoma is understandable: this is the most common cause of discomfort in the weeks following a varicose vein operation, and subcutaneous heparin is associated with increased haematoma formation.[15] Lack of evidence of a risk of DVT is discussed further below.

The responses to a question about other specific methods of thromboembolic prophylaxis are shown in Table 3. With regard to mechanical methods of

Table 1. Factors which influenced surgeons in their use of subcutaneous heparin prophylaxis, for unilateral varicose operations, and for bilateral operations

	Unilateral operation	Bilateral operation
Special risk (e.g. previous DVT)	195	18
Obesity	95	96
Older patients	63	72
Recurrent varicose veins	40	46
Inpatient status	26	32
Younger patients	11	14
All patients	3	14
Day cases	3	6

Table 2. Reasons given for NOT using heparin prophylaxis in bilateral varicose vein operations

Concern about bleeding/bruising	40
No evidence of DVT risk	35
Rapid mobilization	30
Elastic compression effective	13
1–2 doses heparin 'not worth it'	2
More than two surgeons operating	1
'Don't do bilateral operations'	13

Table 3. Other 'specific methods of antithrombotic prophylaxis' used at the time of varicose vein surgery

Antiembolism stockings	48
Compression bandage	21
Elevation	11
Dextran 70	4
Stop smoking	1
Intravenous fluids	1

prophylaxis, anti-embolism stockings or calf pumps are impractical during varicose vein surgery, and foot pumps are also inconvenient. There is no good evidence about whether applying compression *after* operation provides worthwhile prophylaxis against DVT, but all surgeons responding to the questionnaire used some kind of bandage or stocking at the end of a varicose vein operation (most commonly crepe bandages – 52%). In addition, most advised anti-embolism stockings (55%), other stockings (15%), or various kinds of bandage (28%) in the days that followed. Advising patients to mobilize early is common practice, and tilting the operating table head down may help to reduce the risk of DVT.[21] How far any of these methods would be construed as 'demonstrable prophylaxis' in a medicolegal context is uncertain. Certainly, a written record of their use would be important in supporting the contention that specific DVT prophylaxis had been attempted.

Recently, two studies have supported the belief that DVT is uncommon after operation for varicose veins. Bohler *at al.*[22] performed duplex scanning and ascending phlebography on 100 patients before, and 10–21 days after, varicose vein surgery, and observed no cases of postoperative DVT. In a larger series, yet to be published, Coleridge Smith's group at the Middlesex hospital have found no DVTs on duplex scanning after 200 operations for varicose veins (Coleridge-Smith, personal communication). These studies show that the incidence of DVT after varicose vein surgery bears no comparison with that demonstrated after abdominal and pelvic surgery,[3–7,15] and this is in tune with clinical experience. In a personal series of several thousand varicose vein operations, with a strict regime of early postoperative mobilization, Rivlin observed that thromboembolism was very rare (Rivlin, personal communication). Recently, Miller *et al.*[23] have reported a series of 997 patients having varicose vein surgery, of whom four developed proven venous thromboembolism: the incidence was 0.2% during the latter part of their series in which the postoperative compression regime was changed, and advice on early mobilization was more explicit.

There seems no case to recommend subcutaneous heparin prophylaxis for fit young people having expeditious surgery for unilateral varicose veins, and mobilizing early therafter. Controversy is likely to continue about prophylaxis for patients in whom other risk factors are present, such as prolonged operations (over 30 minutes, which means almost all bilateral procedures), and obesity, even though these factors emanate from studies of abdominal and pelvic surgery, and not varicose vein surgery (which is clearly different). Patients with a past history of venous thromboembolism and those taking the contraceptive pill are at special risk, and all possible precautions, including subcutaneous heparin, would seem wise: this was the practice of virtually all surgeons responding to the questionnaire.

CONCLUSIONS

The traditional belief that varicose veins confer a special risk of DVT, and their inclusion high on lists of risk factors are only justified in the context of major surgery. There is no evidence to suggest that varicose veins pose a risk of DVT to people in their normal daily lives. For those with varicose veins and phlebitis, there is only a significant risk of DVT if veins are affected above the knee – particularly the long saphenous. For those having varicose vein surgery the risk of DVT is very small: simple measures for prophylaxis, such as early mobilization, seem sensible, but subcutaneous heparin may be reserved for cases with additional risk factors.

REFERENCES

1. Thromboembolic Risk Factors (THRIFT) Consensus Group: Risk of and prophylaxis for venous thromboembolism in hospital patients. *Br Med J* **305**: 567–574, 1992
2. European Consensus Statement: *Prevention of Venous Thromboembolism*. London: Med-Orion, 1992.
3. Kakkar VV, Howe CT, Nicolaides AN: Deep vein thrombosis of the leg: is there a 'high risk' group? *Am J Surg* **120**: 527–530, 1970
4. Nicolaides AN, Irving D: Clinical factors and the risk of deep vein thrombosis. In: Nicolaides AN (Ed) *Thromboembolism: Aetiology, Advances in Prevention and Management* pp. 193–204. Lancaster: Medical and Technical Publishing, 1975
5. Clayton JK, Anderson JA, McNicol GP: Preoperative prediction of postoperative deep vein thrombosis. *Br Med J* **2**: 910–912, 1976
6. Lowe GDO, Osborne DH, McArdle BM *et al.*: Prediction and selective prophylaxis of venous thrombosis in elective gastrointestinal surgery. *Lancet* **i**: 109–112, 1982
7. Sue-Ling HM, Johnston D, McMahon MJ: Pre-operative identification of patients at high risk of deep venous thrombosis after elective major abdominal surgery. *Lancet* **i**: 1173–1176, 1986
8. Jorgensen JO, Hanel KC, Morgan AM, Hunt JM: The incidence of deep vein thrombosis in patients with superficial thrombophlebitis of the lower limbs. *J Vasc Surg* **18**: 70–73, 1993
9. Lutter KS, Kerr TM, Roedersheimer LR *et al.*: Superficial thrombophlebitis diagnosed by duplex scanning. *Surgery* **110**: 42–46, 1991
10. Skillman JJ, Kent KC, Porter DH, Kim D: Simultaneous occurrence of superficial and deep thrombophlebitis in the lower extremity. *J Vasc Surg* **11**: 818–824, 1990
11. Bergqvist D, Jarozewski H: Deep vein thrombosis in patients with superficial thrombophlebitis of the leg. *Br Med J* **292**: 658–659, 1986
12. Edwards EA: Thrombophlebitis of varicose veins. *Surg Gynecol Obstet* **66**: 236–245, 1938
13. Galloway JMD, Karmody AM, Mavor GE: Thrombophlebitis of the long saphenous vein complicated by pulmonary embolism. *Br J Surg* **56**: 360–361, 1969
14. Plate G, Eklof B, Jensen R, Ohlin P: Deep venous thrombosis, pulmonary embolism and acute surgery in thrombophlebitis of the long saphenous vein. *Acta Chir Scand* **151**: 241–244, 1985
15. Clagett GP, Anderson FA, Heit J: Prevention of venous thromboembolism. *Chest* **108** (Suppl): 312–333. 1995
16. Morris GK: Prevention of venous thromboembolism: a survey of methods used by orthopaedic and general surgeons. *Lancet* **ii**: 572–574, 1980
17. Bergqvist D: Prophylaxis against postoperative venous thromboembolism: a survey of surveys. *Thromb Haemost* **2**: 69–73, 1990
18. Jones DR: Audit of attitudes to and use of postoperative thromboembolic prophylaxis in a regional health authority. *Ann Roy Coll Surg Engl* **73**: 219–222, 1991
19. Caprini JA, Arcelus JI, Hoffmann K *et al.*: Prevention of venous thromboembolism in North America: results of a survey among general surgeons. *J Vasc Surg* **20**: 751–758, 1994
20. Campbell WB, Ridler BMF: Varicose vein surgery and deep vein thrombosis. *Br J Surg* **82**: 1494–1497, 1995
21. Ashford NS, Ashby EC, Campbell MJ: Posture, blood velocity in the common femoral vein, and prophylaxis of venous thromboembolism. *Lancet* **345**: 419–421, 1995

22. Bohler K, Baldt M. Schuller-Petrovic S *et al.*: Varicose vein stripping – a prospective study of the thrombotic risk and the diagnostic significance of preoperative color coded duplex sonography. *Thromb Haemost* **73:** 597–600, 1995
23. Miller GV, Sainsbury JRC, Lewis WG, Macdonald RC: Morbidity of varicose vein surgery: auditing the benefit of changing clinical practice. *Ann Roy Coll Surg Engl* **78:** 345–349, 1996

Superficial Thrombophlebitis

Jarlis Wesche, Ola D. Saether and Hans O. Myhre

INTRODUCTION

Thrombophlebitis and deep venous thrombosis (DVT) have often been regarded as synonymous. At present the term 'deep venous thrombosis' is used for all forms of thrombosis of the deep veins, whereas the term 'superficial thrombophlebitis' is used for thrombosis of superficial veins associated with inflammatory changes within the venous wall. The incidence of superficial vein thrombophlebitis (SVT) has been suggested to be in the order of one in 240 annually[1] and the condition is usually located to the extremities. Iatrogenic SVT on the upper extremity is usually associated with intravenous infusion, whereas affection of the lower extremities is most often seen in patients with varicose veins. Also veins of the chest wall may be affected by SVT. The purpose of this review is to describe aetiological factors, diagnosis and various treatment modalities of superficial thrombophlebitis.

AETIOLOGY

It is known that SVT is a frequent complication of varicose veins and may in these cases often be induced by a superficial trauma damaging the endothelium. The same mechanism may induce SVT following tight bandaging and the application of plaster casts. The condition can be iatrogenic, and may further present as a manifestation of immunological or haematological disorders as well as malignancies and infectious diseases.[2] The condition is associated with obesity and advanced age. There seems to be a preponderance in women, and SVT is further seen during pregnancy, probably because of venous congestion of the lower extremities and by changes of plasma coagulation factors and platelets. Hypercoagulability is probably also responsible for the increased risk of SVT in the postpartum period and in women taking oral contraceptives.[3,4]

Often SVT is caused by vein punctures or indwelling catheters. The composition of the infusion may increase the risk of SVT being hyperosmolar; like some forms of parenteral nutrition or contrast media used for investigation of the vascular system. Thus, the condition is seen as a complication following sclerotherapy for varicose veins or teleangiectasias. Drugs like pentobarbital and diazepam often cause painful, chemically induced SVT. The risk of SVT is higher in veins with a lower blood flow and therefore higher the more peripheral the injection site, or if the same catheter has been used for more than 2–3 days. The thrombus induced by an intravenous catheter may become infected by microorganisms. This may give rise to suppurative thrombophlebitis and septicaemia.[5,6] In drug addicts SVT may be caused by repetitive trauma, the injection of unsterilized drugs or by using contaminated needles.[7]

Malignant conditions frequently associated with superficial thrombophlebitis are carcinoma of the pancreas, lung, stomach, colon, gallbladder, ovaries and prostate gland as well as leukaemia, various forms of lymphomas and neuroblastoma. In 1865 Trousseau[8,9] described an increased incidence of SVT in patients with gastric carcinoma. Such patients frequently suffered from migratory and recurrent thrombophlebitis. The term migratory phlebitis is used for recurrent attacks of SVT lasting for a couple of days and then resolving, often with recanalization of the thrombus.[10] The condition is also frequently associated with immunological disorders. The clinical picture of thrombotic complications in patients with malignancies may vary from uncomplicated SVT to life-threatening disseminated intravascular coagulation.[11] The disease is then usually in an advanced stage. Although elevation of various coagulation factors, including factor VIII, has been reported in certain forms of carcinoma, the mechanism by which these plasma proteins cause coagulopathy still remains unclear.[4]

In addition, SVT accompanies various immunological disorders. In a population of patients with Buerger's disease, 38% had SVT.[12] Furthermore, SVT is associated with Beçhet's disease,[13] and is seen in systemic lupus, scleroderma and in patients with ulcerative colitis. Mondor's disease describes phlebitis of the anterolateral chest wall and may include the long thoracic, superior epigastric and thoraco-epigastric vein. The disease can occur in both sexes and is regarded as a benign condition which is rarely associated with carcinoma of the breast. Local trauma and muscular strain are regarded as predsiposing factors.[14–16] Also, SVT may be the presenting symptom in certain infectious diseases like psittacosis and secondary syphilis.[3,17]

Haematological disorders like primary thrombocythaemia, polycythaemia vera, sickle-cell disease and chronic myelogenous leukaemia and paroxysmal nocturnal haemoglobinuria as well as homocystinuria are also conditions which have been associated with SVT.[4,18] A variety of conditions associated with increased risk of thrombosis are caused by a specific measurable defect in the proteins responsible for coagulation or fibrinolysis. These conditions are usually cathegorized as hypercoagulable states, the most frequent probably being activated protein C resistance.[19] These abnormalities further include antithrombin deficiency, which is an autosomal dominant, inherited condition with a prevalence in the general population as high as one in 2000.[18] There is considerable variety in the clinical manifestations of thrombotic complications in the latter group of patients. Some may become asymptomatic, whereas others develop SVT, mesenteric vein thrombosis, splanchnic- and cerebral vein thrombosis or Budd–Chiari's syndrome. Protein C and protein S deficiency are also associated with an increased risk of SVT. Patients with lupus anticoagulant and anticardiolipin antibody syndrome are prone to develop thromboembolic events.[20] Although associated with SVT, more serious and recurrent episodes of arterial and venous thrombosis usually dominate the clinical picture. It is known that SVT may also be caused by a variety of disorders of the fibrinolytic system, resulting from alterations in tissue plasminogen activator and quantitative and qualitative abnormalities of plasminogen and fibrinogen.[18] The disorders most frequently associated with SVT are listed in Table 1.

Table 1. Some conditions frequently associated with superficial thrombophlebitis

1. *Varicose veins*

2. *Iatrogenic*
   i.v.   Catheters
   i.v.   Solutions/fluids
   i.v.   Drugs

3. *Malignancies*
   Pancreas
   Lung
   Gastrointestinal
   Ovaries
   Prostate gland

4. *Immunologic disorders*
   Buerger's disease
   Mondor's disease
   Bechet's disease
   Systemic lupus

5. *Infectious diseases*
   Septic thrombophlebitis: (*Klebsiella, Staph. aureus, Candida, Enterobacter* sp.,
   Psittacosis   *Proteus* sp., *Pseudomonas aeruginosa*, enterococci)
   Secondary syphilis

6. *Haematological diseases*
   Thrombocythaemia
   Polycythaemia vera
   Leukaemia, lymphomas

7. *Primary hypercoagulable states*
   Activated protein C resistance
   Antithrombin deficiency
   Protein C and Protein S deficiency
   Lupus anticoagulant
   Anticardiolipin antibody syndrome
   Disorders of the fibrinolytic system

DIAGNOSIS

In patients with varicose veins one should examine whether there has been a local trauma or previous episodes of SVT. In iatrogenic SVT, intravenous infusion of fluid or drugs has usually been performed. In patients with congenital diseases predisposing for SVT, the family history is important. The clinical picture of SVT is usually straightforward. The patient presents with a tender mass following the normal course of a subcutaneous vein. The overlying skin is usually red and hot. The pain can be quite severe and the symptoms may extend along the whole course of the vein. On the lower extremity, varicosities are usually present. Differential diagnoses include DVT and lymphangitis. In the latter condition, swollen lymph nodes in the groin can usually be palpated. Erythema nodosum, acute lipodermatosclerosis and various forms of vasculitis should also be kept in mind.

Furthermore, conditions like cutaneous polyarteritis nodosa or sarcoidal granulomas must be taken into consideration. Patients with HIV-infection and Kaposi's sarcoma may present with hyperalgesic pseudothrombophlebitis. A thorough medical history with regard to weight loss, abdominal pain or back pain is important if carcinoma is suspected, and in Buerger's disease a history of intermittent claudication or foot ulceration can be observed.[2,3]

Methods supplementing the clinical examination may become necessary to verify the diagnosis or to detect complications. Colour-coded duplex ultrasound examination is established as the most reliable non-invasive method for diagnosis of lower extremity venous thrombosis including SVT.[21–23] The picture of SVT is characteristic, since there is no blood flow within the vein, which cannot be compressed by the ultrasound transducer.[24] The deep venous system should be investigated to explore whether DVT is occurring simultaneously. If the proximal part of the thrombosis extends proximally into the iliac veins it may not be followed by duplex scanning, which could be an indication for phlebography.

In patients with SVT who do not have varicose veins, one should screen for malignancies. Such a screening programme may include chest X-ray, abdominal ultrasound or computed tomography (CT)-scanning, and in some instances endoscopy of the gastrointestinal system depending upon the history and the clinical examination. To further explore for haematological and immunological disorders as a cause of SVT, it may become necessary to include such laboratory investigations as erythrocyte sedimentation rate and platelet count as well as testing for activated protein C resistance, antithrombin deficiency and protein C and protein S deficiency. Should these tests be negative, screening for lupus anticoagulant and anticardiolipin antibodies may be indicated, and finally the fibrinolytic system is investigated. If there are clinical signs of Buerger's disease, there may be indication for arteriography to verify the diagnosis.

COMPLICATIONS

For a long time SVT of the lower extremity was generally regarded as a benign and self-limiting disorder. However, several reports have emphasised the risk of associated DVT and pulmonary embolism complicating SVT. This is not surprising since Virchow's triad describing the mechanisms of DVT formation may also be relevant for SVT. Edwards[25] reported that DVT occurred frequently in a group of patients demonstrating clinical signs of SVT. In a group of 40 operated cases of SVT of the lower extremities, propagation into the deep venous system was found in 32%.[26] Therefore, in most cases of clinical SVT of the lower extremities, duplex scanning both of the deep and superficial system should be performed.[21–23] Investigations have indicated an incidence of DVT between 12 and 28% in patients with SVT, with the lowest incidence reported in an investigation mainly based on impedance plethysmography.[27] In recent reports using duplex ultrasound examination of the deep venous system the incidence is between 23 and 28%.[21,22] Most investigations include a total number of patients between 40 and 60, except the study of Lutter and co-workers presenting altogether 186 patients[21,22,27–29] (Table 2).

In one investigation, SVT was frequently associated with DVT in patients without varicose veins.[28] This is in contrast to most reports where the risk of DVT is regarded as lower in this particular subgroup of patients.[20–22,29] The discrepancy between the various reports may be explained by the fact that different methods have been used for diagnosing DVT.

Reports from the literature are not conclusive about whether there is a connection between the anatomical location of SVT and the risk of associated DVT.[30] In one study the incidence of DVT was 17% when SVT was located above the knee, compared with 5% below the knee.[27] However, there was no statistically significant difference between the two groups. Both Jorgensen and Prountjos[22,29] found that the risk of DVT was not associated with any particular location of the SVT. It has been reported that SVT of the long saphenous vein was associated with 35% of complications defined as DVT or pulmonary emboli compared with 16% in patients where the shorter saphenous vein was affected.[21] The incidence of concomitant pulmonary embolism in SVT has been reported to be in the order of 2–6%.[21,26,31–33] Although higher incidences have been published, the application of pulmonary scintigraphy has not been performed systematically, but was often reserved for selected patients suspected of having pulmonary emboli.

Table 2. The incidence of varicosities and DVT in series of patients with SVT

Author	Type of study	Varicose veins		Occult DVT	Diagn. method
(Ref.)	N	no.	(%)	(%)	
Bergqvist and Jaroszewski[28]	pros 56	38/56	(68)	(16)	Phlebography
Skillman et al.[27]	retro 42	39/42	(93)	(12)	Impedance plethysmography
Lutter[21]	retro 186	97/157	(62)	(28)	Duplex ultrasound
Prountjos et al.[29]	pros 57	—	(71)	(20)	Phlebography
Jorgensen et al.[22]	pros 44	41/44	(93)	(23)	Duplex ultrasound

PROPHYLAXIS AND TREATMENT

In patients with SVT due to indwelling catheters and intravenous infusion the obvious treatment is to remove the intravenous cannula and provide the patient with mild analgetics and elastic bandage. Peripheral intravenous cannulas or catheters should be changed every 48–72 hours and hyperosmolar fluids preferably administrated via a central venous catheter. Intravenous lines on the lower extremities should, whenever possible, be avoided. In more severe cases, showing evidence of bacterial or fungal contamination, antibiotics are indicated. In rare cases of suppuration or septicaemia, surgical treatment with excision of the affected vein may become necessary. Movelat cream, which is a combination of a corticosteroid, organoheparinoid and salisylic acid has been shown to reduce infusion-induced phlebitis by nearly half.[34] Using filters during intravenous infusion can reduce the incidence of SVT significantly.[35]

In patients with mild attacks of spontaneous SVT of the lower extremities, the primary treatment is usually elastic bandage and mild analgetics. The patient should be stimulated to walk. In more severe cases, the definition of optimal treatment is a controversial matter regardless of the location of the disease. Based on randomized double-blind controlled trials, some authors recommend anti-inflammatory drugs to decrease pain and shorten the duration of symptoms, but the risk of side-effects should not be neglected.[36,37] Occasionally the pain is severe, necessitating bed rest for a couple of days. It is then probably wise to give heparin subcutaneously until ambulation is possible. Prospective randomized studies have shown that hirudoid, a heparinoid ointment, may shorten the duration of symptoms as well as the period of increased J^{125}-fibrinogen uptake.[38] In contrast, another randomized prospective trial including patients with both spontaneous and infusion-induced SVT, was not able to demonstrate any statistically significant difference between three groups who had been randomized to either hirudoid cream, piroxicam gel or placebo.[39] Ketanserin, a serotonin S_2 antagonist, given as a single injection in a group of SVT has been reported to decrease the subjective symptoms significantly.[40] However, this treatment has not been used to any great extent. In patients with haematological disorders, the underlying condition must be treated whenever possible and anticoagulant treatment may become necessary to prevent further attacks of SVT. In patients with defects of blood- and tissue fibrinolytic activity, systemic treatment by stanozolol or ethyloestrenol has been reported to reduce or even eliminate recurrence of SVT.[41,42]

TREATMENT OF SVT IN VARICOSE VEINS

The role of surgery in patients with SVT of the lower extremities combined with varicose veins has been controversial.[43] Surgical intervention has included phlebotomy with removal of thrombotic material and proximal ligation alone or combined with excision of the inflamed vein. The saphenous vein should be ligated at the saphenofemoral junction and carefully separated from the common femoral vein to make sure that there are no thrombotic material which can be dislodged, thereby giving rise to pulmonary emboli. Surgical therapy for acute SVT with the intention of preventing DVT and pulmonary emboli is controversial, since DVT may not be caused by extension of the thrombus from the superficial vein, but could rather be a complication following bed rest and hypercoagulability.[44] High ligation of

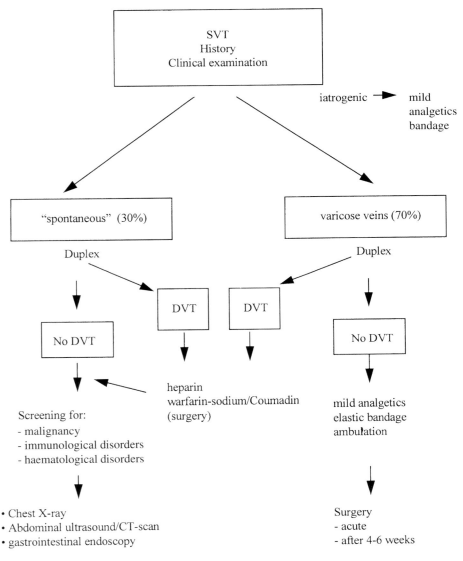

Fig. 1. Flow-chart indicating the management of patients with superficial thrombophlebitis

the saphenous vein or stripping has been recommended in selected cases up to 6 weeks after the acute process, and in a series of 92 patients no thromboembolic complications were reported following such treatment.[45] Husni and Williams[30] reviewed 231 patients with SVT. All the patients with pulmonary embolism including one fatality belonged to the group who was treated conservatively, given analgesics and elastic bandage and who were stimulated to keep walking. Significantly better results were obtained in the two surgical groups including one which was treated by phlebotomy and high saphenous vein ligation followed by anticoagulation, whereas the other group had high ligation and stripping of the saphenous vein. Based on this investigation, it was concluded that, in SVT combined with varicose veins, surgical treatment is preferable. Similar experience was made following review of 163 patients consecutively treated by surgical excision of the thrombosed venous segment.[46] Excision or stripping of varicosities, including the SVT, significantly decreased the symptomatic period and prevented recurrence. It was, therefore, concluded that this was the preferred treatment for SVT in otherwise healthy patients having varicose veins. Plate and co-workers[32] investigated 28 cases of SVT of the long saphenous vein located above the knee level. Propagation of the SVT in proximal direction was noted in 21 patients. However, propagation through the saphenofemoral junction into the common femoral vein was not found in any of the 23 patients who underwent either retrograde phlebography or operative exploration. Signs of SVT extending from the short saphenous vein into the popliteal vein was seen in four cases and two patients had perfusion lung scans consistent with pulmonary embolism. They concluded that high ligation and stripping of the phlebitic vein is the treatment of choice since immediate relief of the symptoms was obtained in all 19 patients treated by this technique. Proximal ligation of the saphenous vein was followed by a prolonged period of pain in four of nine patients. This treatment should therefore be reserved for patients receiving anticoagulation therapy for DVT or pulmonary emboli, since stripping of the saphenous vein may then be complicated by haemorrhage.

REFERENCES

1. Laroche JP: Thrombose veineuse superficielle (veine variqueuse, veine saine) *Actual Vasc Int* **13:** 30–31, 1993
2. Browse NL, Burnand KG, Lea Thomas M: *Diseases of the Veins* pp. 595–601. London: Edward Arnold, 1988
3. Samlaska CP, James WP: Superficial thrombophlebitis II. Secondary hypercoagulable states. *J Am Acad Dermatol* **23:** 1–18, 1990
4. Schafer AI: The hypercoagulable states. *Ann Int Med* **102:** 814–828, 1985
5. McMenamin J, Kennedy D: Infective vasculitides. In Tooke JE, Lowe GD (Eds) *A Textbook of Vascular Medicine* pp. 314–326. London: Arnold, 1996
6. Brook I, Frazier EH. Aerobic and anaerobic microbiology of superficial suppurative trombophlebitis. *Arch Surg* **131:** 95–97, 1996
7. Stuck RM, Doyle D: Superficial thrombophlebitis following parenteral cocaine abuse. *J Am Pediatr Med Ass* **1987:** 351-353, 1987
8. Trousseau A: Phlegmasia alba dolens. *Clin Med Hotel-Dieu Paris* **3:** 94, 1896
9. Moody J, Scott B. Trousseau's syndrome. *Iowa Med* **81:** 303–304, 1991

10. Edwards EA: Migrating thrombophlebitis associated with carcinoma. *N Engl J Med* **240:** 1031–1035, 1949
11. Lesher JL: Superficial migratory thrombophlebitis. *Cutis* **47:** 177–180, 1991
12. Olin JW, Young JR, Graor RA *et al.*: The changing clinical spectrum of thromboangiitis obliterans (Buerger's disease). *Circulation* **82** (suppl IV): IV3-IV8, 1990
13. Koç Y, Gûllû I, Akpek G *et al.*: Vascular involvment in Behçet's disease. *J Rheumatol* **19:** 402–410, 1992
14. Hacker SM: Axillary string phlebitis in pregnancy: A variant of Mondor's disease. *J Am Acad Dermatol* **30:** 636–638, 1994
15. Bejanga BJ: Mondor's disease: analysis of 30 cases. *JR Coll Surg Edinb* **37:** 322–324, 1992
16. Kikano GE, Caceres VM, Sebas JA: Superficial trombophlebitis of the anterior chest wall (Mondor's disease). *J Fam Pract* **33:** 643–644, 1991
17. Jordaan HF: Widespread superficial trombophlebitis as a manifestation of secondary syphilis - a new sign. *South Afr Med J* **8:** 493–494, 1986.
18. Samlaska CP, James WD: Superficial trombophlebitis I. Primary hypercoagulable states. *J Am Acad Dermatol* **22:** 975–989, 1990
19. Djup venetrombos och lungeemboli. *Läkartidningen* **91:** 4403–4411, 1994
20. Blum F, Gilkeson G, Greenberg C, Murray J: Superficial migratory trombophlebitis and lupus anticoagulant. *Int J Dermatol* **3:** 190–192, 1990
21. Lutter KS, Kerr TM, Roedersheimer R *et al.*: Superficial trombophlebitis diagnosed by duplex scanning. *Surgery* **110:** 42–46, 1991
22. Jorgensen JO, Hanel KC, Morgan AM, Hunt JM: The incidence of deep venous thrombosis in pasients with superficial thrombophlebitis of the lower limbs. *J Vasc Surg* **18:** 70–73, 1993
23. Pulliam CW, Barr SL, Ewing AB: Venous duplex scanning in the diagnosis and treatment of progressive superficial thrombophlebitis. *Ann Vasc Surg* **5:** 190–195, 1991
24. Barnes RW: Doppler technique of evaluation of lower extremity venous disease. In: Zwiebel WJ (Ed) *Introduction to Vascular Ultrasonography* pp 339–349 Philadelphia: Grune & Stratton, 1986
25. Edwards EA: Thrombophlebitis of varicose veins. *Surg Gynecol Obstet* **66:** 236–245, 1938
26. Gjöres JE: Surgical therapy of ascending thrombophlebitis in the saphenous system. *Angiology* 13: 241–243, 1962
27. Skillman JJ, Kent KC, Porter DH, Kim D: Simultaneous occurrence of superficial and deep trombophlebitis in the lower extremity. *J Vasc Surg* **11:** 818–824, 1990
28. Bergqvist D, Jaroszewski H: Deep vein thrombosis in patients with superficial thrombophlebitis of the leg. *Br Med J* **292:** 658–659, 1986
29. Prountjos P, Bastounis E, Hadjinikocaou L *et al.*: Superficial venous thrombosis of the lower extremities co-existing with deep venous thrombosis. *Int Angiol* **10:** 63–65, 1991
30. Husni EA, Williams WA: Superficial thrombophlebitis of lower limbs. *Surgery* **91:** 70–74, 1982
31. Hafner CD, Cranley JC, Krause RJ, Strasser ES: A method for managing superficial thrombophlebitis. *Surgery* **55:** 201–206, 1964
32. Plate G, Eklöf B, Jensen R, Ohlin P: Deep venous thrombosis, pulmonary embolism and acute surgery in thrombophlebitis of the long saphenous vein. *Acta Chir Scand* **151:** 241–244, 1985
33. Ternberg JL, Bailes PM Jr, Butcher H Jr: Acute superficial saphenous thrombophlebitis. *Am J Surg* **102:** 691–694, 1961
34. Woodhouse CRJ: Movelat in the prophylaxis of infusion thrombophlebitis. *Br Med J* **1:** 454-455, 1979
35. Bivins B, Rapp R, DeLuca P *et al.*: Final inline filtration; a means of decreasing the incidence of infusion phlebitis. *Surgery* **85:** 388–394, 1979
36. Agus GB, de Angelis R, Mondani P, Moia R: Double-blind comparison of nimesulide and diclofenac in the treatment of superficial thrombophlebitis with telethermographic assessment. *Drugs* **46** (Suppl 1): 200–203, 1993
37. Tomamichel M, Reiner M: Treatment of thrombophlebitis and superficial phlebitis. *Clin Trials J* **20:** 148–157, 1983

38.   Mehta PP, Sagar S, Kakkar VV: Treatment of superficial thrombophlebitis: A randomized double-blind trial of heparinoid cream. *Br Med J* **3:** 614–616, 1975
39.   Bergqvist D, Brunkwall J, Jensen N, Persson NH: Treatment of superficial thrombophlebitis. *Ann Chir Gyn* **79:** 92–96, 1990
40.   de Roose J, Symoens J: Ketanserin in acute superficial thrombophlebitis. *Lancet* **21:** 440–441, 1982
41.   Jarrett EM, Morland M, Browse NL: Idiopathic recurrent superficial thrombophlebitis: treatment with fibrinolytic enhancement. *Br Med J* **1:** 933–934, 1977
42.   Nilsson IM, Hedner U, Isacson S: Phenformin and ethyloestrenol in recurrent venous thrombosis. *Acta Med Scand* **198:** 107–113, 1975
43.   Villavicencio JL, Collins GJ, Youkey JR *et al.*: Nonoperative management of lower extremity venous problems. In: Bergan JJ, Yao ST (Eds) *Surgery of the Veins* pp. 323–345. Philadelphia: Grune & Stratton, 1985
44.   Tournay R: Les thrombophlebites superficielles entaint elles des thrombophlebites des veines profondes? *Phlebologie* **22:** 309–310, 1972
45.   Williams RD, Zollinger RW: Surgical treatment of superficial thrombophlebitis. *Surg Gynecol Obstet* 118: 745–757, 1964
46.   Lofgren EP, Lofgren KA: The surgical treatment of superficial thrombophlebitis. *Surgery* **90:** 49–54, 1981

Inherited Predisposition to Venous Thrombosis

David A. Lane and Katy Hough

INTRODUCTION

It has been pointed out by Allaart and Briet[1] that although there have been reports of familial thrombosis in the literature since the beginning of this century, there was little appreciation of its importance until quite recently. The first deficiency reported as a cause of familial thrombosis was that of antithrombin, known then in 1965 as antithrombin III.[2] Later, it was realized that control of coagulation activation depended upon two principle endogenous anticoagulant pathways (Fig. 1), the

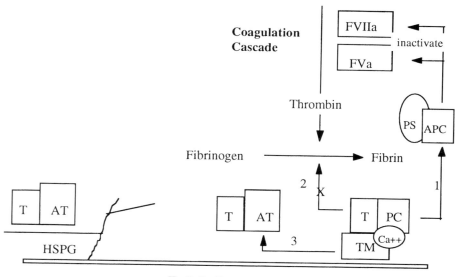

Fig. 1. Representation of the two principle anticoagulant pathways, known to be important in the regulation of coagulation proteinase activity. To the left of the diagram is a simplified view of the inhibition of thrombin (T) by antithrombin (AT) on the endothelial cell surface, mediated by heparan sulphate proteoglycan (HSPG). To the right, are the anticoagulant pathways involving protein C (PC). This protein forms a calcium dependent complex with cell surface thrombomodulin (TM), which generates activated protein C (APC). APC inactivates factor VIIIa (FVIIIa) and factor Va (FVa). Protein S (PS) is a cofactor in this reaction. PS normally forms a complex with C4b-binding protein (not shown) and it is only the free form of PS that acts as a cofactor for APC. Thrombomodulin also prevents the action of thrombin on fibrinogen ('direct anticoagulant action') and accelerates the rate of thrombin-antithrombin complex formation. Adapted from ref. 108.

307

antithrombin-heparan sulphate pathway and the protein C/protein S (PC/PS) pathway. This expanded the possibility of genetic defects being involved in thrombosis to include PC and PS. However, up to 4 years ago the number of thromboses that could be given any genetic explanation was still only ~5%.

A major breakthrough in the study of familial thrombosis has been achieved during the past 2–3 years. First, the concept and method of investigation of activated protein C resistance (APC-R) was introduced and, second, a mutation in the factor V gene (1691 G→A in exon 10, leading to 506Arg to Gln) was identified as the molecular basis for the phenotype of APC-R in the large majority of affected individuals.[3,4] A consequence of this advance has been a conceptual change in how thrombophilia is viewed, which has implications for diagnosis and treatment of the disorder. This review is a summary of a recently published comprehensive account of thrombophilia.[5,6] Another review has also been published recently.[7]

PATHOGENESIS OF THROMBOPHILIA AND DEFINITION OF INHERITED THROMBOPHILIA

Thrombophilia, a tendency towards thrombosis, is generally applied only to patients with atypical thrombosis, those with early age of onset, frequent recurrence, strong family history, unusual, migratory or widespread locations, and severity out of proportion to any recognized stimulus. In fulminant thrombophilia patients thrombose almost continuously but fortunately this is very rare. In most patients thrombosis is episodic, separated by often prolonged asymptomatic periods, suggesting that there is some trigger for each event, perhaps a direct stimulus, a temporary deterioration of intrinsic resistance, or some combination of these factors.

Use of the term inherited thrombophilia acknowledges the presence of an inherited factor that by itself predisposes towards thrombosis but, due to the episodic nature of thrombosis, requires interaction with other components (inherited or acquired) before onset of the clinical disorder. The evolving knowledge of genetic mutation in thrombophilia has moved our view away from a single gene cause, to a model in which genetic and acquired risk factors interact to precipitate the clinical event, see Fig. 2. A genetically based definition has recently been formulated:[5]

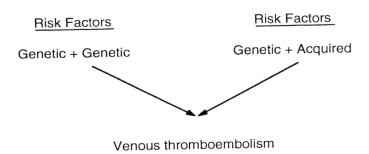

Fig. 2.   Venous thrombosis can be caused by interacting genetic and acquired risk factors.

Inherited thrombophilia is a genetically determined tendency to venous thromboembolism. Dominant abnormalities or combinations of less severe defects may be clinically apparent from early age of onset, frequent recurrence or family history. Milder traits may be discovered only by laboratory investigation. All genetic influences and their interaction are not yet understood.

Currently identified and potential genetic factors predisposing towards thrombophilia are summarized in Table 1. In its footnote are listed some of the many potential interacting acquired risk factors.

Table 1. Deficiencies/abnormalities possibly predisposing towards inherited thrombophilia

Inherited
Antithrombin deficiency
PC deficiency
PS deficiency
APC-R/factor V 506Arg to Gln
Dysfibrinogenaemia
Thrombomodulin defects
Acquired/Inherited (precise relative contribution as yet uncertain)
Hyperhomocysteinaemia
Elevated factor VIII
Elevated fibrinogen?
Potentially Inherited (but firm evidence lacking)[a]
Plasminogen deficiency
Heparin cofactor II deficiency
Elevated histidine rich glycoprotein
Plasminogen activator deficiency?
Elevated plasminogen activator inhibitor?

[a]As discussed in the text, there is as yet no firm evidence that conditions are linked to inherited thrombophilia. The development of thrombosis is thought often to be caused by interaction between genetic and acquired factors, the best recognized of the latter being advancing age, immobilization, major surgery, orthopaedic surgery and neurosurgery, pregnancy, puerperium, use of oestrogen-containing hormones, malignancies and the antiphospholipid syndrome.

CLINICAL MANIFESTATIONS OF INHERITED THROMBOSIS

Clinical manifestation of thrombophilia is most often as deep vein thrombosis (DVT) of the lower limbs, possibly in association with pulmonary embolism. Thrombosis in mesenteric or cerebral veins can also occur, but account for less than 5% of the total episodes in patients with genetic deficiencies. Superficial thrombophlebitis is more frequent in patients with PC or PS deficiency and APC-R than in antithrombin deficient patients.[8–11] There is little current evidence that heterozygous defects of the anticoagulant systems increase the risk of arterial thrombosis.[10,11]

At diagnosis, there is history of thrombosis in 50–60% of individuals with antithrombin, PC and PS deficiencies, with a 50% recurrence rate; the first thrombotic episode occurs as early as before 40 years in approximately 80% of patients.

The risk factors most often found to be associated with the occurrence of thrombosis are pregnancy, puerperium and surgery.[8,9,11,12] In women with antithrombin deficiency, the frequency of thrombosis during pregnancy and the puerperium is between 37% and 44%; in PC or PS deficiency, between 12% and 19%;[13,14] in APC-R, 28%.[15] Thrombotic episodes occur most frequently during the puerperium, accounting for 60–75% of all the episodes complicating pregnancy.[13,14] A retrospective analysis of a large number of antithrombin, PC or PS deficient individuals gave an overall frequency of venous thrombosis complicating surgery of 22%, with no significant differences due to the type of deficiency or surgical procedure.[14] Oral contraceptive use is associated with an increased thrombotic risk, particularly in women with antithrombin deficiency and APC-R.[16–18] Variant, inactive forms of antithrombin, PC and PS have thrombotic risks similar to those of the corresponding quantitative defects. A notable exception is the antithrombin heparin binding site type II subtype (see below for details of subclassification), with a prevalence of thrombosis in these (heterozygous) cases of only 6%, contrasting with 52-68% in patients with other types of antithrombin deficiencies.[19]

Homozygous deficiencies are not often seen. Homozygous antithrombin deficiency is extremely rare and almost exclusively reported in patients with heparin binding site defects. These individuals have a severe thrombotic history of early onset, often affecting arteries.[20] Homozygous type I antithrombin deficiency appears to be incompatible with life.[21] In homozygous PC and PS deficiencies purpura fulminans, due to thrombosis of small vessels with cutaneous and subcutaneous ischaemic necrosis, may occur soon after birth or in the first year of life[22,23] and management of these patients may present great difficulty. Manifestation of disease in homozygotes for APC-R is less than the other deficiencies, some patients remaining asymptomatic despite repeated exposure to acquired risk factors.

EPIDEMIOLOGY OF INHERITED THROMBOPHILIA

The prevalence of hereditary thrombophilia is not yet known and will probably be very difficult to assess accurately. Venous thrombosis is considered to have an overall annual incidence of <1 in 1000, mainly affecting the middle-aged and elderly. In about 50% of patients from families selected on the basis of a high number of unexplained thromboses, an underlying defect will be found (see Table 2).[24] Among unselected consecutive patients with DVT a family history was reported by one out of every four patients.[25]

Investigation of almost 10 000 blood donors has given estimates of the prevalence of deficiencies of PC and antithrombin[26–29] (Table 2) as 1 in 500 and 1 in 5000, respectively. This is in the same range of the findings of a previous study among over 5000 blood donors, where 1 in 250 were considered PC deficient. Assuming that the approximate prevalence of PC deficiency is 1:350, the prevalence of severe (homozygous or compound heterozygous) deficiency will be $1:700 \times 1:700 = 4.9 \times 10^5$. The prevalence of severe antithrombin deficiency is likely to be 100–1000 less than severe PC deficiency. The prevalence of PS deficiency among healthy individuals is still uncertain. The prevalence of APC-R is an order of magnitude higher than the

Table 2. Prevalence of the major thrombophilic clotting abnormalities

	PC deficiency (%)	PS deficiency (%)	Antithrombin deficiency (%)	APC-R (%)
Healthy individuals				
Tait et al. (n=9669)[26,28,29]	0.2[a]		0.02[b]	
Miletich et al. (n=5422)[102]	0.4			
Svensson and Dahlback (n=130)[30]				7
Rosendaal et al. (n=474)[31]				3[a]
Ridker et al. (n=704)[32]				6[a]
Consecutive patients with first DVT				
Heijboer et al. (n=277)[25]	3	2	1	
Koster et al. (n=474)[103]	3[a]	1	1	
Rosendaal et al. (n=471)[31]				20[a]
Thrombophilic patients				
Briet et al. (n=113)[104]	8	13	4	
Scharrer et al. (n=158)[105]	9	6	5	
Ben Tal et al. (n=107)[106]	6	3	7	
Taberno et al. (n=204)[107]	1	1	0.5	
Griffin et al. (n=25)[24]				52

[a]DNA confirmed
[b]Type I Antithrombin deficiency

other inhibitor deficiencies. The estimates for Caucasians range from 3 to 7%.[30–32] The prevalence at birth of homozygous factor V 506 Gln mutation has been estimated at ~1:5000.[31]

Among consecutive patients with objectively confirmed DVT, deficiencies of PC, PS and antithrombin combined account for ~5%. APC-R is present in 20% of consecutive patients with DVT (Table 2).[31,33]

Patients with thrombophilia have a higher prevalence of deficiencies of PC, PS and antithrombin than has been reported among unselected consecutive patients (Table 2). The prevalences for deficiencies of PC, PS and antithrombin are mostly between 5 and 10%, much higher than found in either population studies or series of consecutive unselected patients. It appears that APC-R accounts for half of all cases of hereditary thrombophilia, and clearly emerges from Table 2 as the most important genetic risk factor for hereditary thrombosis, and perhaps for venous thrombosis in general. Because of its high population prevalence, APC-R can be found in patients with other inhibitor deficiency (antithrombin, PC and PS).[34–36] In these circumstances, thrombosis is much more likely and can even occur at a younger age.

MOLECULAR AND GENETIC BASIS OF INHERITED THROMBOPHILIA

Antithrombin deficiency

Antithrombin is a single chain plasma glycoprotein (58 kD) which belongs to the superfamily of the serine protease inhibitors (serpins). It is synthesized in the liver and its concentration in plasma is 2.5 μmol. Antithrombin is the primary inhibitor of thrombin and also inhibits most of the other activated serine proteinases involved in blood coagulation (factor Xa, factor IXa, factor XIa, factor XIIa, kallikrein). It is therefore one of the most important physiological regulators of fibrin formation.

Inactivation of proteinases by antithrombin occurs via the formation of an irreversible 1:1 molar complex, in which Arg393 forms a stabilized bond with the active site of the proteinase. The stable bond forms as the proteinase attempts to cleave the inhibitor Arg 393-Ser 394 bond (this bond is at the reactive centre of antithrombin and is commonly referred to as the P1-P1' bond). Inhibition of most of the blood coagulation proteinases is relatively slow, but can be accelerated at least 1000-fold by the binding of heparin (and heparin-like compounds, such as endothelial cell heparan sulphate, see Fig. 1) to antithrombin. The interaction between heparin and heparin-binding domains of antithrombin results in a conformational change of the protein, which facilitates its interaction with the proteinase. Inactive antithrombin-serine proteinase complexes are rapidly cleared from the circulation. More information on the structure, biochemistry and mechanism of action of antithrombin can be found in a number of recent reviews.[37-39]

cDNA clones of human antithrombin have been isolated and sequenced.[40-42] The gene coding for antithrombin is localized on chromosome 1 between 1q23 and 1q25.[43] It is 13 480 bp long and contains seven exons (1, 2, 3A, 3B, 4, 5, 6);[44] its nucleotide sequence has been recently completed.[45] Several sequence variations or polymorphisms have been described within the human gene,[37-39] including a highly polymorphic trinucleotide repeat sequence in intron 4. The latter, particularly, seems useful for haplotype analysis in the study of recurrent mutations or linkage analysis.[46]

Antithrombin deficiency is a heterogenous disorder. The original subclassification of antithrombin deficiency was based mainly on the results of functional and immunologic assays in plasma. Once more information was available on the actual mutations in the antithrombin gene, the nomenclature was modified[47,48] to include type I antithrombin deficiency (identified by a concordant reduction of both functional and immunological antithrombin) and type II antithrombin deficiency [also identified by a variant antithrombin molecule, which has a defect in the reactive site (II RS), a defect affecting the heparin binding site (II HBS) or multiple functional defects (pleiotropic effect) (II PE)]. From a clinical point of view antithrombin deficiency is heterogenous, see above, with mutations causing type II HBS deficiency being of much less risk than those causing the other subtypes.[19,48]

An antithrombin mutation database is available as a report of the Thrombin and its Inhibitors Subcommittee of the Scientific and Standardization Committee of the International Society on Thrombosis and Haemostasis (SSC ISTH);[48,49] an update will be published in 1997.[50] The number of total and unique identified mutations in the antithrombin gene is shown in Table 3.

PC deficiency

A vitamin K dependent plasma glycoprotein, PC is the precursor of the serine proteinase activated protein C (APC). It is synthesized in the liver as a single chain molecule (62 kDa). Single chain PC is converted into a two chain molecule by

Table 3. Identified gene mutations predisposing towards thrombosis

Gene	Total	Unique	Ref
Antithrombin	256	127	50
Protein C	331	160	60
Protein S	116	90	84
Factor V	Very large	1	4
Fibrinogen	5	5	99
Thrombomodulin	3	3	100, 101

removal of a dipeptide (Arg157 - Thr158) probably in the Golgi. In plasma most of the PC is in the two chain form (41 kD heavy chain and 21 kD light chain); the concentration of PC in plasma is 65 nmol and is reduced during treatment with oral anticoagulants.

Like many other vitamin K dependent proteins, PC is a multimodular protein: the amino terminal light chain contains a γ-carboxyglutamic acid rich domain (Gla-domain) and two epidermal growth factor like domains (EGF domains). The carboxyterminal heavy chain contains the serine proteinase domain.

Thrombin activates PC via cleavage of the Arg169-Leu170 bond – a reaction that can be greatly accelerated by the thrombin-thrombomodulin complex. APC (in complex with PS) inactivates the cofactors, factor Va and VIIIa (see Fig. 1) by specific proteolytic cleavages. Reviews on structural, biochemical and functional aspects of PC are available.[51–53]

Human cDNA clones have been isolated and sequenced[54,55] and the structure of the gene (PROC) has been resolved:[56,57] it contains nine exons and eight introns on 11 kb of genomic DNA. The gene transcript is 1795 bp. It contains a 5' untranslated region of 74 bp, a protein coding region (exons 2-9) and a 3' untranslated region of 294 bp. The gene has been mapped to the chromosome 2q13-q14 region.[58] Several DNA sequence polymorphisms have been identified in the PC gene, both in the promotor region and in the coding region.[59–61]

Deficiency of PC is a heterogenous disorder.[60,62] In type I PC deficiency there is a reduction in both PC activity and PC antigen, while in type II PC deficiency there is evidence for the presence of a variant PC molecule (reduced PC activity, normal PC antigen).

A database of PROC gene mutations has been published on behalf of the Subcommittee on Plasma Coagulation Inhibitors of the SSC ISTH.[60] The numbers of unique and total mutations found in the PC gene are listed in Table 3. Most have been identified in heterozygous individuals, but there are also 18 homozygotes (nine of these had severe clinical symptoms) and 17 compound heterozygotes (eight with severe clinical symptoms). Analysis of PROC gene mutations has not solved an important clinical and epidemiological issue, that of clinically recessive and dominant forms of PC deficiency. The 1995 database lists 14 different mutations that have been found in both these types of PC deficiency. The explanation for the different clinical types has been provided by the finding that genetic risk factors other than PC, such as factor V Arg506 to Gln, can co-exist in families with dominant disease, see Fig. 2.

PS deficiency

PS is a vitamin K dependent plasma glycoprotein (70 kD). It is synthesized in the liver, but also in endothelial cells, megakaryocytes and Leydig cells in the testis. The concentration of PS in plasma is 25 µg/ml and is reduced during treatment with oral anticoagulants.

In addition, PS is a multimodular protein; it contains a γ-carboxyglutamic rich domain, a thrombin sensitive region, four EGF-like domains and a carboxyterminal region which is highly homologous to the sex hormone binding globulin (SHBG). In plasma, PS circulates both free (40%) and in a 1:1 stoichiometric complex with C4b-binding protein (60%). The latter comprises seven identical α-chains (70 kD) and one single β-chain (45 kD) which are linked to each other in the carboxyterminal region by disulphide bonds. The β-chain contains the PS binding site. Two regions in PS have been reported to be involved in binding of the C4b binding protein (Gly605 to Ile 614 and Gly420 to His 434). Only the free form of PS has APC cofactor activity. It has been reported that PS itself also has anticoagulant activity: under well-defined conditions it may inhibit (independently of APC) the activity of both the tenase (IXa-VIIIa) and prothrombinase (Xa-Va) complexes, some reactions being independent of the presence of C4b-binding protein.[63-65] The relative clinical importance of these different functional properties of PS has yet to be established.

In the 1980s cDNAs of human PS were isolated and sequenced.[66-68] Two highly homologous PS genes have been identified and sequenced.[69-71] The *PROS* or *PSα* gene is the active gene; it consists of 15 exons which are spread over 80 kb of genomic DNA and has been mapped to the chromosome 3 p11.1–3 p11.2 region.[72] The *PSβ* gene (a pseudogene) shows 96.5% homology with *PROS* in exon sequences and the positions of the introns are virtually identical to those in the *PROS* gene. Several DNA sequence polymorphisms have been reported in the *PROS* gene.[66,67,73] Some of these have been very useful for tracking PS deficiency through families, for prenatal diagnosis and for evaluating the possibility of allelic exclusion in the case of the study of reverse transcripts of platelet *PROS* mRNA.[74,75]

Two subclassification systems for PS deficiency are still in use; the system proposed by Comp[76] in 1990 (76) and the proposal recommended by the SSC ISTH in Munich, July 1992. Type I deficiencies/defects result in a reduction of total PS antigen (and of free PS antigen and PS activity). Type II, or in Comp's notation type IIb, defines the presence of a functionally variant PS molecule (total PS antigen normal, free PS antigen normal but PS activity reduced). Type III PS deficiency (or in Comp's notation type IIa) is defined by normal total PS antigen but reduced free PS antigen and activity. Duchemin *et al.* reported among type III PS deficiencies an unusual high frequency (22%) of a mutation in codon 460, resulting in the replacement of Ser 460 by Pro in the consensus sequence for the N-linked glycosylation of Asn 458 (PS Heerlen).[77] The frequency of the PS Heerlen allele in the general population is 0.5% and similar in some cohorts of thrombophilic patients (0.7%). Zoller *et al.* have reported that both type I and type III phenotypes can be reflections of the same genotype.[78] In an extension of these studies it has been shown that the variable phenotype within families is caused by an age-related increase in total PS, associated with a rise in C4b-binding protein, which results in changes in total PS, but a stable low level of free PS in affected individuals.[79]

Investigation of PS deficiency at the gene level has progressed relatively slowly because of the structural complexity of the *PROS* gene and an unexpectedly low yield of successful genetic analyses.[80-83] Nevertheless, in the past 2 years our knowledge in this area has increased dramatically (see Table 3) and in 1997 a PS mutation database will be published.[84]

Factor V Arg506 to Gln

Factor V is a single chain plasma glycoprotein (300 000 kD), concentration 20 nmol. It is synthesized in the liver and in megakaryocytes (4 µg/10^9 platelets). Factor V is converted into factor Va by (meizo) thrombin and/or factor Xa, which cleave the Arg709-Ser710, Arg1018-Thr1019 and Arg1545-Ser1546 bonds. Factor Va is composed of an amino terminal fragment (heavy chain 105 kDa) and a carboxy terminal fragment (light chain 74 kDa) non-covalently linked via a tightly bound Ca^{2+} ion. Factor Va serves as a non-enzymatic cofactor in prothrombinase (factor Xa, phospholipids, Ca^{2+}) by increasing the catalytic efficiency approximately 2000-fold.

APC inactivates factor Va by proteolytic degradation of its heavy chain with a first cleavage at Arg506 and subsequent inactivating cleavages at Arg306 and Arg679.[85] Others demonstrated that two random cleavages (mainly at Arg506 and Arg306) are involved and that both contribute to the inactivation of factor Va.[86] Factor V is not only a procofactor in the prothrombinase reaction but also a cofactor in the inactivation of factor VIIIa by APC.[87] A review of the structure and function of human factor V is available.[88]

Human factor V cDNAs have been isolated from HepG2 and (fetal) liver cDNA libraries[89-91] enabling the complete amino acid sequence of factor V to be derived. Factor V consists of 2196 amino acids and is structurally similar to factor VIII. In the factor V gene there are 25 exons and 24 introns which span approximately 80 kb genomic DNA.[92] The factor V gene has been mapped to chromosome 1 (1q21-25) and is closely linked to the antithrombin gene.[93] A number of nucleotide sequence variations in human factor V cDNAs have been identified.[89-91,94,95]

As stated above, in 1994, the single point mutation in the factor V gene was identified as the genetic defect causing the phenotype of APC-R in the vast majority of affected individuals.[4,96,97] It involves a G→A transition of nucleotide 1691 in exon 10, which predicts the synthesis of a variant factor V molecule (factor V 506 Arg to Gln or factor V Leiden).

So far the factor V 506Arg to Gln mutation is the only genetic defect identified in APC-R families. It has a relatively high frequency in Caucasian populations (up to ~6%) but a much lower frequency in the Japanese and other Eastern populations (~0%).[98] The distribution of this mutation amongst the Caucasian populations is best explained by a founder effect and spread by population mobility, rather than by repeated independent mutations.

Future prospects

There are a number of other genetic defects or isolated deficiencies that have been implicated in contributing to the risk of thrombosis in families with thrombophilia and some of these are indicated in Tables 1 and 3. The strongest evidence is available for certain variant fibrinogens[99] and for gene mutation of thrombomodulin,[100,101] (see Table 3). However, for these potential risk factors the evidence is based only on a small number of families and should therefore be regarded as preliminary. There is great current interest in identifying additional genetic risk factors, and those in the lower part of Table 1 are candidates in on-going investigations.

REFERENCES

1. Allaart CF, Briet E: Familial venous thrombophilia. In: Bloom AL, Forbes CD, Thomas DP, Tuddenham EGD (Eds) *Haemostasis and Thrombosis* pp. 1349–1360. Edinburgh: Churchill Livingstone, 1994
2. Egeberg O: Inherited antithrombin III deficiency causing thrombophilia. *Thromb Diath Haemorrh* **13:** 516–530, 1965
3. Dahlback B, Carlsson M, Svensson PJ: Familial thrombophilia due to a previously unrecognized mechanism characterized by poor anticoagulant response to activated protein C: prediction of a cofactor to activated protein C. *Proc Natl Acad Sci USA* **90:** 1004–1008, 1993
4. Bertina RM, Koeleman BP, Koster T *et al.*: Mutation in blood coagulation factor V associated with resistance to activated protein C. *Nature* **369:** 64–67, 1994
5. Lane DA, Mannucci PM, Bauer KA *et al.*: Inherited thrombophilia: Part 1. *Thromb Haemost* **76:** 651–662, 1996
6. Lane DA, Mannucci PM, Bauer KA *et al.*: Inherited thrombophilia: Part 2. *Thromb Haemost* **76:** 824–834, 1996
7. de Stefano V, Finazzi G, Mannucci PM: Inherited thrombophilia: pathogenesis, clinical syndromes and management. *Blood* **87:** 3531–3544, 1996
8. Briet E, Broekmans AW: Hereditary protein S deficiency. In: Bertina RM (Eds) *Protein C and Related Proteins* p. 203. Edinburgh: Churchill Livingstone, 1988
9. Broekmans AW, Conard J: Hereditary protein C deficiency. In: Bertina RM (Eds) *Protein C and Related Proteins*. Edinburgh: Churchill Livingstone, 1988
10. Demers C, Ginsberg JS, Hirsh J *et al.*: Thrombosis in antithrombin-III-deficient persons. Report of a large kindred and literature review. *Ann Intern Med* **116:** 754-761, 1992
11. De Stefano V, Leone G, Mastrangelo S *et al.*: Clinical manifestations and management of inherited thrombophilia: retrospective analysis and follow-up after diagnosis of 238 patients with congenital deficiency of antithrombin III, protein C, protein S. *Thromb Haemost* **72:** 352–358, 1994
12. Zoller B, Svensson PJ, He X, Dahlback B: Identification of the same factor V gene mutation in 47 out of 50 thrombosis-prone families with inherited resistance to activated protein C. *J Clin Invest* **94:** 2521–2524, 1994
13. Conard J, Horellou MH, Van Dreden P *et al.*: Thrombosis and pregnancy in congenital deficiencies in AT III, protein C or protein S: study of 78 women. *Thromb Haemost* **63:** 319–320, 1990
14. De Stefano V, Leone G, Mastrangelo S *et al.*: Thrombosis during pregnancy and surgery in patients with congenital deficiency of antithrombin III, protein C, protein S. *Thromb Haemost* **71:** 799–800, 1994
15. De Stefano V, Mastrangelo S, Paciaroni K *et al.*: Thrombotic risk during pregnancy and puerperium in women with APC-resistance. Effective subcutaneous heparin in prophylaxis in a pregnant patient. *Thromb Haemost* **74:** 793–794, 1995
16. Pabinger I, Schneider B: Thrombotic risk of women with hereditary antithrombin III-, protein C- and protein S-deficiency taking oral contraceptive medication. The GTH Study Group on Natural Inhibitors. *Thromb Haemost* **71:** 548–552, 1994
17. Vandenbroucke JP, Koster T, Briet E *et al.*: Increased risk of venous thrombosis in oral-contraceptive users who are carriers of factor V Leiden mutation. *Lancet* **344:** 1453–1457, 1994

18. Rintelen C, Mannhalter C, Ireland H et al.: Oral contraceptives enhance the risk of clinical manifestations of venous thrombosis at a young age in females homozygous for factor V Leiden. Brit J Haematol 93: 487–490, 1996
19. Finazzi G, Caccia R, Barbui T. Different prevalence of thromboembolism in the subtypes of congenital antithrombin III deficiency: review of 404 cases. Thromb Haemost 58: 1094, 1987
20. Chowdhury V, Lane DA, Auberger K et al.: Homozygous antithrombin deficiency: report of two new cases (99Leuto Phe) associated with arterial and venous thrombosis. Thromb Haemost 72: 198–202, 1994
21. Hakten M, Deniz U, Ozbag G, Ulutin ON: Two cases of homozygous antithrombin III deficiency in a family with congenital deficiency of ATIII. In: Senzinger H, Vinazzer H (Eds) Thrombosis and Haemorrhagic Disorders pp. 177-81, Wurzberg: Scmitt and Meyer GmbH, 1989
22. Branson HE, Katz J, Marble R, Griffin JH: Inherited protein C deficiency and coumarin-responsive chronic relapsing purpura fulminans in a newborn infant. Lancet ii: 1165–1168, 1983
23. Marlar RA, Montgomery RR, Madden RM: Homozygous protein C deficiency. In: Bertina RM (Eds) Protein C and Related Proteins p. 182. Edinburgh: Churchill Livingstone, 1988
24. Griffin JH, Evatt B, Wideman C, Fernandez JA: Anticoagulant protein C pathway defective in majority of thrombophilic patients. Blood 82: 1989–1993, 1993
25. Heijboer H, Brandjes DP, Buller HR et al.: Deficiencies of coagulation-inhibiting and fibrinolytic proteins in outpatients with deep-vein thrombosis. N Engl J Med 323: 1512–1516, 1990
26. Tait RC, Walker ID, Perry DJ et al.: Prevalence of antithrombin III deficiency subtypes in 4000 healthy blood donors. Thromb Haemost 65: 839, 1991
27. Tait RC, Walker ID, Islam SI et al.: Protein C activity in healthy volunteers – influence of age, sex, smoking and oral contraceptives. Thromb Haemost 70: 281–285, 1993
28. Tait RC, Walker ID, Islam SIA et al.: Influence of demographic factors on antithrombin III activity in a healthy population. Br J Haematol 84: 476–480, 1993
29. Tait RC, Walker ID, Reitsma PH et al.: Prevalence of protein C deficiency in the healthy population. Thromb Haemost 73: 87–93, 1995
30. Svensson PJ, Dahlback B: Resistance to activated protein C as a basis for venous thrombosis. N Engl J Med 330: 517–522, 1994
31. Rosendaal FR, Koster T, Vandenbroucke JP, Reitsma PH: High risk of thrombosis in patients homozygous for factor V Leiden (activated protein C resistance). Blood 85: 1504–1508, 1995
32. Ridker PM, Hennekens CH, Lindpaintner K et al.: Mutation in the gene coding for coagulation factor V and the risk of myocardial infarction. N Engl J Med 332: 912–917, 1995
33. Koster T, Rosendaal FR, de Ronde H et al.: Venous thrombosis due to poor anticoagulant response to activated protein C: Leiden Thrombophilia Study. Lancet 342: 1503–1506, 1993
34. Koeleman BP, Reitsma PH, Allaart CF, Bertina RM: Activated protein C resistance as an additional risk factor for thrombosis in protein C-deficient families. Blood 84: 1031–1035, 1994
35. Zoller B, Berntsdotter A, Garcia de Frutos P, Dahlback B: Resistance to activated protein C as an additional genetic risk factor in hereditary deficiency of protein S. Blood 85: 3518–3523, 1995
36. van Boven HH, Reitsma PH, Rosendaal FR et al.: Factor V Leiden (FV R506Q) in families with inherited antithrombin deficiency. Thromb Haemost 75: 417–421, 1996
37. Lane DA, Caso R: Antithrombin: structure, genomic organisation, function and inherited deficiency. Baillière's Clin Haem 2: 961–998, 1989
38. Blajchman M, Austin R, Fernandez-Rachubinski F, Sheffield W: Molecular basis of inherited antithrombin deficiency. Blood 80: 2159–2171, 1992
39. Olds RJ, Lane DA, Mille B et al.: Antithrombin: the principal inhibitor of thrombin. Semin Thromb Haemostas 20: 353–372, 1994
40. Bock SC, Wion KL, Vehar GA, Lawn RM: Cloning and expression of the cDNA for human antithrombin III. Nucl Acids Res 10: 8113–8125, 1982

41. Chandra T, Stackhouse R, Kidd VJ, Woo SLC: Isolation and sequence characterisation of a cDNA clone of human antithrombin III. *Proc Natl Acad Sci USA* **80:** 1845–1848, 1983

42. Prochownik EV, Markam AF, Orkin SH: Isolation of a cDNA clone for human antithrombin III. *J Biol Chem* **258:** 8389–8394, 1983

43. Bock SC, Harris JF, Balazs I, Trent JM: Assignment of the human antithrombin III structural gene to chromosome 1q23-25. *Cytogenet Cell Genet* **39:** 67–69, 1985

44. Bock SC, Marrinan JA, Radziejewska E: Antithrombin III Utah: proline-407 to leucine mutation in a highly conserved region near the inhibitor reactive site. *Biochemistry* **27:** 6171–6178, 1988

45. Olds RJ, Lane DA, Chowdhury V *et al.*: Complete nucleotide sequence of the antithrombin gene: evidence for homologous recombination causing thrombophilia. *Biochemistry* **32:** 4216–4224, 1993

46. Olds RJ, Lane DA, Chowdhury V *et al.*: (ATT) trinucleotide repeats in the antithrombin gene and their use in determining the origin of repeated mutations. *Hum Mutat* **4:** 31–41, 1994

47. Lane DA, Olds RJ, Conard J *et al.*: Pleiotropic effects of antithrombin strand 1C substitution mutations. *J Clin Invest* **90:** 2422–2433, 1992

48. Lane DA, Olds RJ, Boisclair M *et al.*: Antithrombin III mutation database: first update. *Thromb Haemost* **70:** 361–369, 1993

49. Lane DA, Ireland H, Olds RJ *et al.*: Antithrombin III: a database of mutations. *Thromb Haemost* **66:** 657–661, 1991

50. Lane DA, Bayston T, Olds RJ *et al.*: Antithrombin mutation database: 2nd (1997) update. *Thromb Haemost* **77:** 197–211, 1997

51. Esmon CT: The protein C anticoagulant pathway. *Arterioscler Thromb* **12:** 135–145, 1992

52. Esmon CT: Molecular events that control the protein C anticoagulant pathway. *Thromb Haemost* **70:** 29–35, 1993

53. Dahlback B: The protein C anticoagulant system: inherited defects as basis for venous thrombosis. *Thromb Res* **77:** 1–43, 1995

54. Foster D, Davie EW: Characterization of a cDNA coding for human protein C. *Proc Natl Acad Sci USA* **81:** 4766–4770, 1984

55. Beckmann RJ, Schmidt RJ, Santerre RF *et al.*: The structure and evolution of a 461 amino acid human protein C precursor and its messenger RNA, based upon the DNA sequence of cloned human liver cDNAs. *Nucleic Acids Res* **13:** 5233–5247, 1985

56. Foster DC, Yoshitake S, Davie EW: The nucleotide sequence of the gene for human protein C. *Proc Natl Acad Sci USA* **82:** 4673–4677, 1985

57. Plutzky J, Hoskins JA, Long GL, Crabtree GR: Evolution and organization of the human protein C gene. *Proc Natl Acad Sci USA* **83:** 546–550, 1986

58. Patracchini P, Aiello V, Palazzi P *et al.*: Sublocalization of the human protein C gene on chromosome 2q13-q14. *Hum Genet* **81:** 191–192, 1989

59. Reitsma PH, Poort SR, Bernardi F *et al.*: Protein C deficiency: a database of mutations. For the Protein C & S Subcommittee of the Scientific and Standardization Committee of the International Society on Thrombosis and Haemostasis. *Thromb Haemost* **69:** 77–84, 1993

60. Reitsma PH, Bernadi F, Doig RG *et al.*: Protein C deficiency: A database of mutations, 1995 update. *Thromb Haemost* **73:** 876–889, 1995

61. te Lintel Hekkert W, Bertina RM, Reitsma PH: Two RFLPS approximately 7 kb 5' of the human protein C gene. *Nucleic Acids Res* **16:** 11849, 1988

62. Aiach M, Gandrille S, Emmerich J: A review of mutations causing deficiencies of antithrombin, protein C and protein S. *Thromb Haemost* **74:** 81–89, 1995

63. Heeb MJ, Mesters RM, Tans G *et al.*: Binding of protein S to factor Va associated with inhibition of prothrombinase that is independent of activated protein C. *J Biol Chem* **268:** 2872–2877, 1993

64. Heeb MJ, Rosing J, Bakker HM *et al.*: Protein S binds to and inhibits factor Xa. *Proc Natl Acad Sci USA* **91:** 2728–2732, 1994

65. Koppelman SJ, Hackeng TM, Sixma JJ, Bouma BM: Inhibition of the intrinsic factor X activating complex by protein S: Evidence for specific binding of protein S to Factor VIII. *Blood* **86:** 1062–1071, 1995

66. Lundwall A, Dackowski W, Cohen E *et al.*: Isolation and sequence of the cDNA for human protein S, a regulator of blood coagulation. *Proc Natl Acad Sci USA* **83**: 6716–6720, 1986
67. Hoskins JA, Norman DK, Beckmann RJ, Long GL: Cloning and characterisation of a human liver cDNA encoding a protein S precursor. *Proc Natl Acad Sci USA* **84**: 349–353, 1987
68. Ploos van Amstel HK, van der Zanden AL, Reitsma PH, Bertina RM: Human protein S cDNA encodes Phe-16 and Tyr 222 in consensus sequences for the post-translational processing. *FEBS Lett* **222**: 186–190, 1987
69. Edenbrandt CM, Lundwall A, Wydro R, Stenflo J: Molecular analysis of the gene for vitamin K dependent protein S and its pseudogene. Cloning and partial gene organization. *Biochemistry* **29**: 7861–7868, 1990
70. Ploos van Amstel HK, Reitsma PH, van der Logt CP, Bertina RM: Intron-exon organization of the active human protein S gene PS alpha and its pseudogene PS beta: duplication and silencing during primate evolution. *Biochemistry* **29**: 7853–7861, 1990
71. Schmidel DK, Tatro AV, Phelps LG *et al.*: Organization of the human protein S genes. *Biochemistry* **29**: 7845–7852, 1990
72. Watkins PC, Eddy R, Fukushima Y *et al.*: The gene for protein S maps near the centromere of human chromosome 3. *Blood* **71**: 238–241, 1988
73. Diepstraten CM, Ploos van Amstel JK, Reitsma PH, Bertina RM: A CCA/CCG neutral dimorphism in the codon for Pro 626 of the human protein S gene PS alpha (PROS1). *Nucleic Acids Res* **19**: 5091, 1991
74. Formstone CJ, Voke J, Tuddenham EGD *et al.*: Prenatal exclusion of severe protein S deficiency by indirect RFLP analysis. *Thromb Haemostas* **69**: 931, 1993
75. Marchetti G, Legnani C, Patracchini P *et al.*: Study of a protein S gene polymorphism at DNA and mRNA level in a family with symptomatic protein S deficiency. *Br J Haematol* **85**: 173–175, 1993
76. Comp PC: Laboratory evaluation of protein S status. *Semin Thromb Hemost* **16**: 177–181, 1990
77. Bertina RM, Ploos van Amstel HK, van Wijngaarden A *et al.*: Heerlen polymorphism of protein S, an immunologic polymorphism due to dimorphism of residue 460. *Blood* **76**: 538–548, 1990
78. Zoller B, Garcia de Frutos P, Dahlback B: Evaluation of the relationship between protein S and C4b-binding protein isoforms in hereditary protein S deficiency demonstrating type I and type III deficiencies to be phenotypic variants of the same genetic disease. *Blood* **85**: 3524–3531, 1995
79. Simmonds R, Zöller B, Ireland H *et al.*: Genetic and phenotypic analysis of a large (122 member) protein S-deficient kindred provides an explanation for the familial coexistence of type I and type III plasma phenotypes. *Blood* 1997 (in press).
80. Borgel D, Duchemin J, Matheron C *et al.*: Molecular defects responsible for type I and IIa protein S (PS) deficiencies in a panel of 120 French families. *Thromb Haemostas* **73**: 1256, 1995
81. Reitsma PH, Ploos van Amstel HK, Bertina RM: Three novel mutations in five unrelated subjects with hereditary protein S deficiency type I. *J Clin Invest* **93**: 486–492, 1994
82. Gomez E, Poort SR, Bertina RM, Reitsma PH: Identification of eight point mutations in protein S deficiency type I - Analysis of 15 pedigrees. *Thromb Haemost* **73**: 750–755, 1995
83. Simmonds R, Ireland H, Kunz G, Lane DA. Indentification of 19 PROS gene mutations in cases of phenotypic protein S deficiency and thrombosis. *Blood* **88**: 4195–4204, 1996
84. Gandrille S, Borgel D, Ireland H *et al.*: Protein S deficiency: a database of mutations. *Thromb Haemost* 1997 (in press)
85. Kalafatis M, Rand MD, Mann KG: The mechanism of inactivation of human factor V and human factor Va by activated protein C. *J Biol Chem* **269**: 31869–31880, 1994
86. Nicolaes GAF, Tans G, Thomassen MCLGD *et al.*: Peptide bond cleavages and loss of functional activity during inactivation of factor Va and factor Va R506Q by activated protein C. *J Biol Chem* **270**: 21158–21166, 1995
87. Shen L, Dahlback B: Factor V and protein S as synergistic cofactors to activated protein C in degradation of factor VIIIa. *J Biol Chem* **269**: 18735–18738, 1994

88. Jenny RJ, Tracy PB, Mann KG: The physiology and biochemistry of factor V. In: Bloom AL, Forbes CD, Thomas DP, Tuddenham EGD (Eds) *Haemostasis and Thrombosis* pp. 465–476, Edinburgh: Churchill Livingstone, 1994

89. Kane WH, Davie EW: Cloning of a cDNA coding for human factor V, a blood coagulation factor homologous to factor VIII and ceruloplasmin. *Proc Natl Acad Sci USA* **83**: 6800–6804, 1986

90. Kane WH, Ichinose A, Hagen FS, Davie EW: Cloning of cDNAs coding for the heavy chain region and connecting regions of human factor V, a blood coagulation factor with four types of internal repeats. *Biochemistry* **26**: 6508–6514, 1987

91. Jenny RJ, Pittman DD, Toole JJ *et al.*: Complete cDNA and derived amino acid sequence of human factor V. *Proc Natl Acad Sci USA* **84**: 4846–4850, 1987

92. Cripe LD, Moore KD, Kane WH: Structure of the gene for human coagulation factor V. *Biochemistry* **31**: 3777–3785, 1992

93. Wang H, Riddell DC, Guinto ER *et al.*: Localization of the gene encoding human factor V to chromosome 1q21-25. *Genomics* **2**: 324–328, 1988

94. Bayston T, Ireland H, Olds RJ *et al.*: A polymorphism in the human coagulation factor V gene. *Hum Mol Genet* **3**: 2085, 1994

95. Zoller B, Dahlback B: Linkage between inherited resistance to activated protein C and factor V gene mutation in venous thrombosis. *Lancet* **343**: 1536–1538, 1994

96. Greengard JS, Sun X, Xu X *et al.*: Activated protein C resistance caused by Arg506Gln mutation in factor Va. *Lancet* **343**: 1361–1362, 1994

97. Voorberg J, Roelse J, Koopman R *et al.*: Association of idiopathic venous thromboembolism with single point-mutation at Arg506 of factor V. *Lancet* **343**: 1535–1536, 1994

98. Rees DC, Cox M, Clegg JB: World distribution of factor V Leiden. *Lancet* **346**: 1133–1134, 1995

99. Haverkate F, Samama M: Familial dysfibrinogenemia and thrombophilia. Report on a study of the SSC Subcommittee on Fibrinogen. *Thromb Haemost* **73**: 151–161, 1995

100. Ohlin A-K, Marlar RA: The first mutation identified in the thrombomodulin gene in a 45 year old man presenting with thromboembolic disease. *Blood* **85**: 330–336, 1995

101. Ohlin A-K, Marlar RA: Mutations in the thrombomodulin gene associated with thromboembolic disease. *Thromb Haemostas* **73**: 1096, 1995

102. Miletich J, Sherman L, Broze G Jr: Absence of thrombosis in subjects with heterozygous protein C deficiency. *N Engl J Med* **317**: 991–996, 1987

103. Koster T, Rosendaal FR, Briet E *et al.*: Protein C deficiency in a controlled series of unselected outpatients: an infrequent but clear risk factor for venous thrombosis (Leiden Thrombophilia Study). *Blood* **85**: 2756–2761, 1995

104. Briet E, Engesser L, Brommer EJP *et al.*: Thrombophilia: its causes and a rough estimate of its prevalence. *Thromb Haemost* **58**: 39, 1987

105. Scharrer I, Hach-Wunderle V, Heyland H, Kuhn C: Incidence of defective tPA release in 158 unrelated young patients with venous thrombosis in comparison to PC-, PS-, ATIII-, fibrinogen-, and plasminogen deficiency. *Thromb Haemost* **58**: 72, 1987

106. Ben Tal O, Zivelin A, Seligsohn U: The relative frequency of hereditary thrombotic disorders among 107 patients with thrombophilia in Israel. *Thromb Haemost* **61**: 50–54, 1989

107. Tabernero MD, Tomas JF, Alberca I *et al.*: Incidence and clinical characteristics of hereditary disorders associated with venous thrombosis. *Am J Hematol* **36**: 249–254, 1991

108. Bourin MC: Thrombomodulin: a novel proteoglycan. PhD Thesis, Swedish University of Agricultural Sciences, Uppsala 1990

Surgery for Deep Venous Thrombosis

Jesper Swedenborg and Staffan Törngren

SURGERY FOR DEEP VENOUS THROMBOSIS

Surgery for deep venous thrombosis (DVT) in the acute stage is mainly restricted to thrombectomy of iliofemoral venous thrombosis (IFVT). For late sequelae of IFVT cross-over bypass directing the venous emptying to the contralateral side, when outflow obstruction occurs, has been suggested. In recent years percutaneous methods with thrombolysis and recanalization by stenting of the chronically occluded iliac vein have also been suggested.

PATHOGENESIS OF ILIOFEMORAL VENOUS THROMBOSIS

Iliofemoral venous thrombosis constitutes about 10% of all cases of lower leg venous thrombosis. It is usually considered to be primary in the iliofemoral venous segment but could also be a consequence of an ascending thrombotic process originating in the lower leg (Fig. 1). In the former the thrombosis may secondarily extend distally. The differentiation between primary and secondary IFVT is mainly based on history and clinical examination. A primary IFVT often starts with groin pain followed several days later by swelling of the limb and a marked phlebitic reaction can often be palpated in the groin. The secondary thrombosis starts with pain in the calf followed by progressive swelling of the leg.

The narrow segment caused by the crossing of the right iliac artery with the left femoral vein is an important pathogenic aspect and explains why IFVT is much more common on the left side than the right.[1-3] A narrow segment alone cannot explain the occurrence of IFVT since it has been shown in autopsy materials that a large percentage of normal individuals have severely stenosed left iliac veins, sometimes even with webs inside the vein.[4]

Hypercoagulability is often a component in the development of IFVT. A large proportion of patients has been shown to have some sort of coagulation abnormality, mostly impaired fibrinolytic activity.[5] Resistance towards activated protein C (APC) has in recent years been demonstrated as an important risk factor for DVT.[6] Whether APC resistance is as important for IFVT as it is for other forms of DVT remains to be shown.

Pregnancy carries multiple risks for IFVT since it both induces a hypercoagulable state with increased risk of thrombosis[7] and an impaired flow through the iliac vein due to compression by the pregnant uterus. The risk of DVT is therefore increased several-fold during pregnancy and is calculated to be 0.1–1 per 1000 live births. The

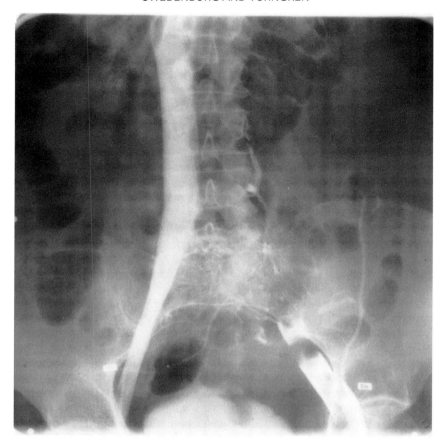

Fig. 1.   Phlebography of left-sided iliofemoral venous thrombosis.

relative proportion of IFVT among all lower leg thrombosis is also increased during pregnancy. External compression can also be caused by tumours and if these are malignant the risk of IFVT is high since lower leg thrombosis is also a paramalignant phenomenon.

In general it can be stated that several factors have to be present in order for IFVT to develop and these prerequisites are fulfilled, e.g. during pregnancy or following trauma in a patient with a stenosed iliac vein.

SECONDARY ILIOFEMORAL VENOUS THROMBOSIS

The secondary ascending thrombosis is a consequence of late treatment of lower leg thrombosis or progression of thrombosis despite treatment. Theoretically, however, the iliofemoral venous thrombosis may be an embolic phenomenon with the narrow left iliac vein acting as a sieve for emboli originating in the lower leg. This would explain why pulmonary emboli are more common after right-sided thrombosis than left-sided ones.[2]

TREATMENT OF ILIOFEMORAL VENOUS THROMBOSIS

The treatment methods include anticoagulation, thrombolysis and surgical thrombectomy. This chapter will deal mainly with surgical thrombectomy but in order to justify such a treatment, it has to be compared with other options.

There are four possible scenarios following any attempt to treat IFVT.

1.   Patent outflow and functioning valves.
2.   Occluded outflow and functioning valves.
3.   Patent outflow and venous valvular insufficiency.
4.   Occluded outflow and venous valvular insufficiency.

1.   If patency of the iliac vein can be restored with a functioning venous system in the leg, a good long-term result can be ensured. Patients with this outcome have not surprisingly been shown to have normal venous function upon testing. This result, however, was mostly obtained in patients undergoing thrombectomy who at the time of surgery had an isolated IVFT. The question arises whether occlusion of the iliac vein without venous valvular insufficiency results in severe long-term symptoms.[8]

2.   Patients with iliac vein occlusion but functioning venous valves in the leg usually have minor symptoms but after careful evaluation many of them are shown to suffer from venous claudication. It has been argued on theoretical grounds that venous distension may predispose to valvular insufficiency and possibly thrombosis.[9] The argument is based on findings in the tibial veins and it has been demonstrated that patients with only outflow obstruction of the iliac vein without venous valvular insufficiency do not have a high degree of recurrent thrombosis.[5,10]

3.   Patients with a patent outflow and venous valvular insufficiency probably have the same risk as patients with primary lower leg thrombosis of developing post-thrombotic syndrome. Outflow patency is most often determined with duplex technique but it can be difficult to differentiate between a patent iliac vein and a large venous collateral. Patients without clinical or physiological signs of outflow obstruction with venous insufficiency in the lower leg can often be dealt with by adequate compression stockings.[11]

4.   Patients who end up with an occluded outflow and venous insufficiency in the lower leg represent the worst group. This group may not only have an impaired reduction in venous pressure upon exercise but may even increase their venous pressure during walking. Since the ambulatory venous pressure is a major determinant for development of post-thrombotic syndrome, these patients are at a high risk of developing venous ulcers.[12] They are problematic to treat and could theoretically be candidates for a Palmas operation or late restoration of flow in the iliac vein by thrombolysis and stenting.

Anticoagulant treatment of iliofemoral venous thrombosis

Although it is not the purpose of this article to review anticoagulant treatment this will be briefly mentioned since it is the basis against which other methods must be compared. The sequelae which every treatment of venous thrombosis must try to prevent are: pulmonary embolism, post-thrombotic syndrome and venous gangrene. It has been demonstrated several years ago that heparin and warfarin reduce the number of pulmonary emboli in patients with venous thrombosis.[13] It has since long been considered that IFVT results in a high degree of post-thrombotic syndrome and therefore a more radical treatment than anticoagulation alone has been judged to be of importance to prevent this complication.[14] Recent studies, however, indicate that anticoagulation alone results in a high degree of recanalization of the iliac vein segment.[10] Furthermore the clinical course of patients following extensive DVT is relatively benign provided that initial anticoagulant treatment is followed by treatment with compression stockings and that the patients are regularly supervised.[11]

Surgical thrombectomy of iliofemoral venous thrombosis

The main goal of the treatment is to prevent a post-thrombotic syndrome by restoring patency of the iliac vein. Prevention of pulmonary embolism may be an added benefit but it should be remembered that surgery in common with thrombolysis carries a small risk of inducing pulmonary embolism. Post-thrombotic syndrome takes many years to develop and therefore the patient should have a long-life expectancy in order for surgery to be justified as treatment for IFVT.

Surgical treatment of IFVT was initially suggested by Homan but he suggested division of the vein rather than thrombectomy.[15] Mahorner was the first to advocate thrombectomy in the treatment of IFVT.[16] Today the procedure is performed with an 8–10F venous thrombectomy catheter from the groin and in order to remove the lower leg thrombus, compression with an Esmarch bandage from the foot and upwards is done. This is performed in order to remove the clot from the valve-bearing veins in the leg. It is often possible to clear the leg by this procedure since the thrombus in the leg is loose, soft and jelly-like, in contrast to the firm and wall-adherent primary thrombus in the iliac vein. Angiography is an important adjunct to surgical thrombectomy, both to ensure that the venous thrombectomy catheter really enters the vena cava and that it does not divert into a large collateral vein and also to ensure a good end result. Since the thrombus in the iliac vein is wall adherent several withdrawals of the thrombectomy catheter are required to clear the iliac vein.

The risk of pulmonary embolism during the procedure originally received much attention and temporary occlusion via the contralateral iliac vein was used by some centres. Placement of caval filters has also been suggested. Authors reporting on pulmonary embolism have, however, not found an increased incidence of pulmonary embolism during the surgery, both by clinical observation and pulmonary scintigram.[17,18] Therefore filters or temporary occlusion of the vena cava are not recommended during the procedure but many authors recommend an increased end expiratory pressure during the thrombectomy procedure in order to decrease venous return during the thrombectomy.

An arteriovenous fistula (AVF) in the groin is generally recommended (Fig. 2). Although no formal comparison has been made of the results after thrombectomy with and without AVF, series using AVF generally report better long-term results.[19] The AVF is usually constructed by dividing the saphenous vein and anastomosing its proximal end to the formal artery. The AVF usually is closed after 1–3 months. Previously this was done by secondary surgery which was often difficult in the scarred tissue with venous collaterals but today it is recommended that endovascular techniques with coiling should be used in order to close the AVF.[20] The AVF may contribute to swelling of the leg, particularly if there is a recurrence of the iliac vein thrombus. In such cases the AVF sometimes has to be closed immediately after a recurrent venous thrombosis.

Several series have reported results after iliofemoral venous thrombectomy, for review see Eklöf and Kistner.[21] The combined immediate patency rate of the iliac vein is 80–90%. There are very few comparative studies and only one randomized study. Plate *et al*.[22] randomized patients with iliofemoral venous thrombosis and followed them for 5 years. The short-term results were significantly better in the surgical group with superior iliac vein patency and lesser venous reflux.[22] After 5 years, however, the significant difference between surgically and medically treated patients had largely vanished, but iliac vein patency based on radionuclide venography was

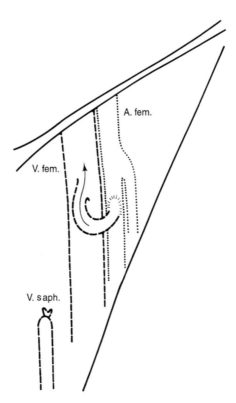

Fig. 2.   Construction of an arteriovenous fistula after venous thrombectomy.

superior in the surgical group. Ambulatory venous pressure was also significantly lower in the surgical group.[23] There was no major difference in clinical results between the two groups. In this study pregnant women, who constitute a large proportion of young patients with isolated IFVT, were not included and many patients had died at 5-year follow-up because of the associated malignancy that triggered the IFVT.

In a comparative study by Törngren and co-workers pregnant women undergoing thrombectomy were compared with selected controls who had been treated with anticoagulation alone. Although not randomized this study may be viewed as a case control study. There was no difference in the late outcome between the groups, neither clinically nor regarding patency of the iliac vein or other parameters reflecting venous insufficiency.[10] It was notable in this study that a major portion of the patients treated with anticoagulation alone had recanalized their iliac veins and also that the clinical symptoms were rather mild in this group. This is in contrast to earlier reports stating that IFVT causes a high percentage of severe post-thrombotic syndrome.[14] This study contradicts the common concept that young patients with isolated iliac vein thrombosis and an expected long survival time should be the ideal candidates for iliofemoral venous thrombectomy.

Gänger et al. have also made a comparative study, although not randomized, and their conclusion was that patients who were operated on within 3 days of onset of symptoms benefited from surgery. They also concluded that surgery usually failed when the thrombosis extended from the iliofemoral level down to the popliteal-crural level.[24] Since the major determinant for late morbidity probably is function of the venous valves, this study may also cast doubt on the rational for venous thrombectomy.

It is often stated that surgery has to be performed within 3–5 days of onset of symptoms. In the case of primary IFVT, this poses a problem since the patients usually present initially with only groin pain which is followed after a few days by leg swelling. The definite diagnosis is in the majority of cases not established until leg swelling occurs and this may coincide with distal extension of the thrombus. Another major problem is that surgery should mainly be restricted to patients with an expected lengthy survival since the post-thrombotic syndrome takes many years to develop.

The risks with surgical treatment are mainly pulmonary embolism, infection, bleeding and increased leg swelling when an AVF is used. The risk of pulmonary embolism is probably rather low and Kistner et al. have demonstrated that there were no added defects on pulmonary scintigrams after surgery where no protective measures had been taken to avoid PE. There were quite a few defects indicating that PE had occurred already preoperatively.[18]

Since thrombectomy is done from the groin, there is a definite risk of infection, particularly if reoperations have to be done for recurrent thrombosis. Leg swelling may be accentuated after the construction of an AVF. As stated above this is particularly troublesome if recurrent iliac vein thrombosis occurs.

Thrombolytic treatment of iliofemoral venous thrombosis

Thrombolytic treatment can be either systemic or catheter directed. Although systemic thrombolytic therapy has been advocated for acute DVT, it usually fails in the treatment of IFVT.[25,26] The reason for this is probably that very little of the drug reaches the thrombus and therefore catheter-directed thrombolysis has been advocated.[27] In this procedure the thrombolytic agent is delivered into the thrombus and complete lysis of IFVT has been reported in about two-thirds of the patients. This procedure has also been combined with PTA and/or stenting of the narrow segment of the iliac vein. In the material reported by Semba and Dake one-fifth of the patients were dead at follow-up due to malignancy which again points to the fact that the underlying disease and the expected survival of the patient have to be carefully evaluated.[27]

Catheter-directed thrombolysis with or without angioplasty or stenting of the narrow segment in the iliac vein is a promising technique which probably will increase in the future. It is, however, contraindicated in many instances, the most important being pregnancy or puerperium.

SUMMARY AND CONCLUSIONS

The initial enthusiasm for venous thrombectomy in the USA rather soon turned into a negative attitude against the procedure. In Europe, IFVT is very popular but the lack of randomized and controlled studies is striking. In the only randomized study few significant results could be shown on the long-term basis, nor in a case control study of women operated during pregnancy or puerperium. In the days of evidence-based medicine, venous thrombectomy can hardly be recommended for all patients with IFVT. The question may, however, not be *if* surgical thrombectomy is effective but *for whom* it is effective – i.e. some subgroup may benefit from the operation. If patients with total leg thrombosis could be cleared from their thrombosis they would certainly benefit the most but it is questionable that this could be achieved by surgery.

REFERENCES

1. Cockett FB, Thomas M: The iliac vein compression syndrome. *Br J Surg* **52:** 816, 1965
2. Mavor GE, Galloway JMD: Ilio-femoral venous thrombosis. Pathological consideration and surgical management. *Br J Surg* **56:** 45–52, 1969
3. May R, Thurner J: The cause of the predominantly sinistral occurrence of thrombosis of the pelvic veins. *Angiology* **8:** 419, 1957
4. Nexus D, Fletcher EWL, Cockett FB, Thomas ML: Compression and band formation at the mouth of the left common iliac vein. *Br J Surg* **55:** 369–374, 1968
5. Törngren S, Bremme K, Hjertberg R et al.: Blood coagulation variables in patients with ilio-femoral venous thrombosis. *Thromb Haemorrh Dis* **4:** 25–29, 1991
6. Dahlbäck B: New molecular insights into the genetics of thrombophilia. Resistance to activated protein C caused by Arg 506 to Gln mutation in factor V as a pathogenic rise factor for venous thrombosis. *Thromb Haemost* **74:** 139–148, 1995
7. Hellgren M, Blombäck M: Studies on blood coagulation and fibrinolysis in pregnancy, during delivery and in the puerperium. *Gynecol Obstet Invest* **12:** 141–154, 1981
8. Swedenborg J, Hägglöf R, Jacobson H et al.: Results of surgical treatment for ilio-femoral venous thrombosis. *Br J Surg* **4:** 43–48, 1986

9. Rutherford RB: Pathogenesis and pathophysiology of the post-thrombotic syndrome. Clinical implications. *Semin Vasc Surg* **9:** 21–25, 1996

10. Törngren S, Hjertberg R, Rosfors S *et al.*: The long-term outcome of proximal vein thrombosis during pregnancy is not improved by the addition of surgical thrombectomy to anticoagulant treatment. *Eur J Vasc Endovasc Surg* **12:** 31–36, 1996

11. Milne AA, Ruckley CV: The clinical course of patients following extensive deep venous thrombosis. *Eur J Vasc Surg* **8:** 56–59, 1994

12. Nicolaides AN, Hussein MK, Szendro G *et al.*: The relation of venous ulceration with ambulatory venous pressure measurements. *J Vasc Surg* **17:** 414–419, 1993

13. Barrett DW, Jordan SC: Anticoagulant drugs in the treatment of pulmonary embolism: A controlled trial. *Lancet* **i:** 1309–1312, 1960

14. O'Donnell TF, Browse NL, Burnand KG, Lea Thomas M: The socio-economic effects of an iliofemoral venous thrombosis. *J Surg Res* **22:** 483–488, 1977

15. Homan J: Exploration and division of the femoral and iliac veins in the treatment of thrombophlebitis of the leg. *JAMA* **224:** 179–186, 1941

16. Mahorner H: New Management for thrombosis of the deep veins of extremities. *Am Surg* **20:** 487–498, 1954

17. Plate G, Ohlin P, Eklöf B: Pulmonary embolism in acute iliofemoral venous thrombosis. *Br J Surg* **72:** 912–915, 1985

18. Kistner RL, Ball JJ, Nordyke RA *et al.*: Incidence of pulmonary embolism in the course of thrombophlebitis of the lower extremities. *Am J Surg* **124:** 169–176, 1972

19. Hutschenreiter S, Vollmar J, Loeprecht H *et al.*: Rekonstruktive Eingriff am Venensystem – Spätergebnisse unter kritischer Bevertung funktioneller und gefässmorphologischer Kriterien. *Chirurg* **50:** 555–563, 1979

20. Endrys J, Eklöf B, Neglén P *et al.*: Percutaneous balloon occlusion of surgical arteriovenous fistulae following venous thrombectomy. *Cardiovasc Intervent Radiol* **12:** 226–229, 1989

21. Eklöf B, Kistner RL: Is there a role for thrombectomy in iliofemoral venous thrombosis? *Semin Vasc Surg* **9:** 34–45, 1996

22. Plate G, Einarsson E, Ohlin P *et al.*: Thrombectomy with temporary arterio-venous fistula. The treatment of choice in acute ilio-femoral venous thrombosis. *J Vasc Surg* **1:** 867–876, 1984

23. Åkesson H, Brudin L, Dahlström JA *et al.*: Venous function assessed during a 5-year period after acute iliofemoral venous thrombosis treated with anticoagulation. *Eur J Vasc Surg* **4:** 43–48, 1990

24. Gänger KH, Nachbur BH, Ris HB, Zurbrygg H: Surgical thrombectomy versus conservative treatment for deep venous thrombosis; functional comparison of long-term results. *Eur J Vasc Surg* **3:** 529–538, 1989

25. Comerota AJ, Aldridge SC: Thrombolytic therapy for acute deep vein thrombosis. *Semin Vasc Surg* **5:** 76–81, 1992

26. Hill SL, Martin D, Evans P: Massive vein thrombosis of the extremities. *Am J Surg* **158:** 131–136, 1989

27. Semba CP, Dake MD: Iliofemoral deep venous thrombosis: Aggressive therapy with catheter-directed thrombolysis. *Radiology* **191:** 487–494, 1994

Imaging and Treatment of Extensive Deep Vein Thrombosis with Phlegmasia

A. I. Handa, A. Platts and G. Hamilton

INTRODUCTION

Extensive deep venous thrombosis (DVT) with phlegmasia caerulea dolens (PCD) is rare, and so an exact incidence is difficult to quote. The extent of the thrombosis is variable and PCD arises from acute massive obstruction of the venous drainage of an extremity. The clinical presentation of PCD is typically of limb swelling, cyanosis and pain, and represents the reversible phase of ischaemic venous occlusion. It was first described by Fabricius Hildanus[1] in the sixteenth century. In 1938 Gregoire[2] used the term phlegmasia caerulea dolens, and distinguished it from the non-ischaemic variety. Extensive DVT progresses to venous gangrene in 40–60% of cases[3,4] and may involve skin, subcutaneous tissue or muscle. Thus, PCD may be threatening to both life and limb.

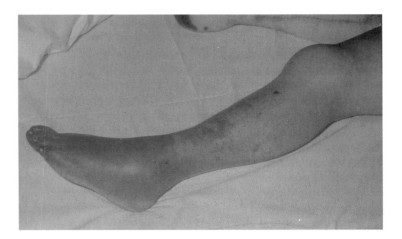

Fig. 1. An example of phlegmasia.

Table 1.   The common underlying causes of phlegmasia

Prothrombotic states	
Primary	*Acquired*
Protein S deficiency	Anticardiolipin antibody
Protein C deficiency	Lupus anticoagulant
Antithrombin III deficiency	Pregnancy and the puerperium
Factor V deficiency	Malignancy
Dysfibrinogenaemias	Immobility
Abnormalities of fibrinolysis	Surgery
Homocystinaemia	Trauma
Hypercholesterolaemia	Myeloproliferative disorders
	Drug related, e.g. HRT
	Klinefelter's syndrome

PATHOPHYSIOLOGY

Essentially there is a complete, or nearly complete, thrombotic occlusion of microvascular collaterals and venous drainage in PCD. Multiple obstructions to the main venous drainage of a limb do not appear to produce significant obstruction to the venous circulation.[5] Studies in canines show that all the veins at the root of a limb have to be ligated to develop changes consistent with venous gangrene.[6] Thus, in PCD there is patency of a number of major or collateral veins of an extremity, and in venous gangrene the venous outflow is completely occluded. This accounts for the reversibility of the ischaemia in PCD.

Change in venous outflow results in alteration of the normal forces governing fluid flow in the capillary system. Following Starling's law,[7] fluid is driven out of the capillary at the arterial end by hydrostatic pressure, and then reabsorbed at the venous end due to colloid oncotic pressure. With occlusion of the venous outflow, the hydrostatic pressure at the venous end exceeds the normal oncotic pressure leading to fluid being driven into the interstitium. This leads to interstitial oedema producing pressures of 25–48 mmHg in the interstitium within 1–2 days.[3,8,9] Large volumes of fluid are thus lost into the affected extremity[10] leading to shock secondary to the decreased circulating volume.

Several mechanisms are implicated in the pathophysiology of PCD-associated arterial insufficiency. Venous gangrene with occlusive thrombosis of small arteries[11] has been reported. However, arterial patency has also been confirmed by anatomical dissection at postmortem studies and angiographically. It is likely that some of the arterioles and capillary bed are thrombosed in venous gangrene.

Vasospasm has also been postulated as a mechanism. The failure of any improved tissue perfusion following periarterial sympathectomy or acetylcholine[12] does not support this mechanism. Spasm as suggested by decreased arterial pulse amplitude[9] or arterial flow[9,13] has not been demonstrated in experimental models of venous gangrene. Normal tissue pressure is close to zero, and arteries remain open due to arterial pressure.[14] As the hydrostatic pressure in the vessel falls, the vessel collapses due to wall tension. In PCD, oedema leads to increased tissue pressure and hypotension resulting in decreased hydrostatic pressure in the vessel. Thus, it is likely that the ischaemia in PCD results from collapsed small arteries due to these pressure changes, and thrombosis of the capillary bed.

AETIOLOGY

There are many predisposing factors to thromboembolic disease. An underlying cause is found in nearly 90% of PCD cases.[3,15,16] An underlying malignancy should always be suspected in extensive DVT and is present in approximately one-third of all such patients.[3,15,17] When complicated by venous gangrene, PCD is usually associated with an underlying malignancy,[16–19] and indeed may be the presenting feature of the tumour.[20] A number of prothrombotic states have been identified and may result in extensive DVT. Thus, where no obvious cause has been identified, patients should be investigated for antithrombin III, protein S, protein C or plasminogen deficiency.[21,22] Anticardiolipin antibody or the lupus anticoagulant may also be detected.[23] Factor V Leiden mutation (resistance to activated protein C) has

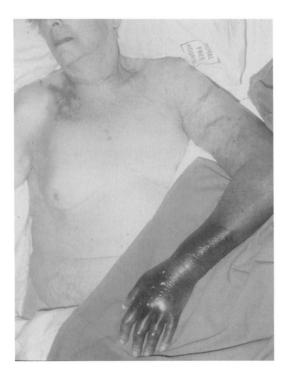

Fig. 2. An example of phlegmasia in the upper limb.

also been demonstrated in recurrent thromboembolism.[24,25] Plasminogen activator inhibitor (PA1-I) in plasma has also been implicated in thrombotic disease.[26]

Anatomical causes such as thoracic outlet syndrome in the upper limb or iliac vein compression syndrome in the lower limb may result in PCD.[27]

Other predisposing factors include surgery, trauma, radiotherapy, pregnancy and puerperium, or prolonged immobilization; PCD has also been reported as a complication of intravenous drug abuse[28] and insertion of a caval filter.[29] It results in shock from the massive fluid sequestration in the affected limb and requires urgent management with resuscitation.

PROGNOSIS

Extensive DVT with phlegmasia is both limb- and life-threatening. It results in amputation in 20–50% of patients.[3,17,30] It has an associated mortality rate of up to 40%.[3,4,15,31]

There is much debate as to the extent of amputation required ranging from only digital amputation or debridement[17] to above-knee amputations in 60%.[3] The mortality rate appears to increase with a corresponding increase in amputation level.[17] The long-term sequelae in extensive DVT with phlegmasia are uncertain as little information is available from the published literature. Estimates of post-phlebitic complications range from 36 to 60% of patients with PCD.[32]

IMAGING

The clinical diagnosis of DVT is unreliable. However, extensive DVT with phlegmasia is a dramatic presentation leaving little doubt as to the diagnosis. Imaging is necessary to confirm the clinical diagnosis and to ascertain the extent of the thrombosis. The traditional 'gold standard' has been contrast venography.[33] However, it may not always be technically possible. It is uninterpretable in up to 25% of patients.[34,35] Furthermore, it is invasive and costly, and may itself precipitate thrombosis in normal patients.[36] Ascending venography is often of little value due to the non-visualization of an occluded deep system. Descending venography is the method of choice in the lower limbs (via the upper limb) as images of the iliocaval system are frequently impossible to obtain via the contralateral femoral vein. For the upper limb, images are obtained via the contralateral upper limb or the femoral approach if superior venacaval obstruction is clinically suspected.

A variety of non-invasive methods are available, including photophlethysmography, radiolabelled fibrinogen and liquid crystal thermography.[33] These physiological tests may be helpful in selected circumstances, but have the disadvantage of being unable to outline the extent of thrombosis.

Rapid, non-invasive assessment of thrombosis is available with continuous wave or duplex Doppler ultrasonography. This compares favourably with contrast venography as regards cost and accuracy,[37,39] and may be used by the patient's bedside. Doppler ultrasonography has now replaced venography as the gold standard in many hospitals. Others advocate the selection of an appropriate diagnosis modality depending upon local availability, patient factors and cost-effectiveness.[33] The advent of magnetic resonance venography provides a means of good quality, non-invasive imaging. It allows assessment of underlying causes, but has the disadvantage of high cost. In time it may prove to be the investigation of choice.

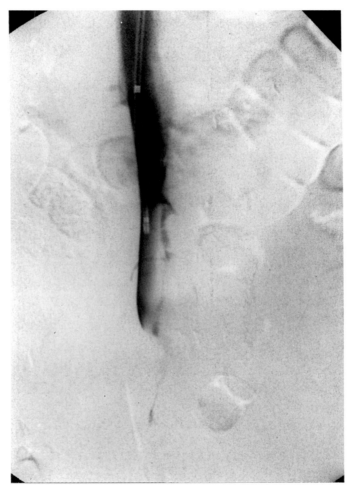

Fig. 3. Descending venogram of the inferior vena cavae showing extensive thrombosis of the lower end and common iliac veins.

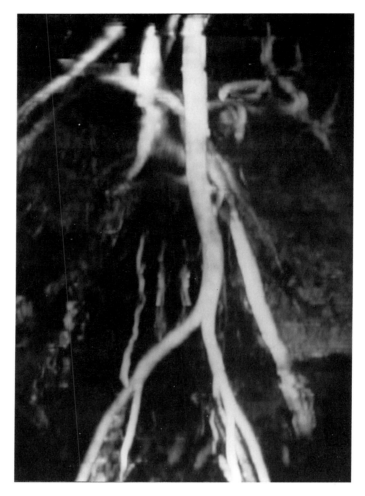

Fig. 4. Magnetic resonance venography of a patient with thrombosis of the common iliac vein on the right with collateral vessels opened up.

TREATMENT

Extensive DVT with PCD presents a therapeutic challenge. Many treatments have been attempted to no avail, including steroids, vasodilator drugs, hyaluronidase and sympathectomy. Treatment aims to stop sequestration of fluid, accompanied by aggressive shock management. This improves tissue perfusion, hence preserving tissue viability. Further, we aim to prevent propagation of the thrombus. Thus, initial management should include intravenous fluids, strict bed rest and high elevation to correct the hypotension and facilitate venous drainage. Intravenous heparin should be commenced with a bolus dose of 10 000 IU, followed by continuous infusion of 30 000 IU over 24 hours.

Definitive treatment can be broadly classified into three categories: conservative, surgical or thrombolysis. Any combination of the three categories may be attempted. Conservative treatment involves the initial resuscitation with intravenous fluid replacement, high elevation and bed rest and formal anticoagulation with intravenous heparin. Following initiation of heparin as above, the activated partial thromboplastin time should be maintained at 1.5–2.5 times the normal value.

The nursing care of these patients is of vital importance including regular observation, pressure area care and strict high elevation. Intravenous antibiotics are indicated if venous gangrene is present. These conservative measures allow successful treatment in a significant proportion of patients with PCD.[4,40] Many of these only require minor amputation or skin debridement after initial conservative treatment.[17] Some authors advocate conservative measures for all patients with uncomplicated PCD or initially for all patients with PCD for the first 6–12 hours.[41] Warfarin therapy should be maintained for 6 months aiming for an international normalized ratio (INR) of 2.0–2.5.

Thrombectomy for extensive DVT with PCD was first performed by Leriche in 1939.[42] Since then it has been advocated both as initial treatment or as secondary to failure of conservative measures.[43] Thrombectomy aims to both improve venous drainage, and hence tissue perfusion, whilst preventing propagation by removing the underlying clot. Early reports for uncomplicated iliofemoral thrombosis were encouraging.[44] However, these have not been reproduced in PCD.[45] Thrombectomy offers rapid clinical improvement,[46] but suffers from the problems of perioperative pulmonary embolism and significant post-thrombotic symptoms.[47]

Furthermore, thrombectomy fails to address the problem of the occluded minor venous channels, and thus has poor results in the setting of venous gangrene complicating PCD.[4,17] In acute iliofemoral venous thromboses, there are marked differences in the approach between the USA and the UK compared with mainland Europe. The European experience reports very favourable results with thrombectomy performed within 10 days.[48] However, the view in the UK and USA is that there is no place for thrombectomy alone and it is reserved for patients where conservative measures have failed, anticoagulation is contraindicated or there is rapid progression to venous gangrene.[4] Thrombectomy has also been advocated in conjunction with regional, catheter-directed thrombolytic therapy[49,50] with improved results. Fasciotomy appears to confer little benefit in the management of PCD,[4,31,51] and is hampered by prolonging wound healing and increases the risk of infection.

Thrombolytic therapy is theoretically the ideal treatment for extensive DVT with PCD. It offers the promise of allowing lysis of the major veins and the small venous channels inaccessible to surgical treatment, whilst maintaining the patency of both the collateral drainage and valvular incompetence. Intra-arterial thrombolysis also opens up the arteriolar channels. Thrombolytic therapy, thus, has the potential to achieve rapid tissue perfusion, maintain valvular function (thereby reducing the post-thrombotic sequelae)[52] and to uncover underlying venous anatomical abnormalities, allowing their secondary treatment with either angioplasty or stent placement.[53]

These potential benefits have to be balanced against the contraindications to thrombolysis and its well described risks of pulmonary embolism and bleeding complications.[54] Thrombolytic therapy may be delivered systemically via the intravenous route or be catheter-directed via the venous or intra-arterial routes. Systemic delivery as first line treatment[55] has lost favour due to the unacceptably high bleeding complications. Transvenous catheter-directed thrombolysis has shown greater promise with complete lysis in 72% and partial lysis in a further 20% in a study by Semba and Dake.[53]

Thrombolytic therapy has more often been reserved as second-line treatment after a failure of conservative measures. In PCD, one centre reviewed the literature showing poor results in venous gangrene with conservative, surgical or thrombolytic treatment.[4] Low dose intra-arterial thrombolysis in PCD has been reported as a useful adjunct to intravenous catheter-directed therapy.[57] This directs the agent directly to the capillary bed, where it is most effective, and results in rapid clinical improvement of the patient. Further experience with this may prove it to be the treatment of choice.

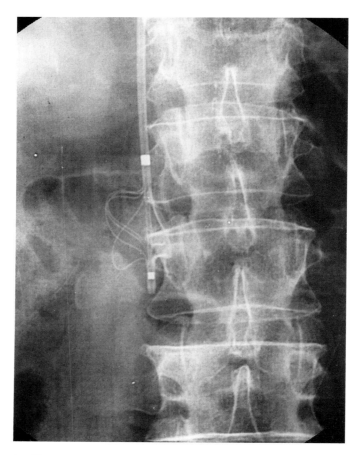

Fig. 5.   Temporary caval filter *in situ* in the inferior vena cavae of a patient undergoing thrombolytic therapy for phlegmasia.

Temporary vena caval filter placement has been advocated[56,57] prior to the commencement of thrombolytic therapy due to its associated high risk of pulmonary embolism in PCD.

Mechanical thrombolysis by the thrombolyser has been reported[52] in two cases of DVT where systemic thrombolysis has failed. This method requires further evaluation and its theoretical risks of pulmonary embolization remain high.

CONCLUSIONS

Extensive DVT with PCD is a rare condition and most surgeons will only be presented with it on a few occasions in their working life. The mortality and morbidity rates have remained high over the last half century, despite the advances in imaging and treatment options available.

Doppler ultrasonography appears to have replaced contrast venography in centres where it is readily available as the first line in investigation. Contrast venography will continue to be utilized in many hospitals either as first line or as an adjunct to identify the extent of thrombosis.

There is no consensus on the best treatment for PCD due to the lack of any large series of patients in any one centre. Systemic thrombolysis is unlikely to remain a treatment option given its bleeding complications, and catheter-directed intravenous therapy requires further evaluation. Intra-arterial thrombolysis offers an encouraging development and more numbers are needed to define its role.

The best initial management for PCD remains unchanged as fluid resuscitation, bed rest, elevation, nursing care and intravenous heparin anticoagulation. An underlying cause should be searched for in all patients. Although at present thrombectomy and thrombolysis appear to be reserved as secondary measures, an aggressive multidisciplinary approach as advocated by Comerota et al.[50] will probably provide the best strategy for PCD which continues to pose a serious threat to life and limb.

REFERENCES

1. Hildanus F: De Gangrena et Sphacelo. Cologne: 1593. In: Haimovici H (Ed) Gangrene of the extremities of venous origin. Review of the literature with case reports. *Circulation* **1**: 225–240, 1950
2. Gregoire R: La phlebite bleue. *Presse Med* **46**: 1313–1315, 1938
3. Brackman SK, Vasko JS: Phlemasia caerulea dolens. *Surg Gyn Obstet* **121**: 1347–1356, 1965
4. Weaver FA, Meacham DW, Adkins RB, Dean DH: Phlegmasia caerulea dolens: therapeutic considerations. *South Med J* **81**: 306–312, 1988
5. Haller JA Jr, Mays T: Experimental studies on iliofemoral venous thrombosis. *Am Surg* **29**: 567–571, 1963
6. Fontaine R, deSousa Pereira A: Obliterations et resections veineuses experimentales; contribution a l'etade de la circulation collaterale veineuse. *Rev Chir (Paris)* **75**: 161–200, 1937
7. Starling EH: On the absorption of fluids from the connective tissue spaces. *J Physiol (Lond)* **19**: 312–326, 1896
8. Snyder MA, Adams JT, Schwartz SI: Haemodynamics of phlegmasia caerulea dolens. *Surg Gyn Obstet* **125**: 342–346, 1967

9. Brockman SK, Vasko JS: The pathologic physiology of phlegmasia caerulea dolens. *Surgery* **59**: 997–1007, 1966
10. Perlow S, Killian ST, Katz LN, Asher R: Shock following venous occlusion of a leg. *Am J Physiol* **134**: 755–760, 1941
11. Perhoniemi V, Kaaja R, Carpen O: Venous gangrene of the limb. Pathophysiological and therapeutic considerations. *Ann Chir Gynaecol* **80**: 68–70, 1991
12. Haller JA Jr: Effects of deep femoral thrombophlebitis on the circulation of the lower extremities. *Circulation* **27**: 693–698, 1963
13. Savage JP: The role of reflex spasm in the pathogenesis of venous ischaemia. *Surg Gyn Obstet* **113**: 47–53, 1961
14. Burton AC: On the physical equilibrium of small blood vessels. *Am J Physiol* **164**: 319–329, 1951
15. Hirschman JV: Ischaemic forms of acute venous thrombosis. *Arch Dermatol* **123**: 933–936, 1987
16. Ross RV Jr, Baggenstross AH, Jeurgens JC: Gangrene of lower extremity secondary to extensive venous occlusion. *Circulation* **24**: 549–556, 1961
17. Haimovici H: The ischaemic forms of venous thrombosis. *J Cardiovasc Surg (Torino)* **65**: 164–173, 1965
18. Sutton RAL: Venous gangrene. *BHJ* **i**: 1465–1466, 1966
19. Bulow S, Suger P: Venous gangrene. *Acta Chirurg Scand* **141**: 272–278, 1975
20. Adamson AS, Littlewood TJ, Poston GJ *et al.*: Malignancy presenting as peripheral venous gangrene. *J Ray Soc Med* **81**: 609–610, 1988
21. Cohen DJ, Briggs R, Head HD, Acher CW: Phlegmasia caerulea dolens and its associations with hypercoagulable states: case reports. *Angiology* **40**: 498–508, 1989
22. Lecheek FWG, Knot EAR, Tencute JW, Traas DW: Severe thrombotic tendency associated with type 1 plasminogen deficiency. *Am J Haematol* **30**: 32–35, 1989
23. Buethge BA, Payne DK: Phlegmasia caerulca dolens associated with the lupus anticoagulant. *West J Med* **154**: 211–213, 1991
24. Svensson PJ, Dahlvack B: Resistance to activated protein C as a basis for venous thrombosis. *New Engl J Med* **330**: 517–522, 1994
25. Voorberg J, Roelse J, Koopmank *et al.*: Association of idiopathic venous thromboembolism with single point-mutation at Arg 506 of factor V. *Lancet* **343**: 1535–1536, 1994
26. Wiman B: Plasminogen activator inhibitor 1 (PAI-1) in plasma: its role in thrombotic disease. *Thromb Haem* **74**: 71–76, 1995
27. Petersen MJ, Brewster DC: Iliac vein compression syndrome. *Perspect Vasc Surg* **8**: 91–96, 1995
28. Lo AC, Vasiliyevich JH, Kernstein MD: Parental illegal drug use and limb loss. *J Cardiovasc Surg (Torino)* **31**: 760–762, 1990
29. Arung JE, Kandarpa K: Phlegmasia caerulea dolens, a complication after placement of a bird's nest vena cava filter. *Am J Roentgenol* **154**: 1105–1106, 1990
30. Stallworth JM, Bradham GB, Kietke RR, Price RG Jr: Phlegmasia caerulea dolens: a 10 year review. *Ann Surg* **161**: 802–811, 1965
31. Fogarty TS, Cranley JJ, Krause RJ *et al.*: Surgical management of phlegmasia caerulea dolens. *Arch Surg* **86**: 256–263, 1963
32. Plate G, Einarsson E, Ohlin P *et al.*: Thrombectomy with temporary arteriovenous fistula: the treatment of choice in acute iliofemoral venous thrombosis. *J Vasc Surg* **I**: 867–876, 1984
33. Wheeler HB, Anderson FA Jr: Diagnostic methods for deep vein thrombosis. *Haemostasis* **25**: 6–26, 1995
34. Hull RD, Hirsh J, Carter CJ *et al.*: Diagnostic efficacy of impedance plethysmography for clinically suspected deep vein thrombosis. A randomised trial. *Ann Intern Med* **102**: 21–28, 1985
35. Huisman MV, Ballen HR, Ten Cate JW, Vreeken J: Serial impedance plethysmography for suspected deep venous thrombosis in outpatients. The Amsterdam General Practitioner Study. *N Engl J Med* **314**: 823–828, 1986
36. Bettmann MA, Robbins A, Braun SD *et al.*: Contrast venography of the leg: diagnostic efficacy, tolerance and complication rates with ionic and non-ionic contrast media. *Radiology* **165**: 113–116, 1987

37. Hobson RWII, Mintz BL, Jamil Z, Breotbart GB: Diagnosis of acute deep vein thrombosis. *Surg Clin North Am* **70**: 143–157, 1990

38. Hill SL, Martin D, McDarnald ER Jr, Donato AT: Early diagnosis of iliofemoral venous thrombosis by doppler examination. *Am J Surg* **156**: 11–15, 1988

39. White RH, McGahan JB, Daschbach MM, Hartling RP: Diagnosis of deep vein thrombosis using duplex ultrasound. *Ann Intern Med* **III**: 297–304, 1989

40. Hood DB, Weaver FA, Modiall JG, Yellin AE: Advances in the treatment of phlegmasia caerulea dolens. *Am J Surg* **166**: 206–210, 1993

41. Perkins JMT, Magee TR, Galland JB: Phlegmasia caerulea dolens and venous gangrene. *Br J Surg* **83**: 19–23, 1996

42. Leriche R, Geisendorf W: Resultats d'une thrombectomie precoce avec resection veineuse dans une phlebite grave des deux membres inferreurs. *Presse Med* **47**: 1239, 1939

43. Rutherford RB: Role of surgery in iliofemoral venous thrombosis. *Chest* **89**: 434–475, 1986

44. Haller JA Jr, Abrams BL: Use of thrombectony in the treatment of acute iliofemoral thrombosis in forty-five patients. *Ann Surg* **158**: 561–569, 1963

45. Karp RB, Wylie EJ: Recurrent thrombosis after iliofemoral venous thrombectomy. *Surg Forum* **17**: 147, 1966

46. Qvarfordt P, Eklof B, Ohlin P: Intramuscular pressure in the lower leg in deep vein thrombosis and phlegmasia caerulea dolens. *Ann Surg* **197**: 450–453, 1983

47. Lansing AM, Davis WM. Five year follow-up study of iliofemoral venous thrombectomy. *Ann Surg* **168**: 620–628, 1968

48. Eklof B, Kistner RL. Is there a role for thrombectomy in iliofemoral venous thrombosis? *Semin Vasc Surg* **9**: 34–45, 1996

49. Nachbar BB, Beck EA, Senn A: Can the results of treatment of deep venous thrombosis be improved by combining surgical thrombectomy with regional fibrinolysis? *J Cardiovasc* **21**: 347–352, 1980

50. Comerota AJ, Aldrige SC, Cohen G et al.: A strategy of aggressive regional therapy for acute iliofemoral venous thrombosis with contemporary venous thrombectomy or catheter directed thrombolysis. *J Vasc Surg* **20**: 244–254, 1994

51. Cymes S, Louw JH: Phlegmasia cacrulea dolens: successful treatment by relieving fasciotomy. *Surgery* **51**: 169–176, 1962

52. Marder VJ, Sherry S: Thrombolytic therapy: current status parts 1 and 2. *N Engl J Med* **318**: 1512–1520, 1585–1595, 1988

53. Semba CP, Dake MD: Iliofemoral deep vein thrombosis: aggressive therapy with catheter directed thrombolysis. *Radiology* **191**: 487–494, 1994

54. Goldhaber SZ, Buring JE, Lipnick RJ, Hennekens CH: Pooled analyses of randomised trials of streptokinase and heparin in phlebologically documented acute deep venous thrombosis. *Am J Med* **76**: 393–397, 1984

55. Elliott MS, Immelman EJ, Jeffery P et al.: The role of thrombolytic therapy in the management of phlegmasia caerulea dolens. *Br J Surg* **66**: 422–424, 1979

56. Robinson DL, Tectelbaum GP: Phlegmasia caerulea dolens: treatment by pulse-spray and infusion thrombolysis. *Am J Roentgenol* **160**: 1288–1290, 1993

57. Wlodarczyk ZK, Gibson M, Dick R, Hamilton G: Low dose intra-arterial thrombolysis in the treatment of phlegmasia caerulea dolens. *Br J Surg* **81**: 370–372, 1994

58. Moughabghab A, Socolovsky C, Lemaitne RM et al.: Treatment of ilio-caval thrombosis by mechanical thrombolysis. *Inten Care Med* **21**: 440–442, 1995

Surgery for Inferior Vena Cava Thrombosis in Patients With and Without Previous Filter Placement

Wilhelm Sandmann, Michael Pillny, Ralf Ritter and Klaus Grabitz

What is wanted is not the wish to believe but the wish to find out,
which is the exact opposite.
(Bertrand Russel 1872–1970)

Although the surgical possibilities to remove acute thrombosis from the deep venous system began more than 50 years ago,[1] the majority of reports concentrate on the spontaneous course of the disease managed conservatively.[2–9] The development of surgery for deep venous thrombosis (DVT) has been slow. The natural history of DVT results in defective healing with only partial recanalization of the venous lumen, valve incompetence, secondary varicose veins, recurrent sequelae of thrombosis and pulmonary embolism. However, treatment of those patients early after the onset of symptoms by removal of the thrombi to maintain the patency of the restored lumen seems logical.[10–12] Pulmonary embolization (PE) prevention has been achieved by the insertion of a filter placed into the infrarenal vena cava.[13–15] Instead of removing the source for further embolization a metalic device is placed in one of the most important veins of our circulation. Thrombosis of the inferior vena cava (IVC) is a common complication of the IVC filter, because in many patients with iliofemoral venous thrombosis the IVC becomes involved. Encouraging results with arterial thrombectomy, thromboendarterectomy and bypass have not been paralelled in the venous system with similar techniques. The causes for venous thrombosis, the morphology, natural history and techniques for surgical treatment are very different from arterial occlusive disease. Surgery for DVT and especially for acute thrombosis of the inferior cava is underdeveloped in North America and Europe. Nevertheless, we report our results in this interesting field.

PATIENTS AND METHODS

From January 1982 to June 1996 74 of 526 patients undergoing thrombectomy for DVT underwent thrombectomy for acute thrombosis of the IVC and one patient was treated for a perforation of an IVC-Greenfield filter, which caused an arteriovenous iliac-caval fistula. The mean age was 36.8 (± 12) years and the male/female ratio was the same (1:1).

In 36 patients the diagnosis of IVC thrombosis was established after pulmonary embolism. Acute massive swelling of both legs, oedema of the pelvis and the flanks, pain related to distended tissues, sudden diffuse abdominal or back pain, cyanosis of both legs and pain from movement were the prominent clinical features as well as respiratory insufficiency in those patients, who developed pulmonary embolism. In patients with thrombosis limited to the IVC only, the symptoms were rather mild and could be misleading. For example, we treated two patients who had developed IVC occlusion during the course of chemotherapy for Hodgkin's disease, in which the IVC occlusion was found accidentally when a CT scan was performed to evaluate the retroperitoneal space for completeness of para-aortic lymph node removal. The most impressive features of venous thrombosis occurred in patients with complete occlusion of the iliofemoral and popliteal veins at the time, when the IVC became occluded. Twelve patients, in which IVC occlusion extended above the renal veins had proteinuria and leg oedema, which were attributed to an anticipated nephrotic syndrome until a CT scan was performed. Obviously the thrombotic process could have begun in the renal veins before extending into the IVC. However, this was difficult to prove at the time of the CT scan, because the patients were referred late after onset.

In 18 patients a single episode of pulmonary embolism preceded the treatment for DVT and 18 patients had recurrent pulmonary embolization before being referred for surgical removal of IVC thrombosis. Beforehand, fibrinolysis had been undertaken unsuccessfully in 12 patients and in another two patients thrombectomy performed elsewhere had failed. Seven patients had received an IVC filter elsewhere causing subsequent clinical problems. Risk factors for thrombosis are given in Table 1, but in 24% of the patients we were unable to detect even a single risk factor. Three imaging methods were used routinely to determine the extent of the thrombosis (duplex sonography for the veins in the leg and the pelvis, phlebography for the origin, formation and age of the clots and CT scans with contrast material for evaluation of the pelvic veins and the IVC). In six patients the extent of the thrombosis was limited to the IVC, while 69 patients presented with additional distal venous thrombosis. The thrombotic process was limited to the inferior part of the IVC in 63 patients while in 12 (16%) patients additional suprarenal extension was demonstrated. A floating thrombus (this term is used by radiologists to point out that the proximal end of the thrombus is not fixed to the venous wall and moves in the blood stream depending on flow and respiratory motion) could be demonstrated by fluoroscopy in 49 (65.3%) of the patients. In most of the patients we were able to determine the age of the

Table 1.   Risk factors for thrombosis

	No	%
Previous surgery	25	33
Unknown	18	24
Hormone therapy	17	23
Pregnancy/delivery	13	17
Hypercoagulopathy	11	15
Trauma and surgery	11	15
Trauma	5	7
Malignancy	5	7
Pancreatitis	1	1

thrombosis, but symptoms and clinical findings were more related to the extent, completeness and direction of thrombotic occlusion than to the location of the initial process. However, from phlebographic and CT scanning, IVC thrombosis was estimated not to be older than 10 days in the majority of the patients. In some patients, who were given bedrest, symptoms and findings were masked until mobilization began. From CT and subsequent surgery the IVC occlusion must have been several weeks old. The diagnosis was not made until the thrombotic process progressed distally. Nevertheless, even in those patients the complete removal of thrombi from the IVC was possible.

Operative technique

Surgery was performed under general anaesthesia. The patient was positioned with the head elevated at about 30°. The sterile dressing was prepared to leave the possibility for sternotomy in the event of massive pulmonary embolism, although this procedure never became necessary. In 38 (51%) patients thrombectomy was performed using a combined transfemoral and transabdominal approach, because the IVC and both iliofemoral veins were occluded completely. In 31 (41%) patients with IVC thrombosis extending into the proximal iliac veins only we were able to remove the thrombi by the transperitoneal approach exclusively. In four patients with very old fibrotic thrombosis and acute occlusion of the proximal iliac veins the IVC was replaced by polytetrafluoroethylene (PTFE) tube grafts. In two patients we could not reconstruct the IVC because with acute occlusion of paravertebral collateral veins it became apparent that the IVC was malformed and chronically obstructed (Table 2).

Generally the exposed veins and/or the IVC were temporarily occluded with silicone vessel loops. Except for the IVC, vascular clamps and forceps grasping the vein wall were never used. Thrombi were removed by longitudinal venotomy (i.e. cavotomy) using open thrombectomy, sucking, manual decompression, venous Fogarty catheters and tourniquet application for compressing thrombectomy of the lower limbs.

Inferior vena cava clamps were applied tangentionally and only in those patients, in which interruption of blood flow with vessel loops and balloon catheters was inefficient to control blood loss at the time of the running suture. After removal of the

Table 2. Operative techniques for thrombectomy of IVC

	No	%
Combined transperitoneal with transfemoral thrombectomy		
unilateral	18	24.0
bilateral	20	26.7
Transperitoneal thrombectomy	31	41.3
IVC replacement with PTFE	4	5.3
Explosive laparotomy	2	2.7
Total:	75	100

vessel loops protective anteriovenous fistulae were constructed in both groins in 30 (40%) patients and unilaterally in 34 (45%) patients. For very recent thrombosis, limited to the IVC and the most proximal part of the iliac veins, anteriovenous fistula was considered unnecessary in eight patients. All patients were kept heparinized. If increasing dosages of heparin was not effective, the plasma coagulation profile was assessed and fresh frozen plasma or coagulation factors replaced. A daily heparin count was performed to detect heparin-induced thrombocytopenia.

Of the seven patients admitted after complications following IVC filter placement four were male and three female with a mean age of 49 years. The indications for the application of the filter were single embolic events in three and recurrent PE in four patients, which resulted from thrombosis in the iliofemoral (3), isolated femoral (1), femoro-popliteal-crural (1) and popliteal-crural (1) veins (Table 3). Unsuccessful thrombectomy and unsuccessful fibrinolysis preceeded filter placement in one and two patients respectively, while four had been treated with heparin only. Five patients had developed progressive ascending thrombosis with occlusion of the filter (Fig. 1) and in one patient the thrombus progressed into the suprarenal IVC. Thrombectomy of the iliofemoral and distal veins was performed as a first step, before the IVC was incised and the filter removed in the same setting. In a seventh patient removal of the filter was performed because of perforation into the right common iliac artery. In general, the removal of the filter was not so easy, because the anchoring of the filter hooks led to several perforations in the IVC wall. In cases with tilted and/or migrated filters the branches had to be cut and removed piece by piece in order to avoid further damage to the wall of the IVC. This manoeuvre turned out to be quite demanding, especially in patients with several perforations which the filter hooks had caused by anchoring in the iliac and renal veins. During this 1–5 minute procedure major blood loss can not always be avoided and fast-working autotransfusion devices are really helpful. Replacement of IVC after removal of the filter was avoided by meticulous repair of the perforations using single stitches and monofilamentous absorbable suture material.

After removal of the filter, six patients received a protective temporary femoral ateriovenous fistula in the groin, while the one patient with filter perforation into the right common iliac artery did not, because thrombus was not present.

RESULTS

Despite successful removal of IVC thrombosis in this whole series three (4%) patients died within 30 days of surgery. Death was caused by combined cardiorespiratory failure after severe or several preoperative pulmonary embolisms. Early recurrent occlusion of the IVC occurred in three (4%) patients, of which two underwent successful reoperation with remaining patency of the IVC. In 16 (21.3%) patients an early unilateral rethrombosis in the iliofemoral or femoral region was confirmed by duplex sonography and/or phlebography. Subsequent reoperation was performed in nine patients with success in seven. The overall rate of intra- and postoperative PE was 6.7%. Three (4%) patients developed PE during the primary procedure and in two (17%) PE was diagnosed at the time of reoperation (Table 4).

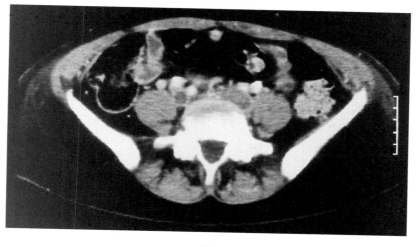

(a)

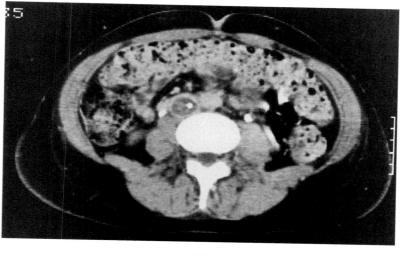

(b)

Fig. 1. Acute bilateral iliofemoral thrombosis, which led to complete thrombotic occlusion of the infrarenal IVC shortly after insertion of a Greenfield filter. (a) CT scan demonstrating complete occlusion of both common iliac veins just below the confluence. (b) CT scan demonstrates complete occlusion of the inferior vena cava with parts of the IVC filter.

Table 3. Removal of IVC filter for complications (8/1993–8/1996)

Case no Male/Female/Age (years)	Previous history and Indication for IVC filter	Position, type and complication of IVC filter	Management of complication	Results
1 F, 57	previous oestrogen therapy 3 weeks bedrest for myocarditis, DVT (femoropopliteal right, popliteotibial left) and PE at mobilization, pulmonary hypertension	subrenal temporary filter, progressive ascending DVT, both external and common iliac veins, IVC below, within and above the filter	removal of IVC filter 3 days after implantation, complete removal of thrombi by transfemoral catheter thrombectomy and transperitoneal approach, protective arteriovenous fistula left groin	uneventfull recovery closure of arteriovenous fistula 3 months later, no further sequelae of DVT and PE, no post-thrombotic syndrome
2 M, 66	5 weeks after tibia repair for traumatic fracture PE from acute popliteal and tibial DVT	subrenal permanent (Greenfield); progressive ascending DVT involving bilateral iliofemoral veins and IVC below the filter, perforation of filter hooks	removal of IVC filter and thrombi by combined transperitoneal and transfemoral route 9 days after filter implantation, repair of IVC damage from filter perforation by direct sutures, protective arteriovenous fistula right groin	except 6 weeks pneumonia uneventfull recovery; closure of arteriovenous fistula 3 months later, mild oedema left ankle
3 M, 69	2 weeks after tibia osteosynthesis and reconstruction of knee ligaments massive PE from left iliofemoral DVT, additionally ruptured symphysis	subrenal temporary filter; progressing ascending bilateral iliofemoral DVT with distal involvement of IVC, unsuccessfull thrombectomy left groin and recurrent[a] PE in another hospital	transfemoral removal of IVC filter 4 days after implantation, bilateral transfemoral thrombectomy without laparotomy, protective arteriovenous fistula left groin	pneumonia from PE; infection left groin debridement and musculocutaneous flap left groin, closure of the arteriovenous fistula after 2 months and reconstruction of the common femoral artery for spurious aneurysm with vein graft, coumadin stopped after 6 months
4 M, 55	14 days history of spontaneous left iliofemoral thrombosis, hospital admission for massive PE, anticoagulation with heparin coumadin after unsuccessfull fibrinolysis	subrenal LGM filter progressing bilateral iliofemoral thrombosis, IVC thrombosis below the filter	removal of IVC filter 4 weeks after implantation; complete removal of thrombi by bilateral transfemoral and transperitoneal route, protective arteriovenous fistula left groin	uneventfull recovery, closure of arteriovenous fistula 3 months later, coumadin terminated 6 months after closure of arteriovenous fistula

5 F, 40	suspected PE from suspected DVT 1 week after hysterectomy	subrenal Kimray-Greenfield recurrent tachycardia and progressive cardiac failure over 3 years filter had tilted and migrated distally, arteriovenous shunt 50% of cardiac output from aortocaval fistula	transperitoneal removal of IVC filter 4 years after implantation, filter had perforated the IVC into the right common iliac artery, suture repair of multiple IVC perforations end-to-end-anastomosis of right common iliac artery	uneventfull recovery with restored patency of the vessels, remaining small arteriovenous fistula from previous cardiac catheterization in the right groin was closed 3 months later, anticoagulation terminated
6 Female, 40	multiple recurrent DVT after cardiac catheterization for tetralogy of Fallot, 14 days before admission another cardiac catheterization, 8 days later iliofemoral DVT right paradioxical embolization into the left popliteal artery, fibrinolysis and aspiration of femoralis	subrenal temporary IVC filter after unsuccessfull venous thrombectomy in another hospital thrombosis progressed to complete iliobifemoral and IVC occlusion	combined transfemoral and transabdominal removal of filter and thrombi 14 days after implantation, protective arteriovenous fistula right groin, revision for early occlusion of arteriovenous fistula	paradox embolization into the left internal carotid artery, right side hemiparesis, closure of arteriovenous fistula 3 months later, neurologically incomplete recovery
7 Male, 37	recurrent DVT and PE 15 years ago, stopped coumadin by himself, new upon old DVT and PE, laparotomy three films for unexplainable abdominal pain	subrenal Greenfield progressive bilateral ascending iliofemoral thrombosis, tilting of IVC filter, two hooks anchoring in the left renal vein, two had perforated into the retroperitoneum, thrombi within filter and IVC causing incomplete occlusion	bilateral transfemoral removal of iliofemoral thrombosis, transperitoneal removal of filter and thrombi, arteriovenous fistula both groins (right side with thrombectomized greater saphenous vein, left side with accessory saphenous vein)	successfull thrombectomy for IVC and left pelvis and leg, remaining chronic occlusion right leg, recurrent occlusion right external iliac vein despite open arteriovenous fistula, intermittent cardiac failure from high volume output, refused to have arteriovenous closure of left side no further sequelae, massive oedema right leg led to early operative closure of arteriovenous fistula

a LGM

Table 4.   Complications after thrombectomy

Pulmonary embolism	5
intraoperative	3
postoperative	0
postoperative after recurrent thrombectomy	2
Wound infection	12
Wound haematoma	10
Lymphatic fistula	3
Amputation	2
Heparin induced thrombocytopenia (HIT)	3

In two of seven patients, who had the IVC filter removed, recurrent PE was suspected during or after filter removal. One patient suffered from paradoxical embolization into the internal carotid artery, which unfortunately was detected too late for appropriate treatment. All patients survived the operation after filter removal and the IVC has remained patent since then (Figs 2, 3).

After a mean follow-up of 44 (± 35) months, 63 patients are alive and 12 are lost to follow-up. According to CT scanning and phlebography/duplex ultrasound examination rethrombosis of the IVC was found in three patients. A further seven patients had developed recurrent iliofemoral thrombosis on one side, while only one patient suffered from bilateral iliofemoral rethrombosis.

A further uneventful course without post-thrombotic syndrome (PTS) was confirmed in 11 (17%) of 63 re-examined patients. Twenty-five (41%) demonstrated light oedema at the end of the day without wearing elastic stockings and 19 (30%) patients had developed moderate oedema. Severe post-thrombotic syndrome was observed in eight (12%) patients, of which five (8%) presented with a crural ulcer.

DISCUSSION

Despite the potential advantages of surgical thrombectomy for treatment of acute DVT over other treatment options, surgery is still only recommended by internists for patients with phlegmasia coerulea dolens and impending venous gangrene. Ginsberg in his latest review article about mangement of venous thromboembolism did not even mention the possibilities of surgical removal of the embolic source.[16] Toglia and Weg obviously did not know that surgical methods have been developed to remove the embolizing thrombosis from the deep veins even in pregnant women and postpartum, but instead recommended in pregnant women for prevention of recurrent PE the prescription of warfarin which is a teratogenic drug.[17] Partsch in his overview on the diagnosis and treatment of DVT devotes less than half a page to thrombectomy for acute DVT and questions its efficacy because of high mortality and failure rates.[9] He points out the lack of reports which compare surgical management with other treatment modalities, but how should those studies be initiated if such prejudgement and ignorance exists? Milne and Ruckley followed the clinical course of 83 patients with 86 affected limbs and stated in their summary 'The post-

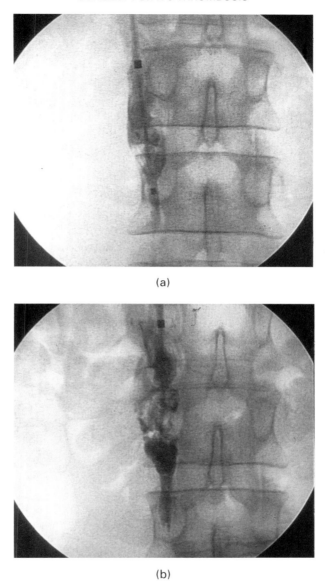

(a)

(b)

Fig. 2. Temporary IVC filter inserted through the internal jugular vein in a 59-year-old male patient. The filter was inserted elsewhere shortly after pulmonary embolism, which occurred during unsuccessful transfemoral thrombectomy for iliofemoral venous thrombosis following knee trauma. (a) Filter partially thrombosed without significant reduction of IVC lumen. (b) Filter completely thrombosed with additional partial thrombosis of the IVC causing further embolization. The filter was successfully withdrawn after successful bilateral transfemoral catheter thrombectomy of both iliofemoral veins and the IVC. The adjunctive arteriovenous fistula in the left groin was closed surgically 3 months later; the venous system is still patent 2 years later without development of postphlebitis syndrome.

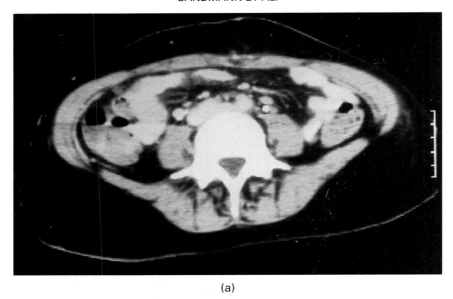

(a)

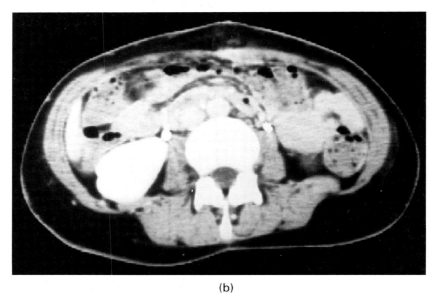

(b)

Fig. 3.   Postoperative CT scan after transfemoral and transperitoneal thrombectomy of IVC and both iliofemoral veins (the same patient as in Fig. 1). (a) Patent and normal configurized common iliac veins are visible. (b) The IVC is patent without any signs of residual thrombosis.

thrombotic syndrome does not carry the poor prognosis reported in earlier studies'.[8] In the detailed description of their clinical material the authors could demonstrate that long-term conservative treatment can reduce the severity of symptoms, but even after a total length of 12–135 months follow-up severe swelling not controlled by compression stockings remained in 23 (25%) patients, Lipodermatosclerosis, skin changes and varicose veins were observed in 29 (35%) and venous ulcers recurred in six (7.2%) patients, thus demonstrating the spontaneous course of the disease is not life-threatening but obviously not benign. Duplex studies following the spontaneous course of the disease revealed that development of deep vein valve incompetence is a progressive process over more than 5 years although the total group of 24 patients in the publication of van Haarst *et al.*[7] was too small to draw any significant conclusions from the correlation between symptoms and valve incompetence. As bedrest and successful surgical thrombectomy do have the same initial effect, i.e. reducing the oedema, more objective criteria must be used to evaluate the success of operative treatment in the early phase. De Weese[18] insisted on postoperative venography to prove the results of thrombectomy. Today, we, like others are using more non-invasive studies, mainly duplex ultrasound in the acute post-operative phase and additional photoplethysmography and venous occlusion plethysmography for follow-up. De Weese obtained complete restoration of the venous lumen in only 30% of the patients, but the operative techniques have been substantially refined since and our knowledge concerning helpful adjuncts to maintain patency of the deep venous system has improved sustantially.[19] Comerota *et al.*[20] were disappointed with standard anticoagulation therapy and systemic fibrinolysis in patients with iliofemoral DVT and embarked on a multidisciplinary aggressive approach using the combination of local catheter-directed fibrinolysis and surgical thrombectomy plus arteriovenous fistula in 12 cases. They described good success rates in their material although the thrombus extended in four patients into the IVC.

We have described our experience with thrombectomy and adjunctive temporary arteriovenous fistula in 185 patients, who had been treated from 1977 to 1986.[21] In 26% of the patients the DVT extended from the crural into the common iliac veins, 42.9% had iliofemoral DVT and in 8.7% the process was limited to the iliac veins. Femoropopliteal DVT was only present in 14.3%. The IVC was involved in 7.1%. In 68 patients, recent pulmonary embolism had occurred before referral for surgery and a total of 196 extremities were involved. The early patency rate after thrombectomy was 96%. After a mean follow-up of 43 (± 23) months 35% of the patients were completely free of symtoms and findings, 34% complained of moderate symptoms, which could be related to peripheral venous hypertension. Only 14% of the patients had developed secondary varicose veins and four patients (2.5%) suffered from crural ulcer. In comparison with the material presented by authors favouring conservative treatment, the late outcome in our series seems to be significantly better especially as our indications relate to a selected group of patients with more extensive and more severe types of DVT.

Patients in whom the DVT involves not only the iliofemoral veins but also the IVC present the most critical subgroup of acute DVT, because the chances for spontaneous recanalization and preservation of valvular competence are rather minimal with conservative treatment. Even the development of collaterals does not resolve the problems of venous hypertension and postphlebitic syndrome in the long run. Despite the extension of the thrombotic process a crural ulcer was observed in only 7.2%. The overall success rate is significantly different from patients treated with heparin and compression alone, and taking into account the much more extended thrombosis and the high incidence of recent acute pulmonary embolism before referal to surgery the chances to develop a severe post-thrombotic syndrome and recurrent pulmonary embolism without surgery were quite high. In this regard thrombectomy in combination with a temporary protective arteriovenous fistula was not only helpful to remove the source of potential or further pulmonary embolism but also restored patency of the deep venous system effectively. In this regard the quite liberal insertion of IVC filters does not seem to be very logical. Reports about early and late complications of IVC filter placement are increasing (Table 5).[14,22–31] The IVC filter placement is not a harmless procedure and despite the fact that many filters have been deployed, proof of the efficacy of this procedure is still missing. As the removal of these devices is not easy and further follow-up of our patients did not reveal any contraindication against anticoagulation one must question even more the indications for filter placement. Although non-invasive haemodynamic studies and valvular function from this series will be reported separately we would like to point out that the vein valves are not necessarily destroyed by thrombectomy. In a previous report competent vein valves were demonstrated by Doppler ultrasound and plethysmography in 44% of the patients.[21]

Finally the main advantage of thrombectomy over other treatment modalities comes from the completeness of thrombus removal. Remaining thrombi after conservative treatment are still a weak area for recurrent thrombosis and a potential source for further pulmonary embolism. The more complete the thrombi can be removed, the less likely is it that recurrencies will occur. In this regard intraoperative angioscopy and on-table phlebography have been shown to be very helpful.[32] Even in patients with unsuccessful fibrinolysis, subsequent thrombectomy can be successful in terms of lumen restoration and avoidance of pulmonary embolism.[33,34]

SUMMARY

We report our experience in 75 patients undergoing IVC surgery. In 74 patients thrombectomy with temporary adjunctive arteriovenous fistula was performed for acute thrombosis of the IVC and in most cases the iliofemoral veins as well. One patient without DVT had removal of an IVC filter, which was found to be perforated into the right common iliac artery causing myocardial failure from arteriovenous shunting. Immobilization and hypercoagulable status were the predominant risk factors for DVT. Acute pulmonary embolism was confirmed in 48% of the patients and 24% suffered from recurrent PE before venous thrombectomy was considered. Surgery was performed under general anaesthesia. There were three (4%) postoperative deaths and three (4%) early recurrencies of IVC thrombosis. Sixteen (21.3%) patients developed an early recurrence of distal venous thrombosis, of which seven were rethrombectomized successfully. The overall intra- and postoperative PE rate related to the procedures was 5.7%. In seven patients IVC filters placed

Table 5. Complications after placement of IVC filter

Authors Year	Patients No	Time interval (months)	Type of	Frequency of IVC-thrombosis %	Tilting %	Penetration %	Migration %	Fracture No	PE %
Lang et al. 1994[22]	60	up to 57	Greenfield	13	25	33	5	2	8
Greenfield et al. 1994[14]	113	>12	TGF	1	–	–	–	–	3.5
Millward et al. 1994[23]	50		LGM	28	–	–	–	–	6
McCowan et al. 1992[24]	16	14	Nitinol	25	–	31	6	2	0
Bull et al. 1992[25]	26	12	Günther	20	–	20	73	–	3.8
McCowan et al. 1990[26]	30	13	Amplatz	23	–	10	0	–	7.0

previously and elsewhere had to be removed at the time of thrombectomy because of clinical complications. Patency of IVC was restored and all patients of this subgroup were long-term survivers. After a mean follow-up of 44 months in the total series clinical outcome was quite convincing and favourable to the concept of surgery compared with reports about conservative or fibrinolytic treatment in the literature.

REFERENCES

1. Lawen A: Weitere Erfahrungen über operative Thrombenentfernung bei Venenthrombose. *Arch Klin Chir* **193**: 723, 1938
2. Van Ramshorst B, van Bemmelen PS, Hoeneveld H, Eikelboom BC: The development of valvular incompetence after deep vein thrombosis: A follow-up study with duplex scanning. *J Vasc Surg* **19**: 1059–1066, 1994
3. Beebe HG, Bergan JJ, Bergqvist D *et al.*: Classification and grading of chronic venous disease in the lower limbs – A consensus statement *VASA* **24**: 313–318, 1995
4. Labropoulos N, Delis K, Nicolaides AN *et al.*: The role of the distribution and anatomic extent of reflux in the development of signs and symptoms in chronic insufficiency. *J Vasc Surg* **23**: 504–510, 1996
5. Comerota AJ, Katz ML, Greenwald LL *et al.*: Venous duplex imaging: Should it replace hemodynamic tests for deep venous thrombosis? *J Vasc Surg* **11**: 53–61, 1990
6. Eichlisberger R, Frauchiger B, Widmer Mth *et al.*: Spätfolgen der tiefen Venenthrombose: ein 13-Jahres Follow-up von 223 Patienten. *VASA* **23**: 234–243, 1994
7. Van Haarst EP, Liasis N, van Ramshorst B, Moll FL: The development of valvular incompetence after deep vein thrombosis: A 7-year follow-up study with duplex scanning. *Eur J Vasc Endovasc Surg* **12**: 295–299, 1996
8. Milne AA, Ruckley CV: The clinical course of patients following extensive deep venous thrombosis. *Eur J Vasc Surg* **8**: 56–59, 1994
9. Partsch H: Diagnose und Therapie der tiefen Venenthrombose. *VASA* **46** (Suppl): 1996
10. De Weese JA. Thrombectomy for acute iliofemoral venous thrombosis. *J Cardiovasc Surg* **5**: 703, 1964
11. Edwards WH, Sawyers JL, Foster JL: Iliofemoral venous thrombosis: Reappraisal of thrombectomy. *Ann Surg* **171**: 961, 1970
12. Sandmann W, Nüllen H, Lerut J, Kremer K: Akute Thrombose der tiefen Bein- und/oder Beckenvenen mit Embolisierung, Stenosierung oder Verschluß: Chirurgische Therapie und postoperative Klappenfunktion. *Langenbecks Arch Chir* **352**: 527, 1980
13. Greenfield LJ, Michna BA: Twelve-year clinical experience with the Greenfield vena caval filter. *Surgery* **104**: 706–712, 1988
14. Greenfield LJ, Proctor MC, Cho KJ *et al.*: Extended evaluation of the titanium Greenfield vena caval filter. *J Vasc Surg* **20**: 458–465, 1994
15. Messmer JM, Greenfield LJ: Greenfield caval filters: Long-term follow-up study. *Radiology* **156**: 613–618, 1985
16. Ginsberg JS: Drug therapy: Management of venous thromboembolism. *N Engl J Med* **335**: 1816–1828, 1996
17. Toglia MR, Weg JG: Venous thromboembolism during pregnancy. *N Engl J Med* **335**: 108–114, 1996
18. De Weese JA: Iliofemoral venous thrombectomy. In: Bergan JJ, Yao JST (Eds) *Venous Problems* pp. 421–435. Chicago: Year Book Medical Publishers, 1978
19. Kniemeyer HW, Sandmann W, Schwindt C *et al.*.: Thrombectomy with arteriovenous fistula for embolizing deep venous thrombosis: an alternative therapy for prevention of recurrent pulmonary embolism. *Clin Invest* **72**: 40–45, 1993
20. Comerota AJ, Aldridge SC, Cohen G *et al.*: A strategy of aggressive regional therapy for acute iliofemoral venous thrombosis with contemporary venous thrombectomy or catheter-directed thrombolysis. *J Vasc Surg* **20**: 244–254, 1994

21. Kniemeyer HW, Merckle R, Stühmeier K, Sandmann W: Chirurgische Therapie der akuten und embolisierenden tiefen Beinvenenthrombose – Indikation, Technisches Prinzip, Ergebnisse. *Klin Wochenschr* **68**: 1208–1216, 1990
22. Lang W, Weingärtner M, Sturm M, Schweiger H: Cavafilter zur Prophylaxe der Lungenembolie: Ist die Implantation noch gerechtfertigt? *Zentralbl Chir* **119**: 625–630, 1994
23. Millward SF, Petersen RA, Moher D *et al.*: LGM (Vena-Tech) vena caval filter: experience at a single institution. *J Vasc Intern Radiol* **5**: 351–356, 1994
24. McCowan TC, Ferris EJ, Carver DK, Molpus WM: Complications of the Nitinol vena caval filter. *JVIR* **3**: 401–408, 1992
25. Bull PG, Mendel H, Schlegl A: Günther vena caval filter: Clinical appraisal. *JVIR* **3**: 395–399, 1992
26. McCowan TC, Ferris EJ, Carver DK, Baker ML: Amplatz vena caval filter: Clinical experience in 30 patients. *Am J Roentgenol* **155**: 177–181, 1990
27. Kniemeyer HW, Sandman W, Bach D *et al.*: Complications following caval interruption. *Eur J Vasc Surg* **8**: 617–621, 1994
28. Vollmar J: Considerations on the question: V. cava interruption or reconstruction? In: May R, Weber J (Eds) *Pelvic and Abdominal Veins, Progress in diagnostics and therapy* pp. 333–335. Oxford: Excerpta Medica, 1981
29. Harris EJ, Kinney EV, Harris EJ *et al.*: Phlegmasia complicating prophylactic percutaneous inferior vena caval interruption: A word of caution. *J Vasc Surg* **22**: 606–611, 1995
30. Kröger K, Rudofsky G: Rezidivthrombosen bei einer 32jährigen Schwangeren mit permanentem Cava-Filter. *VASA* **24**: 385–388, 1995
31. Goldman KA, Adelman MA: Retroperitoneal caval filter as a source of abdominal pain. *Cardiovasc Surg* **2**: 85–87, 1994
32. Wack C, Wölfle KD, Weber H *et al.*: Diagnostischer Stellenwert der Angioskopie bei der venösen Thrombektomie. *VASA* **24**: 135–140, 1995
33. Stiegler H, Hiller W, Arbogast H *et al.*: Thrombektomie nach erfolgloser Lysetherapie tiefer Bein-Beckenvenenthrombosen: ein sinnvolles Verfahren? *VASA* **21**: 280–288, 1992
34. Stiegler H, Hiller E, Arbogast H *et al.*: Langzeitergebnisse nach erfolgloser Lyse und sekundärer Thrombektomie tiefer Bein-Beckenvenenthrombose: eine kritische Analyse. *VASA* **22:** 33–43, 1993

Low Molecular Weight Heparins for Deep Vein Thrombosis

David Bergqvist

INTRODUCTION

Heparin was incidentally discovered by the medical student Jay McLean[1] and named by Howell and Holt.[2] During the 1930s and 1940s intensive research made heparin chemistry known and led to the development of a pharmacological substance with anticoagulant properties to be used in clinical situations for prevention and treatment of venous thromboembolism. The Swedish chemist Erik Jorpes and cardiac surgeon Clarence Crafoord made important early contributions.[3,4] Heparin was a prerequisite for the development of cardiac and vascular surgery, and later made haemodialysis and organ transplantation possible. In 1976 several groups defined the biochemical basis for the anticoagulant effects of heparin.[5-7] Soon after, results from *in vitro* and *in vivo* studies in animal models suggested that it might be possible to obtain an antithrombotic with less haemorrhagic effect by using low molecular weight fractions instead of unfractionated heparin.[8,9] The observations stimulated the pharmaceutical industry to develop low molecular heparin preparations and to evaluate them clinically. By now there is a large number of investigations on low molecular weight heparins (LMWHs) both for prevention and treatment of venous thromboembolism.

PREPARATION OF LOW MOLECULAR WEIGHT HEPARINS

Both heparin and LMWHs are glucosaminoglucans. Through fractionation of the raw heparin from pig intestinal or bovine lung tissue, it is possible to obtain LMWHs of well defined molecular weights, but this type of production is extremely inefficient because of a low yield. The methodology used today is, therefore, various ways to fragment large molecules by controlled depolymerization (Table 1). The various commercial LMWHs differ in production, and also in a number of chemical, physical and pharmacological aspects.[10,11] Most, if not all, of the differences appear to be due to differences in molecular weight.[12] The clinical relevance of these differences is not clear at present. To show clinically important differences in prophylaxis or treatment would probably require large randomized trials and manufacturers have given this problem low priority. On the other hand, the differences in production, molecular weight distribution, pharmacodynamic properties and anticoagulant profile have led regulatory authorities to regard every LMWH as an exclusive pharmacological substance with its own documentation and approval.

Table 1.   Comparison of various LMWH preparations

INN	Manufacturer	Production methodology	Mean molecular weight and range (daltons)	antiXa: antilla ratio
Ardeparin	Wyeth	Peroxidation cleavage	4600 (5500–6500)	1.9
Dalteparin	Pharmacia–Upjohn	Nitrous acid depylomerization	5700 (2000–9000)	4.0
Certiparin	Sandoz	Isoamylnitrate digestion	5100 (4500–8000)	2.0
Enoxaparin	Rhône–Poulenc Rorer	Benzylation followed by hydrolysis	3800 (3500–5500)	3.6
Nadroparin	Sanofi	Fractionation, nitrous acid depolymerization	4500	4.4
Parnaparin	Alfa Wassermann	Peroxidation cleavage	4500	2.4
Reviparin	Knoll	Nitrous acid digestion	3900 (3500–4500)	3.5
Tinzaparin	Novo Lövens	Heparinase (from flavobacterium heparinum) digestion	4500 (3000–6000)	1.5

INN: International non-proprietory name

MECHANISMS OF ACTION

The heparin molecule has a unique pentasaccharide sequence with high affinity to antithrombin III (Fig. 1).[13–15] The pentasaccharide can be obtained by synthesis.[15] About one-third of the heparin and LMWH molecules contain this unit. The major anticoagulant effect of heparin depends on its interaction with antithrombin III, creating a conformational change which, in turn, accelerates the inactivation of the serine proteases (e.g. factor IIa, IXa and Xa). To inhibit thrombin (IIa), a ternary complex is formed between heparin, antithrombin III and thrombin, and this requires a heparin molecule of at least 18 saccharide units, which means around 5400 molecular weight or more (the pentasaccarides and at least 13 additional units).[13,16] Heparin molecules with fewer than 18 saccharides cannot inactivate thrombin, though factor Xa is still effectively inhibited. The commercially developed LMWHs have mean molecular weights between 3800 and 5700 (Table 1), and they are relatively more potent in inactivating factor Xa than thrombin. The relationship between *ex vivo* measured inhibitory effects on IIa and Xa activities on the one hand and clinical antithrombotic and antihaemostatic effects on the other remains controversial.

Unfortunately, the various manufacturers have different dose recommendations in factor Xa inhibitor units and one LMWH (enoxaparin) is moreover dosed in mg (1 mg

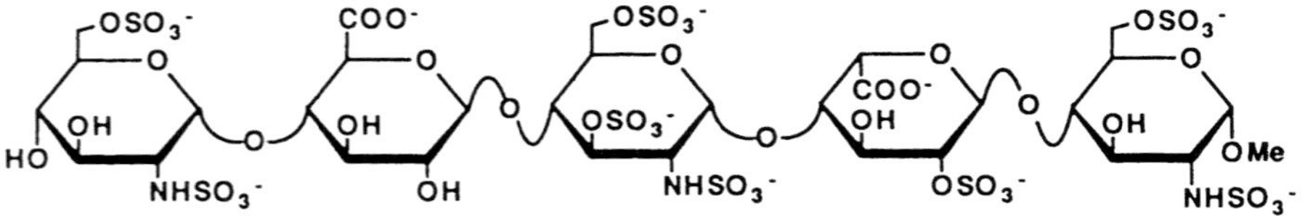

Fig. 1. The sequence of the antithrombin kind of pentasaccharide of the heparin molecule.

corresponds to 100 antiXa units). This situation may cause confusion, and there is an ongoing debate how to best standardize LMWHs.[17,18]

Both unfractionated heparin (UFH) and LMWHs bind to several plasma, platelet and vessel wall matrix proteins, though LMWHs bind with a 70–90% lower affinity.[19] The relatively higher concentration of free LMWH may explain the more predictable anticoagulant response, the lesser resistance to anticoagulant effects, as well as better plasma recovery of LMWHs compared with UFH; LMWHs do not bind to endothelial cells in culture or at least bind to a much lower degree than UFH. Endothelial cell factors are affected to various degrees by LMWHs (for review see ref. 20). So, tissue factor pathway inhibitor (TFPI) is released[21] which is interesting in that TFPI has a marked thromboprophylactic effect in a rabbit model.[22] At least part of the heparin effect could be mediated through TFPI release but whether TFPI contributes to the antithrombotic activity of LMWHs is uncertain. Prostacyclin release does not seem to be stimulated,[23] and whether fibrinolysis is activated remains controversial.[20]

Binding affinity to platelets increases with increasing molecular weight.[24] The proaggregatory effect of heparins is probably related to direct binding to platelets. The LMWH fractions induce less reactivity of platelets than does UFH.[25] The lesser effect on platelet function *in vitro* has been one suggestion why LMWHs appear to have a somewhat smaller risk for haemorrhagic side-effects than UFH.

It is known that LMWHs are associated with significantly lower lipolytic activity or mobilization of free fatty acids than UFH.[26–30] During a 1-year period of dialysis, patients on LMWH had unchanged plasma triglyceride levels whereas those on UFH had a 36% increase.[31]

PHARMACODYNAMICS

The pharmacodynamics of LMWH differ in many respects from those of UFH. The decreased affinity and binding of LMWHs to plasma proteins, endothelial cells and macrophages accounts for at least some of the differences. After subcutaneous injection, the bioavailability is considerably higher (between 90 and 100% vs 20–30%) and the biological half-life two to four times longer.[32–35] The biological half-life varies depending on the function measured. The antithrombin activity disappears faster than the factor Xa Inhibitor.[33] The elimination of UFH from blood is supposed to be a combination of endothelial cell binding and internalization, metabolism in the reticuloendothelial system and excretion via the kidneys;[36] LMWHs are excreted unchanged through the kidneys.[37] The half-life of LMWHs is increased in patients with impaired renal function.[38]

There are statistical differences between various commercial LMWHs concerning pharmacodynamic profile in plasma anti-Xa activity, total body clearance, renal excretion and elimination half-life.[39] Whether or not these differences have clinical implications is so far not known.

The UFH can be totally neutralized by an equimolar amount of protamine sulphate. The IIaI and APTT activities of LMWH can also be totally inhibited, whereas there is some XaI activity left (about 20% after intravenous injection and 35–40% after subcutaneous) (Fig. 2).[40,41] The differentiated neutralization may be

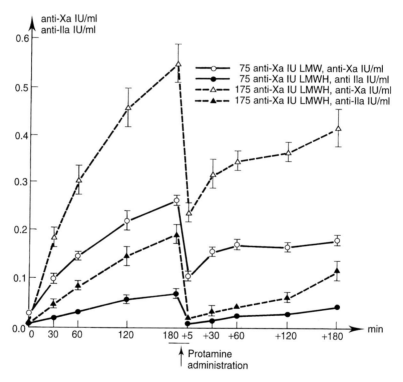

Fig. 2. Mean (±SEM) anti-Xa activity (open symbols) in IU/ml for the two subcutaneous groups receiving a prophylactic dose (75 anti-Xa IU/kg, straight line) and a treatment dose (175 anti-Xa IU/kg, dotted line), respectively. Both were neutralized with intravenous infusion of 1 mg protamine sulphate (PS)/100 anti-Xa IU of LMWH over 10 min. The plus sign denotes the samples taken after neutralization. The maximum acitivity was observed 180 min (0.26 and 0.55 anti-Xa IU) after LMWH injection. PS incompletely neutralized the anti-Xa activity to 0.10 and 0.23 anti-Xa IU for the two doses. The activity measured as anti-IIa completely neutralized in the 75 anti-Xa IU/kg group and almost completely in the 175 anti-Xa IU/kg group (<10% remained). Throughout the continuing observations a gradual and substantial return of activity was seen in both the anti-Xa and the anti-IIa activities. (From ref. 41, with permission.)

sufficient to inhibit bleeding.[42,43] After neutralization of subcutaneously injected LMWHs there is a gradual return of XaI activity, IIaI activity and APTT activity, indicating continuous absorption of LMWHs from the subcutaneous depot.[41]

CLINICAL STUDIES ON LMWHS AND VENOUS THROMBOEMBOLISM

By now there is a large number of studies showing that LMWHs are both safe and effective for prevention and treatment of venous thromboembolism. The documentation has been further analysed in reviews and meta-analyses. In the majority, if not all, of the meta-analyses the LMWHs have been considered as one pharmacological substance, which they are not. Because of variations in study design and populations studied, comparisons between various trials must be made with caution, and actually there may be greater differences between some studies on one LMWH than between other studies using different LMWHs.

Most investigations deal with effects on deep vein thrombosis (DVT), because this problem is relatively easy to study. Because pulmonary embolism, especially fatal, is infrequent relevant trials need much larger sample sizes.

Development of the post-thrombotic syndrome is a long-term process. It is difficult to design prospective studies to evaluate effects on frequency and course, both logistically and regarding sample size. Moreover, there is a background of non-thrombotic venous insufficiency in the relevant age groups.[44]

Prophylaxis against deep vein thrombosis

The effect of LMWHs to prevent postoperative venous thromboembolism is documented in a large number of original articles and summarized in reviews and meta-analyses.[45-51] Once-daily LMWHs have a prophylactic effect against postoperative DVT in all types of surgical procedures, where it has been investigated. The best effect relative to UFH is seen in patients undergoing hip surgery; in randomized studies in general surgery it is more controversial.[46] The effect of LMWHs have been similar to both adjusted-dose heparin and low-intensity warfarin (INR 2.0 to 3.0), both of which, however, are unpractical for prophylaxis in that they require laboratory monitoring. The preventive effect is better than that of dextran.[52-54]

One placebo-controlled study was large enough on its own to show a significant reduction of total mortality,[55] the relative reduction in fatal pulmonary embolism (FPE) being of similar size (around 50%), although not significant. In one study scintigraphically diagnosed asymptomatic pulmonary embolism was less frequent with LMWH than with UFH.[56] The clinical relevance of these findings is not known, but some of the reviews indicate a preventive effect on symptomatic and FPE.[45,49,50] The effect is similar to, or better than, UFH in low dose two or three times daily, which by itself clearly reduces postoperative FPE.[57] Several studies have shown LMWHs to prevent proximal DVT more effectively than UFH.[58-60] Although the optimal dose of LMWH has still to be settled, data from a recent randomized study seems to motivate a differentiation between a low dose in intermediate risk surgery and a high dose in high risk surgery.[61] This means approximately 2500 XaI units or

20 mg (mg refers to enoxaparin) and 5000 units or 40 mg, respectively, which is the recommendation in a recent European consensus document.[62] A once daily dose of 2500 Xa I units of dalteparin for 90 days has a preventive effect on upper extremity thrombosis in cancer patients with venous access devices.[63]

When the first injection of LMWHs should be given is a matter for debate. In the early studies, the first dose was given approximately 2 hours before surgery. In some studies on LMWH, it was shown that a similar, or even better, effect was obtained if the first injection was given on the evening prior to surgery.[58,64] This is clinically practical, because it is difficult to ensure that the first dose is really administered 2 hours prior to surgery.[64,65] One controversial issue concerning the start of prophylaxis has emanated from surgeons who are reluctant to start prophylaxis before surgery, because of fear of bleeding problems. Several studies have actually shown that a good prophylactic effect is obtained also when starting within the first 24 hours after operation,[66,67] but this does not fully eliminate the risk of bleeding.[68] The only way to solve the controversy between pre- and postoperative start of prophylaxis would be to perform a study designed as a prospective, randomized trial; at least one of these studies is under way. A recent review concluded that any loss of efficacy of delay of prophylaxis until after surgery was unlikely to be clinically significant.[69]

One problem which is not yet fully evaluated is the duration of prophylaxis. Three doses of LMWH is not enough to prevent proximal DVT after hip surgery,[70] and in the vast majority of studies prophylaxis has been given for 1–2 weeks. An interesting observation was made in a study by Scurr et al.[71] where they found that the risk period to develop DVT continued after departure from hospital in a substantial number of patients, and it is known that fatal pulmonary embolism can occur up to several weeks postoperatively.[72,73] This has led to the question whether prolonged prophylaxis may be indicated in some situations and at least after hip surgery there are several factors which indicate an increased risk during several weeks.[74] In four randomized studies it has been shown that LMWH prophylaxis continued after hospitalization for the first postoperative month significantly reduces the frequency of venographically detected DVT compared with prophylaxis during hospitalization alone (1–2 weeks) (Table 2). Also symptomatic, clinically relevant thromboembolism can be reduced.[75]

Another matter for discussion has been the risk of combining LMWHs with epidural/spinal puncture for anaesthesia. The debate was started by Tryba,[79] who reported on a patient with irreversible neurological deficit because of spinal haematoma. Analysis of available literature and data from the manufacturers' files

Table 2. Prolonged prophylaxis in elective hip surgery (frequency of DVT in %)

	No. of patients	LMWH	Placebo	Period (days)
[a]Bergqvist et al.[75]	262	18	33	0–30
[a]Planes et al.[76]	173	7	19	10–31
[b]Dahl et al.[77]	227	19	32	0–35
		12	26	7–35
[b]Danish study[78]	216	4	12	8–37

[a] Enoxaparin
[b] Dalteparin

shows that this complication is extremely rare (one or two in at least a million patients where the combination has been used), and there is no evidence that it is increased by LMWHs.[79,80–82]

The documentation on prophylaxis in non-surgical situations is less extensive than on postoperative prophylaxis. There are some high risk groups for DVT where LMWHs have been shown effective in prospective randomized trials, such as stroke,[83] spinal cord injury,[84] multiple trauma,[85] elderly medical inpatients[86] and patients with lower leg injury immobilized by plaster casts.[87]

Treatment of deep vein thrombosis

For decades, the initial treatment of DVT has been UFH, which requires monitoring of the effect with measurements of APTT and dose adjustment. Regarding LMWHs we are still in a process of modification. Initially, continuous infusion of LMWHs with XaI monitoring was compared with UFH.[88,89] The next step was subcutaneous injection twice-daily of LMWH, still with XaI monitoring,[90] followed by twice-daily injections without monitoring.[91–93] The most recent development is one weight-adjusted subcutaneous injection of LMWH daily (175–200 XaI units/kg bodyweight) without monitoring, which is a major step forward in the treatment of DVT.[94,95] A plasma level of 0.4–0.8 XaI units/ml is both effective and safe.[96] Totally there are several meta-analyses and reviews on LMWH treatment.[96,97–100] In comparison with UFH, LMWHs reduce thrombus extension on repeat phlebography. To study changes of thrombus size on repeat phlebography methodologically is difficult, and a scoring system is often used.[101,102] A reduction in thrombus size may mean thrombolysis but could also be an effect of embolization. Also LMWHs seem to reduce the frequency of recurrences, mortality and major bleedings.[96,98] A summary from the meta-analysis by Lensing et al.[98] is given in Table 3.

Because of the possibility of instituting treatment with subcutaneous injections of LMWH it has become of interest with outpatient treatment. There are now two randomized studies comparing outpatient twice-daily unmonitored injections of LMWH with inhospital continuous infusion of UFH with APTT-monitoring.[103,104] The measured effects were similar (Table 4) although the proper comparison should in

Table 3. Comparison between UFH and LMWH as initial treatment of DVT. Data from the meta-analysis by Lensing et al.[98]

	No. of patients (studies)	LMWH %	UFH %	Risk reduction %	Positive
Recurent symptomatic thromboembolism	1086 (5)	3.1	6.6	53	<0.01
Venographic improvement	992 (9)	63	52	21	<0.001
Major bleeding	1512 (10)	0.8	2.8	68	<0.005
Mortality	1086 (5)	3.9	7.1	47	<0.04

Table 4.   Outpatient subcutaneous LMWH versus UFH in infusion – two randomized
comparative studies

| | Levine et al.[103] | | Koopman et al.[104] | |
	LMWH	UFH	LMWH	UFH
No. of patients (n)	247	253	202	198
Recurrence (n)	13	17	14	17
Major bleeding (n)	5	3	1	4
Mortality (n)[a]	11	17	14	16
Mean hospital stay (days)	1.1	6.5	2.7	8.1

[a] Levine *et al.* 3 months; Koopman *et al.* 6 months

my opinion have been twice-daily subcutaneous injections of UFH. Although this requires monitoring, a shorter hospital stay might have been possible also among UFH patients.

In some patients where it is not possible to use oral anticoagulation or this is contraindicated, long-term heparin is necessary. Three small randomized series comparing LMWHs with warfarin and UFH have shown equal efficacy.[105–107] In the UFH study[105] there was a tendency for LMWH to give rise to fewer osteoporotic complications.

Low molecular weight heparin during pregnancy

Oral anticoagulants are contraindicated during pregnancy because of teratogenicity and the risk of fetal bleeding. Therefore heparin is used for long periods and, besides requiring frequent injection, there is a risk of developing osteoporosis with ensuing fractures. The prerequisites for clinical application of LMWHs were no transplacental passage to the fetal circulation and little risk for osteoporosis. Several experimental and clinical studies have shown that the placental barrier is not crossed.[108,109] Although there is a dose- and time-dependent induction of osteoporosis in rats,[110] the clinical problem is small and bone-density scans have shown normal mineral mass in women after delivery. Moreover, the antithrombotic effect has been satisfactory.[111,112]

Health economic aspects

Health economic analyses of various therapeutic and prophylactic options have become increasingly important. A number of studies concerning prophylaxis versus postoperative thromboembolism are consistent in showing that, in addition to reducing FPE with various types of prophylaxis, there is health care money to be saved. A few studies have compared the alternative prophylactic strategies UFH and LMWH.[49,113–117] In most, the use of LMWH leads to a net saving per patient. In a sensitivity analysis it was shown that the price level of the pharmacological substances is of relatively great importance for the conclusion to be valid.[49] Ambulant treatment of venous thromboembolism in a significant number of patients would seem to be beneficial from an economic point of view. This concept must, however, be prospectively evaluated, using adequate health economic methodology.

Side-effects

The most obvious potential side-effect is haemorrhage. One problem with perioperative haemorrhagic complications is the heterogenecity in classification, and there is no consensus on how to classify or quantify bleedings. Studies analysing bleeding should therefore be double-blind to avoid bias. From a biostatistical point of view the majority of prophylactic and therapeutic studies have been designed to discover differences in efficacy and only exceptionally to analyse potential differences in bleeding.[61,118] There is a relation between dose and bleeding risk, although it is probably not related in any simple way to the factor XaI activity. An increased frequency of postoperative bleeding complications was observed in early studies on LMWHs, where the dose was set too high, according to present knowledge.[119-121] With today's recommended doses the risk for bleeding is low, similar to placebo in orthopaedic surgery and somewhat higher in general surgery.[45,46,50] Major bleeding complications or blood transfusion requirements are lower than after low dose UFH[118,122] and possibly lower than after dextran.[53] In one study on knee arthroplasty, there were more wound haematomas with LMWH than with warfarin.[68]

Haematomas at injection site seem to be less frequent than with UFH.[64] The presence of malignant disease seems to diminish the risk of bleeding complications after surgery compared with patients operated on for benign conditions when dalteparin is used for prophylaxis.[61]

Thrombocytopenia is a rare complication to heparin treatment or prophylaxis. Thrombocytopenia is considered an immune response which clinically may give rise to the white clot syndrome, sometimes with devastating thrombotic complications. Although rare with LMWHs,[67,122] thrombocytopenia does occur.[123] In a study on total hip replacement, mild thrombocytopenia (100×10^9/litre to normal range) was found in 12% and moderate ($20-100 \times 10^9$/litre) in less than 1% of the patients.[67] In a randomized prophylactic study on hip arthroplasty, enoxaparin induced less thrombocytopenia associated with thrombotic events and less heparin-dependent IgG antibodies than UFH.[124] In treatment situations data are still too sparse. In cases of heparin-induced thrombocytopenia, LMWHs have been successfully used to replace UFH, but there are patients with cross-reactions.[125]

Osteoporosis, allergic reactions and skin necrosis are very rare side-effects.

Transient elevations of aminotransferases are well known after UFH administration[66] and they are also seen with LMWHs[66,67] but with no clinical relevance.

FUTURE ASPECTS

Some examples of problems that should be further evaluated are:

1. the value of long-term prophylaxis, that is after hospitalization, in various risk groups: the optimal duration must be established;
2. the clinical relevance of differences in chemical and pharmacodynamic properties;
3. the relative effectiveness of various commercial LMWHs;

4. the necessity of LMWH prophylaxis in patients undergoing laparoscopic procedures;
5. the value of LMWHs in emergency general surgery;
6. pre- or postoperative start of prophylaxis;
7. the value of combining LMWHs with mechanical prophylaxis;
8. the patient compliance if LMWH prophylaxis and treatment are transferred to an ambulant basis;
9. the quality of life of ambulant treatment with LMWHs;
10. the reduction in mortality when DVT treatment is instituted with LMWHs;
11. the effect of LMWHs to treat pulmonary embolism;
12. once or twice daily injections for optimal treatment;
13. the risk for osteoporosis during long-term treatment.

ACKNOWLEDGEMENTS

Swedish Medical Research Council 00759, Swedish Heart and Lung Foundation.

REFERENCES

1. McLean J: The thromboplastic action of cephalin. *Am J Physiol* **41**: 250–270, 1916
2. Howell WH, Holt E: Two near factors in blood coagulation. *Am J Physiol* **47**: 328–341, 1918
3. Jorpes E: The chemistry of heparin. *Biochem J* **29**: 1817, 1935
4. Crafoord C: Preliminary report on postoperative treatment with heparin as a preventive of thrombosis. *Acta Chir Scand* **79**: 407–426, 1937
5. Höök M, Björk I, Hopwood J, Lindahl U: Anticoagulant activity of heparin, separation of high-activity and low-activity heparin species by affinity chromatography on immobilized antithrombin. *FEBS Lett* **66**: 90–93, 1976
6. Andersson L-O, Barrowcliffe TW, Holmer E *et al.*: Anticoagulant properties of heparin fractionated by affinity chromatography on matrix-bound antithrombin III and by gel filtration. *Thromb Res* **9**: 575, 1976
7. Lam LH, Silberg JA, Rosenberg RD: The separation of active and inactive forms of heparin. *Biochem Biophys Res Commun* **69**: 570–577, 1976
8. Carter CJ, Kelton JG, Hirsh J *et al.*: The relationship between the haemorrhagic and antithrombotic properties of low molecular weight heparin in rabbits. *Blood* **59**: 1239–1245, 1982
9. Esquivel CO, Bergqvist D, Björck C-G, Nilsson B: Effect of heparin and a heparinoid on platelet activity and microvascular haemostasis *in vivo*. *Eur Surg Res* **14**: 154, 1982
10. Hoppensteadt DA, Haas S, Breddin HK, Fareed J: Modulation of laboratory parameters after therapeutic and prophylactic administration of sandoparin. *Semin Thromb Hemost* **19**: S31–S35, 1993
11. Collignon F, Frydman A, Caplain H *et al.*: Comparison of the pharmacokinetic profiles of three low molecular mass heparins – dalteparin, enoxaparin and nadroparin – administered subcutaneously in healthy volunteers (doses for prevention of thromboembolism). *Thromb Haemost* **73**: 630–640, 1995
12. Østergaard PB, Nilsson B, Bergqvist D *et al.*: The effect of low molecular weight heparin on experimental thrombosis and haemostasis – the influence of production method. *Thromb Res* **45**: 739–749, 1987
13. Lindahl U, Bäckström G, Höök M *et al.*: Structure of the antithrombin-binding site of heparin. *Proc Natl Acad Sci USA* **76**: 3198–3202, 1979

14. Rosenberg RD, Lam L: Correlation between structure and function of heparin. *Proc Natl Acad Sci USA* **76**: 1218–1222, 1979
15. Choay J, Pettou M, Lormeau J *et al.*: Structure–activity relationship in heparin, a synthetic pentasaccharide with high affinity for antithrombin III and eliciting high anti-factor Xa activity. *Biochem Biophys Res Commun* **116**: 492–499, 1983
16. Rosenberg RD, Jordan RE, Favreau LV, Lam LH: Highly active heparin species with multiple binding sites for antithrombin. *Biochem Biophys Res Commun* **86**: 1319–1324, 1979
17. Hemker HC: A standard for low molecular weight heparins? *Haemostasis* **19**: 1–4, 1989
18. Gray E, Heath AB, Mulloy B *et al.*: A collaborative study of proposed European Pharmacopein. Reference preparations of low molecular mass heparin. *Thromb Haemost* **74**: 893–899, 1995
19. Young E, Wells P, Holloway S *et al.*: *Ex vivo* and *in vitro* evidence that low molecular weight heparins exhibit less binding to plasma proteins than unfractionated heparin. *Thromb Haemost* **71**: 300–304, 1994
20. Bergqvist D, Siegbahn A: Effects of heparin on the vessel wall and blood cellular elements. *Vasc Med Rev* **4**: 221–233, 1993
21. Hoppensteadt DA, Jeske W, Fareed J, Bermes EW: The role of tissue factor pathway inhibitor in the mediation of the antithrombotic actions of heparin and low-molecular-weight heparin. *Blood Coagul Fibrinol* **6**: S57–S64, 1995
22. Holst J, Lindblad B, Bergqvist D *et al.*: Antithrombotic properties of a truncated recombinant tissue factor pathway inhibitor ($rTFPI_{1-161}$) in an experimental venous thrombosis model. *Haemostasis* **23**(Suppl): 112–17, 1993
23. Brunkwall J, Mätzsch T, Bergqvist D: The effect of unfractionated and low-molecular-weight heparin on the release of prostacyclin from the arterial wall. *Blood Coagul Fibrinolysis* **1**: 641–645, 1990
24. Horne MK, Chao ES: The effect of molecular weight on heparin binding to platelets. *Br J Haematol* **74**: 306–312, 1990
25. Salzman EW, Rosenberg RD, Smith MH *et al.*: Effect of heparin and heparin fractions on platelet aggregation. *J Clin Invest* **65**: 64–73: 1980
26. Persson E, Nordenström J, Hagenfeldt L: Plasma lipolytic activity after subcutaneous administratin of heparin and a low molecular weight heparin fragment. *Thromb Res* **46**: 697–704, 1987
27. Myrmel T, Larsen TS, Reikerås O: Lipolytic effect of low molecular weight heparin (Fragmin) and heparin/dihydroergotamin in thromboprophylactic doses during total hip replacement. *Scand J Clin Lab Invest* **52**: 741–745, 1992
28. Bengtsson G, Olivecrona T, Höök M *et al.*: Interaction of lipoprotein lipase with native and modified heparin-like polysaccharides. *Biochem J* **189**: 625–633, 1980
29. Persson E. Nordenström J, Nilson-Ehle P, Hagenfeldt L: Lipolytic and anticoagulant activities of a low molecular weight fragment of heparin. *Eur J Clin Inv* **15**: 215–220, 1985
30. Olivecrona T, Bengtsson-Olivecrona G, Østergaard P *et al.*: New aspects on heparin and lipoprotein metabolism. *Haemostasis* **23**: S150–S160, 1993
31. Schroeder J, Stibbe W, Armstrong VW: Comparison of low molecular weight heparin to standard heparin in hemodialysis/hemofiltration. *Kidney Int* **33**: 890–896, 1988
32. Bergqvist D, Hedner U, Sjörin E, Holmer E: Anticoagulant effects of two types of low molecular weight heparin administrated subcutaneously. *Thromb Res* **32**: 381–391, 1983
33. Mätzsch T, Bergqvist D, Hedner U, Østergaard PB: Effects of an enzymatically depolymerized heparin as compared with conventional heparin in healthy volunteers. *Thromb Haemost* **57**: 97–101, 1987
34. Boneau B, Dol F, Caranobe C *et al.*: Pharmacokinetics of heparin and related polysaccharides. *Ann NY Acad Sci* **556**: 282–291, 1989
35. Bendetowicz V, Béguin S, Caplain H, Hemker HC: Pharmacokinetics and pharmaco-dynamics of a low molecular weight heparin (Enoxaparin) after subcutaneous injection, comparison with unfractionated heparin- A three-way cross-over study in human volunteers. *Thromb Haemost* **71**: 305–313, 1994
36. Albada J, Nieuwenhuis HK, Sixma JJ: Pharmacokinetics of standard and low molecular weight heparin. In: Lane DA, Lindahl U (Eds) *Heparin*. London: Arnold, 1989

37. Palm M, Mattson C: Pharmacokinetics of heparin and low molecular weight heparin fragment (Fragmin®) in rabbits with impaired renal or metabolic clearance. *Thromb Haemost* **58:** 932–935, 1987

38. Cadroy Y, Pourrat J, Baladre MF: Delayed elimination of enoxaparin in patients with chronic renal insufficiency. *Thromb Res* **63:** 385–390, 1991

39. Eriksson BI. Söderberg K, Widlund L *et al.*: A comparative study of three low-molecular weight heparins (LMWH) and unfractionated heparin (UH) in healthy volunteers. *Thromb Haemost* **73:** 398–401, 1995

40. Harenberg J, Gnasso A, de Vries JX *et al.*: Inhibition of low molecular weight heparin by protamine chloride *in vivo*. *Thromb Res* **38:** 11–20, 1985

41. Holst J, Lindblad B, Bergqvist D *et al.*: Protamine neutralization of intravenous and subcutaneous LMWH (tinzaparin, Logiparin). An experimental investigation in healthy volunteers. *Blood Coagul Fibrinolys* **5:** 795–803, 1995

42. Diness V, Østergaard P: Neutralization of a low-molecular-weight heparin (LHN-1) and conventional heparin by protamine sulphate in rats. *Thromb Haemost* **56:** 318–322, 1986

43. Hirsh J, Fuster V: Guide to anticoagulant therapy. Part I, heparin. *Circulation* **89:** 1449–1468, 1994

44. Lindhagen A, Bergqvist D, Hallböök T: Deep venous insufficiency after postoperative thrombosis diagnosed with ^{125}I-labelled fibrinogen uptake test. *Br J Surg* **71:** 511–515, 1984

45. Bergqvist D: Review of clinical trials of low molecular weight heparins. *Eur J Surg* **158:** 67–78, 1992

46. Nurmohammed MT, Rosendaal FR, Büller HR *et al.*: Low-molecular-weight heparin versus standard heparin in general and orthopaedic surgery, a meta-analysis. *Lancet* **340:** 152–156, 1992

47. Leizorovicz A, Haugh MC, Chapuis F-R *et al.*: Low molecular weight heparin in prevention of perioperative thrombosis. *Br Med J* **305:** 913–920, 1992

48. Kakkar VV: Efficacy and safety of clivarin® and other LMWHs in general surgery, a meta-analysis. *Blood Coagul Fibrinolysis* **4:** S23–S27, 1993

49. Anderson DR, O'Brien BJ, Levine MN *et al.*: Efficacy and cost of low-molecular-weight heparin compared with standard heparin for the prevention of deep vein thrombosis after total hip arthroplasty. *Ann Intern Med* **119:** 1105–112, 1993

50. Jørgensen LN, Wille-Jørgensen P, O Hauch: Prophylaxis of postoperative thrombo-embolism with low molecular weight heparins. *Br J Surg* **80:** 689–704, 1993

51. Imperiale TF, Speroff T: A meta-analysis of methods to prevent venous thrombo-embolism following total hip replacement. *J Am Med Assoc* **271:** 1780–1785, 1994

52. Mätzsch T, Bergqvist D, Fredin H, Hedner U: Low molecular weight heparin compared with dextran as prophylaxis against thrombosis after total hip replacement. *Acta Chir Scand* **156:** 445–450, 1990

53. The Danish enoxaparin study group: Low molecular weight heparin (enoxaparin) vs dextran-70. The prevention of postoperative deep vein thrombosis after total hip replacement. *Arch Intern Med* **151:** 1621–1624, 1991

54. Reiertsen D, Larsen S, Størkson R *et al.*: Safety of enoxaparin and dextran-70 in the prevention of venous thromboembolism in digestive surgery. A play-the-winner-designed study. *Scand J Gastroenterol* **28:** 1015–1020, 1993

55. Pezzuoli G, Serneri GGN, Settembrini P *et al.*: Prophylaxis of fatal pulmonary embolism in general surgery using low-molecular weight heparin Cy 216, A multicentre, double-blind, randomized, controlled, clinical trial versus placebo (STEP). *Int Surg* **74:** 205–210, 1989

56. Eriksson BI, Kälebo P, Anthmyr BA *et al.*: Prevention of deep-vein thrombosis and pulmonary embolism after total hip replacement. Comparison of low-molecular-weight heparin and unfractionated heparin. *J Bone Jt Surg* **73A:** 484–493, 1991

57. Collins R, Scrimgeour A, Yusuf S *et al.*: Reduction in fatal pulmonary embolism and venous thrombosis by perioperative administration of subcutaneous heparin. Overview of results of randomized trials in general, orthopaedic, and urologic surgery. *N Engl J Med* **318:** 1162–1173, 1988

58. Planes A, Vochelle N, Mazas F et al.: Prevention of postoperative venous thrombosis, A randomized trial comparing unfractionated heparin with low molecular weight heparin in patients undergoing total hip replacement. Thromb Haemost **60**: 407–410, 1988

59. Leyvraz PF, Bachmann F, Hoek J et al.: Prevention of deep vein thrombosis after hip replacement, randomised comparison between unfractionated heparin and low molecular weight heparin. Br Med J **303**: 543–548, 1991

60. The German Hip Arthroplasty Trial (GHAT) Group: Prevention of deep vein thrombosis with low molecular-weight heparin in patients undergoing total hip replacement. Arch Orthop Trauma Surg **111**: 110–120, 1992

61. Bergqvist D, Burmark US, Flordal PA et al.: Low molecular weight heparin started before surgery as prophylaxis against deep vein thrombosis, 2500 versus 5000 XaI units in 2070 patients. Br J Surg **82**: 496–501, 1995

62. Nicolaides AN, Bergqvist D, Comerota AJ et al.: European Consensus Statement. Prevention of venous thromboembolism. Int Angiol **11**: 151–159, 1992

63. Monreal M, Alastrue A, Rull M et al.: Upper extremity deep venous thrombosis in cancer patients with venous access devices – prophylaxis with a low molecular weight heparin (Fragmin). Thromb Haemost **75**: 251–153, 1996

64. Bergqvist D, Mätzsch T, Burmark US et al.: Low molecular weight heparin given the evening before surgery compared with conventional low dose heparin in the prevention of thrombosis after elective general abdominal surgery. Br J Surg **75**: 888–891, 1988

65. Mätzsch T, Bergqvist D, Burmark US et al.: The influence of surgical trauma on factor XaI- and IIaI-activity and heparin concentration after a single dose of low molecular weight heparin. Blood Coagul Fibrinolysis **2**: 651–657, 1991

66. Colwell CW, Spiro TE, Trowbridge AA et al.: Use of enoxaparin, a low-molecular-weight heparin, and unfractionated heparin for the prevention of deep venous thrombosis after elective hip replacement. J Bone Jt Surg **76A**: 3–14, 1994

67. Spiro TE, Johnson GJ, Christie MJ et al.: Efficacy and safety of enoxaparin to prevent deep venous thrombosis after hip replacement surgery. Ann Intern Med **121**: 81–89, 1994

68. Hull RD, Raskob G, Pineo G et al.: A comparison of subcutaneous low-molecular-weight heparin with warfarin sodium for prophylaxis against deep-vein thrombosis after hip or knee implantation. N Engl J Med **329**: 1370–1376, 1993

69. Kearon C, Hirsh J: Starting prophylaxis for venous thromboembolism postoperatively. Arch Intern Med **155**: 366–372, 1995

70. Warwick D, Bannister GC, Glew D, Mitchelmore A: Perioperative low-molecular-weight heparin. Is it effective and safe? J Bone Jt Surg **77B**: 715–719, 1995

71. Scurr J. Coleridge-Smith P, Hasty JH: Deep venous thrombosis, a continuing problem. Br J Med **297**: 28, 1988

72. Bergqvist D, Lindblad B: A 30–year survey of pulmonary embolism verified at autopsy, an analysis of 1274 surgical patients. Br J Surg **72**: 105–108, 1985

73. Lindblad B, Sternby NH, Bergqvist D: Incidence of venous thromboembolism verified by necroscopy over 30 years. Br Med J **302**: 709–711, 1991

74. Bergqvist D: The post-discharge risk of venous thromboembolism after hip replacement – the role of prolonged prophylaxis. Drugs **52** (Suppl 7): 55–59, 1996

75. Bergqvist D, Benoni G, Björgell O et al.: Low-molecular-weight heparin (enoxaparin) as prophylaxis against venous thromboembolism after total hip replacement. N Engl J Med **385**: 696–700, 1996

76. Planes A, Vouchelle N, Fagola M: Persistence of the risk of deep venous thrombosis after hospital discharge in patients undergoing total hip replacement. Lancet **348**: 224–228, 1996

77. Dahl OE, Andreasson G, Müller C: The effect of prolonged thromboprophylaxis with dalteparin on the frequency of deep vein thrombosis (DVT) and pulmonary embolism (PE) 35 days after hip replacement surgery (HRS). Thromb Haemost **73**: 1094(abstract), 1995

78. Lassen MR, Borris LC: On behalf of the Danish Prolonged Prophylaxis Study Group: Prolonged thromboprophylaxis with low molecular weight heparin (Fragmin) after elective total hip arthroplasty – a placebo-controlled study. Thromb Haemost **73**: 1104(abstract), 1995

79. Tryba M und die Teilnehmer des Workshop über hämostaseologische Probleme bei

Regionalanaesthesien: Haemostaseologische Voraussetzungen zur Durch-führung von Regionalanaesthesien. *Regional Anaesthesie* **12:** 127–131, 1989

80. Bergqvist D, Lindblad B, Mätzsch T: Low molecular weight heparin for thrombo-prophylaxis and epidural/spinal anaesthesia – is there a risk? *Acta Anaesthesiol Scand* **36:** 605–609, 1992

81. Wolf H: Experience with regional anaesthesia in patients receiving low molecular weight heparins. *Semin Thromb Hemost* **19:** S152–S159, 1993

82. Vandermeulen AP, Van Aken H, Vermylen J: Anticoagulants and spinal-epidural anesthesia. *Anesth Analg* **79:** 1165–1177, 1994

83. Prins MH, Gelsema R, Sing AK: Prophylaxis of deep venous thrombin with a low molecular weight heparin (Kabi 2165/Fragmin) in stroke patients. *Haemost* **19:** 245–250, 1989

84. Green D, Lee MY, Lim AC *et al.*: Prevention of thromboembolism after spinal cord injury using low-molecular-weight heparin. *Ann Intern Med* **113:** 571–574, 1990

85. Geerts WH, Jay RM, Code KI *et al.*: A comparison of low-dose heparin with low-molecular-weight heparin as prophylaxis against venous thromboembolism after major trauma. *N Engl J Med* **335:** 701–707, 1996

86. Dahan R, Houlbert D, Caulin C *et al.*: Prevention of deep vein thrombosis in elderly medical in-patients by a low-molecular weight heparin, a randomized double-blind trial. *Haemost* **16:** 159–164, 1986

87. Spannagel U, Kujath P: Low molecular weight heparin for the prevention of thromboembolism in outpatients immobilized by plaster cast. *Semin Thromb Hemost* **19:** S131–S141, 1993

88. Bratt G, Törnebohm E, Granqvist S *et al.*: A comparison between low molecular weight heparin (Kabi 2165) and standard heparin in the intravenous treatment of deep venous thrombosis. *Thromb Haemost* **54:** 813–817, 1985

89. Albada J, Niuwenhuis HK, Sixma JJ: Treatment of acute venous thromboembolism with low molecular weight heparin (Fragmin). *Circulation* **80:** 935–940, 1989

90. Bratt G, Åberg W, Johansson M *et al.*: Two daily subcutaneous injections of Fragmin as compared with intravenous standard heparin in the treatment of deep venous thrombosis (DVT). *Thromb Haemost* **64:** 506–510, 1990

91. Coll Eur Multic Study: A randomised trial of subcutaneous low molecular weight heparin (CY 216) compared with intravenous unfractionated heparin in the treatment of deep vein thrombosis. *Thromb Haemost* **65:** 251–256, 1991

92. Prandoni P, Lensing A, Büller HR *et al.*: Comparison of subcutaneous low-molecular-weight heparin with intravenous standard heparin in proximal deep-vein thrombosis. *Lancet* **339:** 441–445, 1992

93. Lopacuik S, Meissner J, Filipecki S *et al.*: Subcutaneous low molecular weight heparin versus subcutaneous unfractionated heparin in the treatment of deep vein thrombosis, a Polish multicenter trial. *Thromb Haemost* **68:** 14–8, 1992

94. Hull DH, Raskob GE, Pineo GF *et al.*: Subcutaneous low-molecular-weight heparin compared with continuous intravenous heparin int the treatment of proximal-vein thrombosis. *N Engl J Med* **326:** 975–982, 1992

95. Lindmarker P, Holmström M, Granqvist S *et al.*: Comparison of once-daily subcutaneous Fragmin® with continuous intravenous unfractionated heparin in the treatment of deep vein thrombosis. *Thromb Haemost* **72:** 186–190, 1994

96. Leizorovicz A, Simonneau G, Decousus H, Boisse JP: Comparison of efficacy and safety of low molecular weight heparins and unfractionated heparin in the initial treatment of deep venous thrombosis, a meta-analysis. *Br Med J* **309:** 229–304, 1994

97. Tapson VF, Hull RD: Management of venous thromboembolic disease. The impact of low-molecular-weight heparin. *Clin Chest Med* **16:** 281–294, 1995

98. Lensing AWA, Prins MH, Davidson BL, Hirsh J: Treatment of deep venous thrombosis with low-molecular-weight heparins. *Arch Intern Med* **155:** 601–607, 1995

99. Dalsgaard Nielsen J, Landorph A: Lavmolekylært heparin versus ufraktioneret heparin ved behandling af dyb venetrombose – en metaanalyse. *Ugeskr Læger* **156:** 5844–5849, 1994

100. Siragusa S, Cosmi B, Piovella F *et al.*: Low-molecular-weight heparins and unfractionated

heparin in the treatment of patients with acute venous thromboembolism, results of a meta-analysis. *Am J Med* **100**: 269–277, 1996

101. Marder VJ, Soulen RL, Atichartakarn VM *et al.*: Quantitative venographic assessment of deep vein thrombosis in the evaluation of streptokinase and heparin therapy. *J Lab Clin Med* **89**: 1018–1029, 1997

102. Arnesen H, Heilo A, Jakobsen E *et al.*: A prospective study on streptokinase and heparin in the treatment of deep vein thrombosis. *Acta Med Scand* **203**: 457–463, 1978

103. Levine M, Gent M, Hirsh J *et al.*: A comparison of low-molecular-weight heparin administrered primarily at home with unfractionated heparin administered in the hospital for proximal deep-vein thrombosis. *N Engl J Med* **334**: 677–681, 1995

104. Koopman MMW, Prandoni P, Piovella F *et al.* for the Tasman Study Group: Treatment of venous thrombosis with intravenous unfractionated heparin administered in the hospital as compared with subcutaneous low-molecular-weight heparin administered at home. *N Engl J Med* **334**: 682–687, 1996

105. Monreal M, Lafoz E, Olive A *et al.*: Comparison of subcutaneous unfractionated heparin with a low molecular weight heparin (Fragmin®) in patients with venous thrombo-embolism and contraindications to coumarin. *Thromb Haemost* **71**: 7–11, 1994

106. Pini M, Aiello S, Manotti C *et al.*: Low molecular weight heparin versus warfarin in the prevention of recurrences after deep vein thrombosis. *Thromb Haemost* **72**: 191–197, 1994

107. Das SK, Cohen AT, Edmondson RA *et al.*: Low-molecular-weight heparin versus warfarin for prevention of recurrent venous thromboembolism. A randomized trial. *World J Surg* **20**: 521–527, 1996

108. Andrew M, Boneu B, Cade J *et al.*: Placental transport of low molecular weight heparin in the pregnant sheep. *Br J Hematol* **59**: 103–108, 1985

109. Mätzsch T, Bergqvist D, Bergqvist A *et al.*: No transplacental passage of standard heparin or an enzymatically depolymerized low molecular weight heparin. *Blood Coagul Fibrinol* **2**: 273–278, 1991

110. Mätzsch T, Bergqvist D, Hedner U *et al.*: Effects of low molecular weight heparin and unfragmented heparin on induction of osteoporosis in rats. *Thromb Haemost* **79**: 92–96, 1990

111. Wahlberg TB, Kher A: Low molecular weight heparin as thromboprophylaxis in pregnancy. *Haemostasis* **24**: 55–56, 1994

112. Fejgin MD, Lourwood DL: Low molecular weight heparins and their use in obstetrics and gynecology. *Obstet Gynecol Surv* **49**: 424–431

113. Bergqvist D, Lindgren B, Mätzsch T: Comparison of the cost of preventing postoperative deep vein thrombosis with either unfractionated or low molecular weight heparin. *Br J Surg* **83**: 1548–1552, 1996

114. Drummond M, Aristides M, Davies L, Forbes C: Economic evaluation of standard heparin and enoxaparin for prophylaxis against deep vein thrombosis in elective hip surgery. *Br J Surg* **81**: 1742–1746, 1994

115. Menzin J, Richner R, Huse D *et al.*: Prevention of deep-vein thrombosis following total hip replacement surgery with enoxaparin versus unfractionated heparin, a pharmaco-economic evaluation. *Ann Pharmacother* **28**: 271–275, 1994

116. Borris LC, Lassen MR, Jensen HP *et al.*: Perioperative thrombosis prophylaxis with low molecular weight heparins in elective hip surgery. *Int J Clin Pharmacol Ther* **32**: 262–268, 1994

117. Heaton D, Pearce M: Low molecular weight versus unfractionated heparin. A clinical and economic appraisal. *PharmacoEconomics* **8**: 91–99, 1995

118. Kakkar VV, Cohen AT, Edmonson RA *et al.*: Low molecular weight heparin versus standard heparin for prevention of venous thromboembolism after major abdominal surgery. *Lancet* **341**: 259–265, 1993

119. Bergqvist D, Burmark US, Frisell J *et al.*: Low molecular weight heparin once daily compared with conventional low-dose heparin twice daily. A prospective double-blind multicentre trial on prevention of postoperative thrombosis. *Br J Surg* **73**: 204–208, 1986

120. Koller M, Schoch U, Buchmann P *et al.*: Low molecular weight heparin (Kabi 2165) as

thromboprophylaxis in elective visceral surgery. A randomized, double-blind study versus unfractionated heparin. *Thromb Haemost* **56:** 243–246, 1986

121. Schimdt-Hübner U, Bünte H, Freise G *et al.*: Clinical efficacy of low molecular weight heparin in postoperative thrombosis prophylaxis. *Klin Wochenschr* **62:** 349–353, 1984

122. Wolf H: Low-molecular-weight heparin. *Med Clin North Am* **78:** 733–743, 1994

123. Lecompte T, Luo SK, Stieltjes N *et al.*: Thrombocytopenia associated with low-molecular-weight heparin. *Lancet* **338:** 1217, 1991

124. Warkentin T, Levine M, Hirsh J *et al.*: Heparin indured thrombocytopenia in patients treated with low-molecular-weight heparin or unfractionated heparin. *N Engl J Med* **332:** 1330–1335, 1995

125. Leroy J, Leclerc MH, Delahousse B *et al.*: Treatment of heparin-associated thrombo-cytopenia and thrombosis with low molecular weight heparin (CY216). *Semin Thromb Hemost* **11:** 326–329, 1985

Management of Axillary Vein Thrombosis

J. R. Rochester and J. D. Beard

INTRODUCTION

Axillary vein thrombosis is becoming an increasingly common clinical problem secondary to the dramatic increase in the use of subclavian cannulae for venous access. The incidence has increased from 1.3 to 4% of all deep venous thromboses over the last 30 years[1,2] giving a prevelance of 1:25 000 of the population per year. Cases have been reported in all age groups from neonates to the elderly with no sexual predominance.

Patients present with swelling of the arm (74%) (Fig. 1), discomfort, ache or pain (26%),[3] and less commonly weakness and tingling.[1] In women up to 22% develop unilateral breast swelling.[1] On physical examination 68% will have discolouration of the limb with cyanosis, 32% a palpable thrombosed vein in the axilla and all patients will have prominent venous collaterals around the shoulder girdle.[3]

In a recent review 40% of cases were secondary to subclavian catheters, 24% neoplasms, 18% 'primary', 6% hypercoagulable states, 6% trauma and 3% congestive cardiac failure, 'primary' thrombosis indicating that no obvious direct cause is apparent after initial evaluation.[2] The outcome of treatment is dependent on the aetiology rather than the management[4] but an aggressive approach is still required if long-term sequelae are to be avoided, particularly in the 'primary' group.

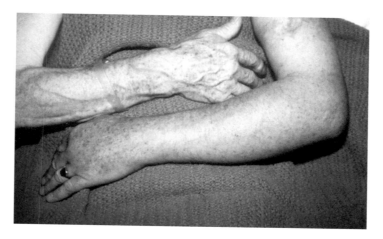

Fig. 1. Acute left axillary vein thrombosis leading to swelling and cyanosis of the arm.

INVESTIGATION

Once the diagnosis is clinically suspected routine investigation with full blood count, urea and electrolytes, thrombophilia screen, clotting studies and chest X-ray are undertaken. These investigations will identify the underlying cause of the thrombosis in about 80% of cases and provide base line results prior to anti-coagulation and/or thrombolysis. The other 20% of cases are almost all 'primary' axillary vein thromboses. In the absence of a contraindication the patient should be anticoagulated with heparin and nursed with the affected arm elevated on pillows at shoulder height. Initiation of heparin within 7 days of the onset of the thrombosis carries a better prognosis than delayed heparinization.[1,5] The heparin does not cause resolution of the thrombosis but reduces the risk of extension into the collaterals, neither does it eliminate the risk of pulmonary embolism. In a review of ten studies, 48% of emboli occured in fully anticoagulated patients.[2]

Historically, axillary vein thrombosis was considered to be a benign self-limiting disease, however, it is now evident that this is not the case. Axillary vein thrombosis may lead to septic thrombophlebitis, superior vena cava obstruction, loss of central venous access, major long-term upper limb disability, venous gangrene, extravasation of infusate, pulmonary embolization and death.[2]

The diagnosis may be confirmed by duplex scanning via the supraclavicular fossa. This is a good 'first line' investigation; however, the extensive collaterals around the shoulder girdle can be mistaken for flow in the axillary and subclavian veins leading to a false negative result in up to 25% of patients.[6] Duplex may also give additional information about the cause of extrinsic compression, although magnetic resonance imaging gives better resolution of structures such as fibrous bands. In the majority of patients venography should be performed using digital subtraction imaging through a catheter placed via the basilic vein and advanced into the distal axillary vein.[4] If the cephalic vein is used the majority of the contrast bypasses the axillary vein via venous collaterals and, even with digital subtraction, good definition of the thrombosis and any underlying venous lesion is poor.[4] The catheter should not be withdrawn until a decision has been made whether to proceed with thrombolysis. Venography demonstrates the extent of the thrombus and the collateral venous drainage (Fig. 2), treatment depends on the aetiology of the thrombosis and co-morbidity.

TREATMENT

Catheter-induced thrombosis

Catheter-induced thrombosis is related to the size of the catheter and has an increased incidence with PVC catheters, duration of catheter placement, catheter infection, hyperosmolar infusate and multiple attempts at placement. Up to 35% of patients with long-term catheters will develop thrombosis[2] and a much higher proportion with have non-occlusive 'sleeve thrombosis' around the catheter.

Treatment is traditionally by anticoagulation and removal of the catheter and in

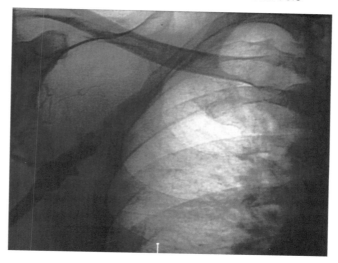

Fig. 2.   Venogram of a patient with axillary vein thrombosis showing complete occlusion of the axillary vein down to the cephalic vein and virtually no collaterals indicating the acute nature of the occlusion.

some series this results in complete resolution of symptoms with no long-term sequelae in 100% of patients.[4,7] However, there is an increasing number of patients in whom the maintainance of long-term central venous access, for total parenteral nutrition or chemotherapy, is essential and removal of the catheter may severely compromise overall patient management. In these patients it may be desirable to accept the increased risk of rethrombosis in order to preserve the catheter. The use of thrombolysis in these patients is not well reported in the literature. Renal dialysis patients who have previously had subclavian venous lines on the side of a forearm dialysis fistula may have a subclinical stenosis of the axillary vein which is unmasked by the high flow through the fistula leading to significant venous oedema of the arm or a secondary venous thrombosis. Appropriate screening for the occult axillary vein stenosis prior to fistula formation will avoid unnecessary morbidity.

Thrombolysis

In patients with 'primary' thrombosis or thrombosis secondary to external compression of the axillary vein, management with anticoagulation alone results in residual symptoms in up to 70% of patients. In these groups thrombolysis has been shown to be effective if it is initiated before organization of the thrombus which usually starts to occur at 5 days.[1,2,5] The basilic vein catheter is advanced into the axillary vein to deliver a 2 mg bolus of recombinant tissue plasminogen activator (rt-PA) directly into the thrombus followed by an infusion of 0.5 mg per hour. The successful use of both urokinase and streptokinase has also been reported.[8-13] Repeat venography via the infusing catheter is used to monitor the progression of lysis. Once lysis is complete the patient should be maintained on heparin via the basilic vein catheter and warfarinized.

All patients should have post-thrombolysis venography to ensure complete lysis and identify lesions of the axillary vein which require further active management if the risk of rethrombosis is to be reduced (Fig. 3).

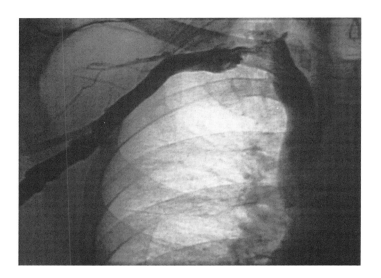

Fig. 3. Venogram of the same patient as Fig. 2 following sucessful thrombolysis showing a residual complex stenosis of the vein as it passes over the first rib.

Balloon venoplasty and stenting

Two different lesions may be identified on post-lysis venography, an intrinsic lesion that is within the lumen of the vein and extrinsic compression of the vein by structures or tumours of the thoracic outlet. Intrinsic and extrinsic lesions may co-exist and correction of both are required for optimum outcome.

Intrinsic lesions may be either a web like stenosis at the inner border of the first rib at the site of the subclavian semi-lumar valve (Fig. 4),[9–11,13] or synaechae secondary to recanalization of organized thrombus. In the absence of a co-existant extrinsic lesion these patients may be managed by percutaneous transluminal venoplasty either via the brachial vein or from the groin.[14,15] The angioplasty balloons need to be closely matched to the size of the native vein and are typically 12 mm or more in diameter. Dilatation with an undersized balloon leads to early restenosis detected on duplex scanning (Fig. 5, left scan) or by rethrombosis. Inflation pressures of around 12 atmospheres for 1–2 minutes are used, commonly the balloon will be 'waisted' at lower pressures (Fig. 6). If the patient feels severe pain during inflation the time is reduced as this may herald imminent rupture of the vein.[14] In a proportion of patients the stenosis reccurs on balloon deflation and in these cases insertion of a wall stent has proved sucessful in the long-term, (Figs 7 and 8).[16] Patients who have been managed percutaneously can be followed up non-invasively by duplex scanning of the axillary vein (Fig. 5, right scan).

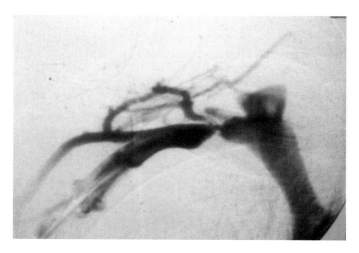

Fig. 4. Venogram of the axillary vein after sucessful thrombolysis showing a residual 'web' at the site of the semi-lunar valve at the inner border of the first rib.

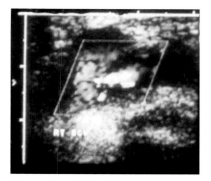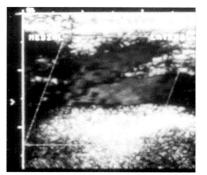

Fig. 5. Supraclavicular colour coded duplex scan of the axillary vein showing a tight stenosis of the proximal axillary vein at follow-up (left-hand image), and resolution after venoplasty to 14 mm (right-hand image).

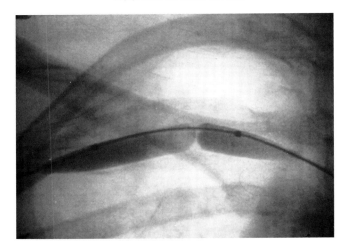

Fig. 6. 'Waisting' of the venoplasty balloon at 8 atmospheres inflation pressure, a pressure of 12 atmospheres abolished the stenosis with no recurrence of the stenosis on duplex at 18-month follow-up.

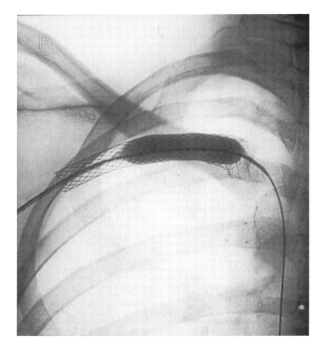

Fig. 7. Venoplasty of a wall stent placed across a resistant stenosis in the axillary vein.

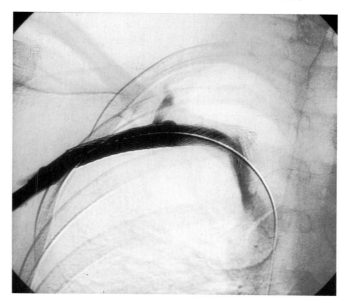

Fig. 8. Completion venogram of a deployed wall stent in the axillary vein with complete resolution of the stenosis.

Surgical treatment

If the lesion cannot be crossed with a guidewire from above or below or there is co-existing extrinsic compression of the vein then surgery may be indicated. Reviewing the literature there have been many procedures described for subclavian occlusion and external compression, all the series are small and the long-term outcome variably reported. It is probably true to say that there is great potential for failure and venous surgery for axillary vein thrombosis should not be undertaken lightly. In patients with catheter-induced thrombosis, where the prognosis with anticoagulation and removal of the catheter is reported as excellent and in patients with advanced malignancy surgery is probably only indicated in exceptional cicumstances. The majority of the literature on the operative management of axillary vein thrombosis concentrates on patients with 'primary' thrombosis who are often young fit adults with the most to gain from resolution of symptoms.

Three aspects of surgical treatment need consideration, adequate decompression of the thoracic outlet, which has received the most attention in the past, recanalization of the native subclavian vein and if recanalization is not possible venous bypass surgery. The timing of surgery is still a matter of debate. Traditionally patients are managed with anticoagulation and only offered surgery if they remain symptomatic or re-present with recurrent thrombosis. However, some authors favour immediate correction of anatomical lesions at the first presentation.[17]

Surgical exposure

Two surgical approaches can be made to the axillary vein, supraclavicular and trans-axillary. In the supraclavicular approach an incision is made parallel with and 2 cm above the medial half of the clavicle and developed down to the sternocleidomastoid and scalene fat pad. The clavicular fibres of sternocleidomastoid are divided and the scalene fat pad mobilized and retracted superiomedially. The anterior scalene muscle is now exposed with the phrenic nerve running on its anterior surface in the upper part of the dissection and passing inferiomedially to lie medial to it as it passes into the thorax. Once the phrenic has been identified the anterior scalene may be divided in its lower third. The subclavian vessels lie just deep to the muscle and a McDonald's dissector can be used to protect the vessels during muscle division. The subclavian vein is exposed running over the first rib and the dissection can be developed into the thorax or axilla to enable the venous surgery to be performed.

The advantage of this approach is that there is good exposure of all the possible anatomical variations that may occur at the thoracic outlet and if more proximal access is needed the incision may be extended to include a sternotomy; there is also good access to the jugular vein should venous bypass be needed.

In the transaxillary approach the patient is positioned on the table with the arm abducted at 120 degrees. A transverse incision is made low in the axilla adjacent to the third rib and developed down to the thoracic wall, the intercostobrachial vessels are divided and the nerve divided if unduly stretched. The dissection is developed up the thoracic wall to the first rib where the fascia separating the axilla from the neck is opened to expose the subclavian vessels. Exposure of the proximal subclavian vein is poor and as the intrinsic lesions within the vein are often at the inner border of the first rib, adequate exposure can only be obtained by first rib resection. If more proximal control is required the transaxillary approach is not appropriate. The axillary approach is very useful in patients with thoracic outlet syndrome but it does not provide the exposure of the axillary and jugular vein that is needed for patients with venous obstruction.

Surgical thrombectomy and venoplasty

With the development of percutaneous thrombolysis, venoplasty and stenting, the place of operative thrombectomy and venoplasty is being challenged. However, in combination with thoracic outlet decompression for patients with proven intrinsic and extrinsic venous lesions or when lysis is not effective because of late presentation or referral, it is still a useful procedure.

In patients with a 'web' across the vein in the position of the semilunar valve simple venotomy, excision of the webb and primary closure of the vessel has been reported to give good results although numbers are small.[17–19] The preferred option in the literature is closure of the venotomy with a saphenous vein patch as this allows closure of a vein with perivascular fibrosis and/or extensive synaechae without the risk of residual stenosis.[3,4,15,17,20] In many reports on surgery for axillary vein thrombosis the first rib has been excised as part of the surgical procedure along with division of various 'fibrous bands'. It is therefore difficult to comment on surgical treatment which does not include first rib resection and thoracic outlet decompression. In patients with persistent symptoms postoperatively it is of comfort (to the surgeon, but no help to the patient) to know the thoracic outlet has been adequately decompressed.

Venous bypass

In patients with an occluded axillary vein, recurrent thromboses or severe symptoms, venous bypass may be considered. Repeat venography just prior to surgery is vital to define the exact anatomy of the collateral venous drainage and to determine the inflow and outflow to the bypass. If there are well-formed collaterals extra caution should be exercised before proceding with surgery as a venous bypass is unlikely to increase significantly venous drainage in these patients and may compromise the existing collaterals.

If the occlusion spares the cephalic–axillary vein junction then the cephalic vein can be used as the venous graft preserving the continuity between the two veins. The outflow vessel is often the internal jugular vein either on the ipsilateral side if the brachiocephalic vein is not involved in the occlusion or the contralateral jugular vein if it is. Involvement of both brachiocephalic veins to give superior vena cava syndrome is outside the scope of this article. If the cephalic axillary vein junction is involved in the occlusion then a brachial to jugular bypass is required and either cephalic or long saphenous vein may be used. In order to increase the short-term patency rate a number of authors have added forearm fistulas to the operation to increase blood flow in the graft.[21,22] In one reported case the bypass failed but symptoms resolved because of increased venous collaterals, presumably stimulated by the high flow fistula.[21] There are no reports of a fistula being used in isolation for this purpose. If a fistula is used symptoms may not fully resolve untill after closure of the fistula at 6 weeks.[22] Most reports of venous bypass are of single or a small number of case reports; of 24 patients from the literature 15 were improved symptomatically but not all grafts in these patients remained patent.[11,15,21,22,23]

SUMMARY

Axillary vein thrombosis is a rare disorder of multiple aetiology with a rising incidence secondary to the increased use of central venous catheters. Catheter-induced thrombosis can be managed by removal of the catheter and full anticoagulation and in the majority of cases this gives excellent results. Apart from patients with advanced malignancy, most other cases need venography with a view to catheter-directed local thrombolysis. Lysis is monitored with regular venography until complete. Post-lysis venography often reveals an intrinsic lesion within the vein which is amenable to percutaneous venoplasty and/or stenting. Patients with complete occlusion of the axillary vein which cannot be crossed with a guidewire, and in whom insufficient collaterals form after a period of conservative treatment with full anticoagulation venous bypass surgery may be considered. Patients with extrinsic compression of the vein require thoracic outlet decompression with or without direct venous surgery.

REFERENCES

1. Coon WW, Willis PW: Thrombosis of axillary and subclavian veins. *Arch Surg* **94:** 657–663, 1967
2. Horattas MC, Wright DJ, Fenton AH et al.: Changing concepts of deep venous thrombosis of the upper extremity. Report of a series and review of the literature. *Surgery* **104:** 561–567, 1988
3. Adams JT, McEvoy RK, DeWeese JA: Primary deep vein thrombosis of the upper extremity. *Arch Surg* **91:** 29–42, 1965
4. Campbell CB, Chandler JG, Tegtmeyer CJ, Bernstein EF: Axillary, subclavian and brachiocephalic vein obstruction. *Surgery* **82:** 816–826, 1977
5. Roos DB: Axillary-subclavian vein occlusion. In: Rutherford RB (Ed) *Vascular Surgery*. Philadelphia: WB Saunders, 1984
6. Pollak EW, Walsh J: Subclavian-axillary venous thrombosis, role of non-invasive diagnostic methods. *South Med J* **73:** 1503–1506, 1980
7. Donayre CE, White GH, Mehringer SM, Wilson SE: Pathogenesis determines late morbidity of axillosubclavian vein thrombosis. *Am J Surg* **52:** 179–184, 1986
8. AbuRahma AF, Sadler D, Stuart P et al.: Conventional versus thrombolytic therapy in spontaneous (effort) axillary-subclavian vein thronbosis. *Am J Surg* **161:** 459–465, 1991
9. Wiles PG, Birtwell AJ, Davies JA, Chennels P: Subclavian vein notch, a phlebographic abnormality associated with subclavian-axillary vein thrombosis. *Br J Hosp Med* **37:** 349–350, 1987
10. O'Leary MR, Smith MS, Druy EM: Diagnostic and therapeutic approach to axillary-subclavian vein thrombosis. *Ann Emerg Med* **16:** 889–893, 1987
11. Becker GJ, Holden RW, Mail JT et al.: Local thrombolytic therapy for 'thoracic inlet syndrome'. *Semin Intervent Radiol* **2:** 349–353, 1985
12. Taylor LM, McAllister WR, Dennis DL, Porter JM: Thrombolytic therapy followed by first rib resection for spontaneous ('effort') subclavian vein thrombosis. *Am J Surg* **149:** 644–647, 1985
13. Landercasper J, Gall W, Fischer M et al.: Thrombolytic therapy of axillary-subclavian venous thrombosis. *Arch Surg* **122:** 1072–1075, 1987
14. Glanz S, Gordon DH, Lipkowitz GS et al.: Axillary and subclavian vein stenosis, percutaneous angioplasty. *Radiology* **168:** 371–373, 1988
15. Molina JE: Surgery for effort thrombosis of the subclavian vein. *J Thorac Cardiovasc Surg* **103:** 341–346, 1992
16. Strandness DE: Interventional management of large venous obstruction. In: Strandness DE, Breda AV (Eds) *Vascular Diseases: Surgical and Interventional Therapy*. Edinburgh: Churchill Livingstone, 1994
17. Aziz S, Straehley CJ, Whelan TJ: Effort related axillosubclavian vein thrombosis. A new theory of pathogenesis and a plea for direct surgical intervention. *Am J Surg* **152:** 57–60, 1986
18. Jackobson JH, Haimov M: Venous revascularisation of the arm, report of three cases. *Surgery* **81:** 599–604, 1977
19. DeWeese JA, Adams JT, Gaiser DL: Subclavian venous thrombectomy. *Cardiovasc Surg Circulation* XLI, XLII (Suppl II): 158–164, 1970
20. Gaylis H: A rational approach to venous thrombectomy. *Surg Gynecol Obstet* **138:** 864–868, 1974
21. Rabinowitz R, Goldfarb D: Surgical treatment of axillosubclavian venous thrombosis, A case report. *Surgery* **70:** 703–706, 1971
22. Hashmonai M, Schramek A, Farbstein J: Cephalic vein cross-over bypass for subclavian vein thrombosis, A case report. *Surgery* **80:** 563–564, 1976
23. Sanders RJ, Haug CE: Management of subclavian vein obstruction. In: Bergan JJ, Kistner RL (Eds) *Atlas of Venous Surgery*. Philadelphia: WB Saunders, 1992

Hyperthrombotic States and Vascular Surgical Emergencies

Jonathan B. Towne

INTRODUCTION

Acute vascular thrombosis is a catastrophic complication which results in limb loss and death, the treatment of which taxes the clinical skills of the surgeon. There are four clinical situations in which this occurs; three involving the arterial system, and one the venous system. First is sudden unexplained thrombosis of medium to large sized arteries typically including the upper or the lower extremity which on occasion can involve renal, mesenteric and cerebral vessels. The second, which is of particular concern to vascular surgeons, is the acute thrombosis of an arterial repair in the perioperative period. These problems are usually evident in the operating room, and all occur in the first 12 hours following surgery. The third is thrombosis of arterial repair at a time remote from the vascular reconstruction, which is the most uncommon occurrence. Finally, are the sudden, unexplained episodes of venous thrombosis which can involve any and all parts of the venous circulation, but most typically involve the lower extremities, and on occasion also involve the upper extremities and the mesenteric venous circulation.

The ability of blood to remain fluid within the intravascular system and to form a thrombus when there is disruption or injury to the endothelial lining is a result of a complex interaction between the various components of the vascular system. These include the endothelium, platelets, plasma, procoagulant factors, and fibrinolytic factors. Any abnormality of these factors can result in either haemorrhage or thrombosis. Since the vascular surgeon deals primarily with ischaemia he generally has to deal with abnormalities on the thrombosis side of the blood coagulation equilibrium. Over the last several decades, there has been an explosion of knowledge regarding the coagulation system, so that our understanding of the various components of the clotting system is much better. With this increased understanding, there has been the identification of several clotting disorders that are secondary to either inherited or acquired deficiency of one of the components of the clotting cascade, resulting in unusual or previously unexplained thrombosis. Early on, the first hypercoagulable states identified were those that involved problems on the procoagulant side. However, within the last decade, problems involving the fibrinolytic systems or anticoagulant side of the clotting cascade, have been identified. In order adequately to treat these unusual thrombotic episodes, some knowledge of these thrombotic syndromes is necessary.

Hypercoagulable states as a cause of unexplained vascular thrombosis is a difficult clinical problem. Most graft failures in the perioperative period are presumed to be on the basis of technical errors in the construction of the anastomosis, problems with the conduit, or poor patient selection. The diagnosis of an abnormal hypercoagulable state is often made only after excluding all these other factors. Although the failure of heparin to prevent clotting in the operative field or the immediate thrombosis of a vascular repair suggests abnormal coagulation, the diagnosis can only be confirmed by the blood coagulation laboratory. The clotting disorder must be detected early in the course of the disease to obtain a favourable outcome. Abnormal thrombosis falls into five general categories: abnormalities in the antithrombin system; abnormalities of the fibrinolytic system; heparin-induced platelet aggregation; lupus anticoagulant; and a miscellaneous category consisting primarily of abnormal platelet aggregation, protein C and protein S deficiencies. More recently activated protein C resistance has been implicated in a high proportion of patients with acute deep venous thrombosis.

ANTITHROMBIN DEFICIENCY

Antithrombin III is an α-globulin manufactured in the liver and perhaps by vascular endothelium, with a molecular weight of approximately 60 000 and a half-life of 2.8 days.[1] It is a serine proteinase inhibitor that binds in equimolar ratios to several enzymes participating in the intrinsic pathway of blood coagulation including thrombin, factor Xa, IXa, and XIa.[1] Heparin significantly accelerates the rate that antithrombin III neutralizes these enzymes, limiting sequential clotting reactions and preventing fibrin formation. In 1965, Egeberg described a family with an inborn defect of antithrombin III,[2] and subsequent work has demonstrated the genetic transmission of this disease.[3-6] The frequency of this defect is approximately 1 in 2000 to 1 in 5000 in the general population.[7,8] There are probably at least two types of antithrombin III deficiency. In the classic form both the level of antithrombin III as determined by measuring its protein concentration, as well as its activity level are reduced in the patient's plasma.[9] However, there are other patients in whom the concentration of antithrombin III is normal or even slightly elevated as measured by protein level, but the biologic function as measured by activity tests is abnormal.[10] This suggests that these patients are manufacturing a defective antithrombin molecule. Acquired antithrombin III deficiency can occur in severe liver disease, nephrotic syndrome, hypoalbuminaemia, malnutrition, disseminated intravascular coagulation, and in some patients taking oral contraceptives. Antithrombin III deficiency may be an indicator of significant protein catabolism. Flinn et al. noted low ATIII activity in 16% of patients undergoing vascular surgery.[11] There was low serum albumin (<3.0 mg/dl) in 48% of these patients, which was associated with an increased incidence of early graft failure.

Clinical presentation

Although antithrombin III deficiency is inherited, it is rare for episodes of thrombosis to be clinically manifested before the second decade of life. Despite continuously depressed levels of antithrombin III in these patients, thrombotic episodes are often related to predisposing factors such as operations, childbirth, and infection, and rarely occur spontaneously. This deficiency can cause venous thrombosis with resulting pulmonary embolism, dialysis fistula failure, arterial graft occlusion, and spontaneous arterial occlusion. In our initial report, we identified seven patients with antithrombin deficiencies as a cause of thrombosis.[12] These included patients with spontaneous arterial occlusion of arteries of both the upper and lower extremities, as well as patients who occluded vascular reconstructions in the perioperative period. One unusual patient presented with ischaemia of one arm and both legs secondary to extensive thromboses of the brachial artery and its branches of one arm, and the femoral, popliteal, and tibial systems of both legs. Extensive angiography of the entire aorta and cardiac evaluation failed to reveal a proximal origin of embolic material. What distinguishes these patients from those with thrombotic occlusive disease secondary to atherosclerotic disease is the unique history, distribution of occluded vessels, unusual angiographic findings, and absence of any proximal source of embolic material. Often clot formation in the operative field despite heparin sodium administration, is the first clue that the patient may have an antithrombin deficiency. The presence of multiple thrombi on operative angiograms, is suggestive of a clotting abnormality (Fig. 1).

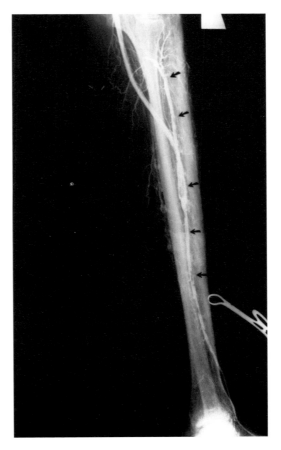

Fig. 1. Operative angiogram of a patient demonstrating numerous areas of thrombus that formed during construction of a femoral anterior tibial graft. (Reprinted from ref. 12, with permission.)

Diagnosis

Results of routine coagulation tests are normal in patients with antithrombin III deficiency. Generally reductions in antithrombin are measured by both immunological (tests which measure the total amount of the protein) and functional (tests which measure the activity of the antithrombin III molecules) assays.

Initially, patients with repeated episodes of venous thrombosis were identified, because of reduced levels of antithrombin III to 50–60% of normal values. Subsequent work identified patients with arterial thrombosis secondary to low antithrombin III levels. Lynch *et al.* demonstrated a correlation between low preoperative plasma functional antithrombin III levels and the occurrence of postoperative thrombotic complications following cardiac and vascular surgery.[13] Thrombotic complications included arterial thrombosis, graft thrombosis, deep vein thrombosis, cerebral vascular thrombosis, spinal infarction, and embolic cortical blindness.

A decrease in antithrombin III levels is the mechanism of the increased thrombotic tendency in patients taking oral contraceptives. Sagar demonstrated that antithrombin III activity was significantly lower in patients taking oral contraceptives than in control patients.[14] During surgery, the antithrombin III activity fell in both the contraceptive and the control groups, but the fall was greater in patients on oral contraceptives. The only patients that developed deep vein thrombosis postoperatively as determined by the I^{125}-fibrinogen test were those taking oral contraceptives. Five of the 31 patients taking oral contraceptives had an antithrombin III activity below 50% and, of these, three developed deep vein thrombosis.

More recent work has demonstrated that the administration of heparin tends to lower the antithrombin level. Conrad *et al.* demonstrated that it is the presence of heparin and not the rate of administration which is the determinant of the decrease in antithrombin III.[15] He noted that both subcutaneous and intravenous heparin cause antithrombin III levels to drop the same amount. Since heparin is dependent on antithrombin for its antithrombotic action, the antithrombin lowering effect of heparin in patients with an already low antithrombin concentration probably indicates that patients are at risk of thrombosis for two reasons. First, heparin is relatively ineffective in patients with low levels of antithrombin III. Second, because heparin binds with antithrombin III, the already low level is decreased even further, possibly to dangerous levels. This is the theoretic basis of paradoxical thrombotic episodes occasionally seen in patients following cessation of heparin. Since heparin administration has decreased the level of antithrombin III, sometimes to significantly dangerous levels, cessation of heparin is followed by a period when the patient is hypercoagulable because the lower antithrombin III level is not counteracted by the heparin. This is the reason that warfarin administration should be overlapped with heparin cessation when treating thrombotic problems. Patients with antithrombin III deficiency on a congenital basis should be on chronic long-term warfarin because of the risk of recurrent thrombotic episodes. In addition to its anticoagulant effect, warfarin increases the level of antithrombin III by as yet an undetermined mechanism. More recently, purified antithrombin III can be obtained by recombinant techniques, which will in the future change the treatment of this deficiency. Antithrombin III concentrate was used as factor-specific replacement by Tengborn and Bergqvist in patients with antithrombin III deficiency.[16] It is now widely available and should be considered when factor specific therapy is indicated.

DEFECTS IN THE FIBRINOLYTIC SYSTEM

The fibrinolytic system has become better understood in recent years and has been found to be the source of coagulation abnormalities. The components of the fibrinolytic system include plasminogen, plasminogen activators, including tissue plasminogen activators (TPA) and urokinase, and inhibitors directed against plasminogen activators, plasmin inhibitors, the most important of which is α-II antiplasmin, and cellular plasmin inhibitors, which have been identified in platelets and endothelial cells.[17,18] The degradation of fibrin is normally carried out by the proteolytic enzyme plasmin, which is formed from the proenzyme plasminogen by the activation action of plasminogen activators such as TPA or urokinase. The process is regulated at many different levels resulting in localized plasmin formation at the fibrin surface. The TPA is the most important activator and is produced and released from vascular endothelium.[19]

Plasminogen is a normal plasma protein consisting of a single polypeptide chain, with a molecular weight of 90 000 to 94 000.[20] Thin layer gel electrofocusing, coupled with immunofixation, can demonstrate up to ten different forms of plasminogen, with each variant having a glutamic acid as its terminal amino acid. Plasminogen is converted to plasmin by activators, many of which are released from endothelial cells. Plasmin is a serine protease, and is an important member of the fibrinolytic systems that acts by cleaving fibrinogen and fibrin.

The biosynthesis of plasminogen and fibrinolytic inhibitors are probably under genetic control. In 1978, Aoki *et al.* reported a patient with recurrent thrombosis who had a hereditary molecular defect of plasminogen.[21] This was followed by reports by Kazama *et al.* in 1981,[22] and Soria *et al.*[23] in 1982. These authors demonstrated that the abnormal plasminogen did not have the functional ability of normal plasminogen, resulting in a discrepancy between the biologic activity and the amount of plasminogen detected in the serum by radioimmunoassay. These patients had normal concentrations of plasminogen antigen, with approximately half of the activity of normal plasminogen. Using electrofocusing techniques coupled with immunofixation and zymograms, they were able to identify ten additional bands, each of which was located on the basic side in close proximity to the corresponding normal band.

Determination of amino acid sequence has demonstrated defects in the arginine 516 valine bond and the substitution of alanine 600 by threonine.[24] The major function of the fibrinolytic system *in vivo* is the limitation of fibrin deposition. A reduction of fibrinolytic activity may provoke a thrombotic tendency by allowing the growth and development of thrombi after the initiating thrombotic event. Most patients with abnormal plasminogen are characterized by a normal antigen concentration and by decreased functional activity. Liu *et al.* reported a plasminogen which was characterized by both low functional activity and low antigen, and called it plasminogen San Antonio.[25]

In a study of patients with unusual and unexplained thrombosis who had an abnormal plasminogen band detected on immunoelectrophoresis, we noted that only one of our initial eight patients demonstrated a decreased functional level of plasminogen, compared with antigenic levels.[26] We felt that this might be related to the assay of functional activity used in the study, or may represent a different form of abnormality than reported in the literature. One of our patients had a low functional plasminogen level at the time of thrombotic activity but when studied 4 months after the institution of warfarin therapy showed an increase in the level of functional plasminogen to 70% of normal. One year later he had normal plasminogen activity. The patient continued to show an abnormal band of plasminogen in the electrophoretic pattern demonstrating persistence of an abnormal plasminogen molecule in the plasma. This patient has had two episodes of pulmonary emboli.

Ikemoto *et al.* reported that the genetic characteristics of this disorder follow an autosomal co-dominant inheritance pattern with the alleles completely expressed.[27] The results of the study of two families in our series are in agreement with this. The clinical history of recurrent phlebitis in one of our patients and his sister supports the genetic aspect of this disease.

The immunoelectrophoresis technique used in our study is quicker, simpler, and less costly than isoelectric focusing, and is more applicable to screening large groups of patients. The significance of the abnormal plasminogen is uncertain. It is present in 10% of the normal population and its presence does not insure that a patient is going to have thrombotic complications. More likely, this abnormal plasminogen results in the relative defect of the fibrinolytic system, which places the patient at increased risk should he be in a thrombosis prone situation. Our data suggests, however, that once a thrombotic episode occurs, it is likely to reoccur emphasizing the need to identify and treat these patients with long-term warfarin therapy.

Clinical presentation

We have noted thrombosis occurring both on the arterial and venous sides of the circulation in patients with abnormal plasminogen. In our initial report of eight patients, the age of onset of the first thrombotic episode ranged from 21 to 57 years. Three patients had venous thrombosis, two had spontaneous arterial thrombosis, two had occlusion of an arterial reconstruction in the early postoperative period, and one patient had separate episodes of both arterial and venous occlusions.

Thrombosis involving the venous systems occurred in four patients, two had complete obstruction of the iliofemoral venous segment and inferior vena cava. One had primarily popliteal vein thrombosis, and the remaining patient had axillary and subclavian vein thrombosis. Two of these patients had concomitant pulmonary emboli, which occurred in one patient after an interval of 4 months. Arterial thrombosis occurred in five patients; two patients presented with spontaneous thrombosis of the iliofemoral segment. Following thrombectomy with Fogarty catheters, there was no evidence of inflow obstruction, and a complete evaluation for the proximal source of the emboli was negative (Figs 3, 4). Postoperative occlusions of arterial reconstructions occurred in two patients.

Six patients had recurrent episodes of thrombosis. There were two patients who had three recurrences and four patients who had two recurrences (Figs 2–4). The

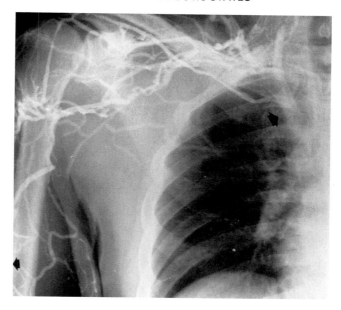

Fig. 2. Venogram demonstrating subclavian and axillary vein thrombosis in a patient who had separate episodes of arterial and venous thrombosis. (Reprinted from ref. 26, with permission.)

interval between thrombotic episodes ranged from 4 to 36 months. Significantly, five of the patients who had recurrent thrombosis were treated with warfarin following the first episode. Recurrent episodes of thrombosis occurred 2 weeks to several months following cessation of warfarin therapy, and recurrent thrombosis did not develop in any patient while on anticoagulation therapy. We subsequently identified four patients who had an abnormal plasminogen as detected by an abnormal arc on immunoelectrophoresis who developed severe thrombosis in the upper extremities.[28] The lack of atherosclerosis in the upper extremities as well as the absence in these patients of any proximal embolic source further demonstrates the sometimes catastrophic consequences which can occur in patients with abnormal plasminogen. In our experience of over 35 patients we have detected over the last 7 years, we have had only one patient develop recurrent thrombosis while on warfarin therapy.

Methods of testing

A complete coagulation profile on each patient should be performed, including tests of platelet aggregation, prothrombin time, partial thromboplastin time, fibrinogen level, and platelet count. Functional assays of antithrombin III and plasminogen α-II antiplasmin, antigenic activities of antithrombin III, plasminogen, α-I antitrypsin, and α-II macroglobulins should be obtained. With immunoelectrophoresis, the

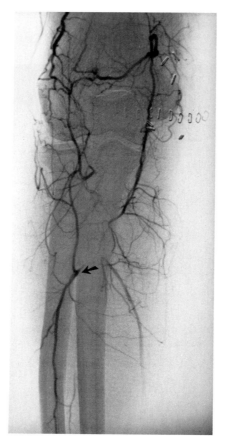

Fig. 3. Arteriogram of a patient who developed brachial artery occlusion and hand ischaemia after cardiac catheterization. The interosseous artery is the only patent major artery in the forearm. (Reprinted from ref. 28, with permission.)

abnormal plasminogen presents as an abnormal band which is separate on the electrophoretic pattern located nearer the anode and distinct from the normal band. We have also noted one patient who had a plasminogen which was separate from the main band but was not confined to a distinct band. Indeed this may represent still another species. Work by several investigators is ongoing to further characterize the molecular defect in these abnormal plasminogens, and to assess the functional impairment. This requires rather sophisticated techniques to determine amino acid sequencing and to test the functional ability of the various components of the plasminogen molecule.

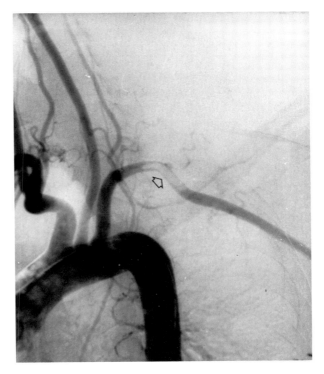

Fig. 4. Non-occluding thrombus of subclavian artery occurring several days after carotid angiography from a femoral approach. (Reprinted from ref. 28, with permission.)

TPA AND ANTI-TPA

With the discovery of the ability to measure TPA, investigators have discovered that the levels of TPA can vary and be related to the occurrence of thrombotic disease.[29] Also, the presence of an anti-TPA which counteracts the effects of TPA has been discovered.[30,31] Several studies have identified patients who are thrombosis prone because of increased levels of anti TPA.[29,30–32] Our knowledge of both the mechanisms and the effect of alterations of these mechanisms are poorly understood at the present time. Wiman first developed the test to measure TPA.[29] In a study of patients with deep vein thrombosis, he noted that 40% of his patients had a reduced fibrinolytic potential which was found to be due to a reduced capacity to release TPA or to an increased plasma level of an anti-TPA, or a combination of these two.[31] He also noted a significant correlation between the plasma anti-TPA and serum triglycerides among patients with myocardial infarction below the age of 45. Obviously this is preliminary data, but it emphasized the need for ongoing investigation to more precisely determine the role of the fibrinolytic system in the pathogenesis of thrombotic disorders.

PROTEIN C

Protein C is a vitamin K dependent proenzyme which is involved in the control of clotting and fibrinolysis. Protein C itself is activated by thrombin, but slowly. This activation is increased up to 20 000-fold when thrombin forms a complex with an endothelial cell membrane called thrombomodulin. Activated protein C, when combined with phospholipids, calcium, and protein S, inactivates the cofactors of the two rate limiting steps of coagulation, factors V_a and VIII_a.[33–35]

Protein S is likewise a vitamin K-dependent factor. It acts as a cofactor for the anticoagulant activity of activated protein C by promoting its binding to lipid and platelet surfaces and thus localizing protein C activity.[36,37] Protein C, in conjunction with protein S, also acts as a profibrinolytic agent by increasing plasmin activity through the inactivation of the major inhibitor of tissue plasminogen activator.[33,34]

Heterozygous protein C deficiency is inherited in an autosomal dominant fashion. In hereditary protein C deficiency, the homozygous state is associated with a very high risk of thrombosis.[38,39] It usually presents as massive venous thrombosis in the neonatal period, which is often fatal. The latter is a severe, fatal thrombotic haemorrhagic complication, predominantly in neonates. The survival of affected infants *in utero* may reflect the protection afforded by maternal transfer of protein C, or to reduced synthesis of other procoagulants by the fetal liver, thus compensating for the deficiency of protein C.

In the heterozygous form, a protein C level of 50% is sufficient to predispose individuals to venous thrombosis.[39] The occurrence of thrombophlebitis in patients who are heterozygous for this deficiency is uncertain. Some kindred have been identified in which there is a very high incidence of venous thrombosis (up to 80%) by the age of 40, and there are others in which the occurrence of thrombosis is sporadic.[40,41] Acquired protein C deficiency can be observed in the acute phase of thrombosis, in patients with disseminating intervascular coagulation, and in patients with liver disease, and postoperative patients.

Protein C deficiency generally manifests with venous thrombosis. This can either be in the form of lower extremity venous thrombosis, oftentimes accompanied by pulmonary embolism, or present as mesenteric venous thrombosis. We recently reported five patients with protein C deficiency – four had deep venous thrombosis of the lower extremity as their initial thrombotic event, and one had mesenteric venous thrombosis with small bowel necrosis.[42] Our patients age range was 28–41 years. Two patients had recurrent lower extremity thrombosis, which was bilateral in one. One patient had only one clinical episode of deep venous thrombosis, but developed venous stasis ulceration suggesting multiple episodes of subclinical phlebitis. One patient had a pulmonary embolus. Green *et al.* evaluated eight consecutive patients with splanchnic venous thrombosis and demonstrated decreases in the levels of antithrombin III and protein C in all.[43] They were unable to document whether the low levels of protein C and antithrombin III were a result or cause of the thrombosis. Two of their patients had had an antecedent history of venous thrombotic problems and in six of the eight patients, evaluated following a period of 1–6 months, a persistent low level of protein C was revealed which would certainly suggest a congenital aetiology. The only case of peripheral arterial thrombosis secondary to protein C deficiency was reported by Coller *et al.*[44] Their patient developed arterial occlusions of both the superficial femoral artery and radial and ulnar arteries. Nelson *et al.* reported a patient who had two episodes of branch retinal arteriolar occlusions secondary to protein C deficiency.[45] These reports indicate that protein C can cause arterial thrombosis, although it is unusual.

Methods of testing

Standard testing includes a radiolabelled Laurell electroimmunoassay to determine human protein C antigen in plasma samples. Normals should be between 70 and 130% of normal activity. In our patients with venous thrombosis, the level of protein C ranged from 34 to 67%. As with the evaluation of all patients with unusual or unexplained thrombosis, there should be simultaneous measurement of antithrombin III and protein S and routine coagulation studies. We evaluated the family of our patient with mesenteric venous occlusion for protein C deficiency, the results of which were compatible with an autosomal dominant-type of transmission. There has not, however, been any thrombotic episodes reported among other members with low protein C levels. Since all family members with low protein C do not develop thrombosis, asymptomatic patients with low levels of protein C should be followed closely and not prophylactically anticoagulated. However, they should be prophylactically anticoagulated preoperatively if major surgery or prolonged immobilization is required. In those who develop thrombotic events, the onset is typically between 15 and 30 years of age. This delay in onset of the first thrombotic episode is not well understood. The fact that protein C rarely causes arterial thrombosis, as contrasted with our experiences with either abnormal plasminogen or antithrombin III abnormalities, is not well understood. It may be that protein C deficiency requires slower moving blood and increased endothelial surface area found in the venous system. However, when protein C deficiency is homozygous, thrombosis is widespread resulting in death in infancy unless this is treated.

Because of the risk of recurrent thrombotic events with the possible sequelae of pulmonary emboli and venous stasis disease, long-term therapy with warfarin is recommended. No loading dose should be administered, as this could precipitate warfarin-associated skin necrosis.[36,37] This occurs 2–5 days following the onset of warfarin therapy and presents as an erythematous patch on the skin that rapidly progresses to a haemorrhagic area that can become gangrenous. There is a predilection for involvement of the breasts, abdomen, buttocks and thighs. The proposed mechanism is one of a transient hypercoagulable state which is created by bolus loading doses of warfarin given to initiate anticoagulation. Because of its short half-life, protein C levels fall faster than factor X and prothrombin levels, and thus the inhibitory effect of protein C on the coagulation cascade is further diminished. If these levels fall to a critical level, the procoagulant effects of the coagulation cascade proceed unabated and thrombosis ensues. Warfarin 5.0 mg by mouth, four times daily should be started to gradually attain a prothrombin time of 1.5–2.0 times control. Heparin and warfarin therapy should overlap by 4–5 days.

PROTEIN S DEFICIENCY

Protein S is also a vitamin K-dependent protein which functions as a cofactor of anticoagulant activity of activated protein C. The liver is the major source of synthesis, although more recently the endothelial cells and megakaryocyte were identified as other sites of synthesis. Protein S functions by expediting the binding of activated protein C to lipid and platelet surfaces. To date, only heterozygous patients with protein S have been reported.[39] Symptomatic patients often have protein S levels 50% of normal, and like protein C deficiency, protein S likewise primarily causes venous thrombosis.[46–48] It has been estimated by some to be the cause of approximately 10% of spontaneous venous thrombosis. Coller *et al.* also reported the only known case history of a protein S deficient patient having arterial occlusive problems.[44] As with patients with protein C problems, the clotting abnormalities tend to be recurrent and therefore it is essential that these patients remain on long-term warfarin therapy. Clark *et al.* emphasized the importance of measuring both free protein S as well as the total which is composed of both a free and bound factor.[49] His patient with mesenteric venous thrombosis had a normal total protein S but a marked decreased level of the free compound. The association of deficiencies in protein C and its cofactor protein S with hypercoagulable states has only been recently appreciated. Data now suggests that the incidence of protein C and protein S deficiencies are more common than either antithrombin III or plasminogen abnormalities. In a recent report evaluating 139 individuals who had at least one major venous thrombotic event, 7% were protein C deficient, 5% were protein S deficient, and only 2% were deficient in plasminogen and 3% deficient in antithrombin III.[34] A majority (79%) however, had no detectable coagulopathy with current testing methods.

HEPARIN-INDUCED THROMBOSIS

Paradoxical thrombotic complications of heparin sodium therapy are an uncommon but potentially limb-threatening and occasionally fatal complication of heparin anticoagulant therapy. Up to 30% of patients may manifest a decrease in their platelet count after starting heparin therapy, but the incidence of significant thrombocytopenia and resulting thrombotic and/or haemorrhagic complications is approximately 5%. Two types of heparin-induced thrombocytopenia are described. Type I or the acute form occurs relatively early and results in a benign course with improvement in the platelet count during continued heparin therapy. Type II or delayed form occurs 5–14 days after the institution of heparin therapy in a patient not previously exposed to heparin, and after 3–9 days in patients with a history of previous heparin therapy. Type II heparin-induced thrombocytopenia is reported to have a 23–60% thrombotic or haemorrhagic complication rate and a 12–18% mortality rate. Early recognition and treatment results in a significant improvement in the associated morbidity and mortality.

In Type I heparin-induced thrombocytopenia the mechanism of action is thought to be a non-immune mediated direct effect of heparin on platelets that causes aggregation. Type II heparin-induced thrombocytopenia is due to an immune mediated (IgG and IgM) platelet aggregation. Heparin is not the antigen against which the antibody is directed. Instead, heparin is thought to bind to the platelet causing the expression of a neoantigen against which the immune response is directed.

Several investigators have identified a chemically-induced, immune thrombo-cytopenia as the cause of the intravascular thrombosis initiated by heparin that usually occurs 4–10 days after continued exposure to the drug.[50–54] This immune factor has been identified as an IgG antibody, which produces agglutination of normal platelets when heparin is added and is seen with both porcine gut as well as beef lung heparin. The thrombi of patients with heparin-induced thrombosis have an unusual greyish-white appearance in contradistinction to the red colour of most thrombi. The white colour is secondary to fibrin platelet aggregates, which can be clearly identified on electron microscopy.

Rhodes et al. demonstrated an IgG-heparin-dependent antibody in the serum of several of their patients by means of the complement lysis inhibitions test.[55] They also demonstrated a residual heparin platelet aggregating effect 12 days to 2 months after recovery from the initial exposure to heparin. In these patients, a 24-hour infusion of heparin caused a mean reduction of platelet count of 197 000 mm³. Since heparin preparations are not pure substances, it is also possible that a high molecular contaminant not eliminated by the extraction procedure may be the cause of the antiplatelet effect. More recent work has demonstrated that the heparin-specific antibodies react with heparin causing the platelet aggregation.[56]

Clinical presentation

We have seen heparin-induced intravascular thrombosis following a wide variety of indications for heparin administration, including thrombophlebitis with and without pulmonary embolus, perioperative heparin prophylaxis in patients prone to develop thrombophlebitis, cardiac surgery, and vascular reconstruction. Platelet aggregation induced by heparin can result from both porcine gut as well as bovine lung heparin. Heparin-induced intravascular thrombosis can affect either the arterial or venous circulation. Both subcutaneous and intravenous heparin administration can produce this phenomenon.[57] Even heparin-coated catheters can cause heparin-induced thrombocytopenia. Laster and Silver reported ten patients who had heparin-coated pulmonary artery catheters and developed heparin-induced thrombocytopenia which persisted despite discontinuation of all other sources of heparin.[58] Although all of their patient also had administration of heparin, it is theoretically possible that the heparin-bonded catheters alone could cause abnormal platelet aggregation. This same group has demonstrated the heparin-induced platelet aggregation can occur in neonates and is a common cause of aortic thrombosis in newborn intensive care units.[59]

Heparin-induced platelet aggregation can occur with the newer forms of low molecular weight heparin, but the incidence is low. The clinical features of this syndrome are often dramatic. Any patient who has thrombotic complications while receiving heparin therapy should have heparin-induced aggregation of platelets considered. This is especially important in patients with arterial occlusions who do not have any other evidence of atherosclerotic vascular disease. At operation, the finding of a white clot at thrombectomy should alert the surgeon to the possibility of a heparin-induced thrombosis. In contrast to several reports in the literature, increased heparin sensitivity rather than increased heparin resistance was seen in several of our patients.[60] We are uncertain as to the cause of this, but presently believe that it is unrelated to the heparin-induced aggregative immune globulin.

Diagnosis

The definitive diagnosis of heparin-induced intravascular thrombosis is obtained by performing platelet aggregation tests. We have noted two patterns of response. The more common is for the patient's platelet poor plasma to aggregate donor platelets upon the addition of heparin indicating the presence of a relatively non-specific platelet aggregating factor in the patient's plasma. The less common pattern seen in one of our patients is for the patient's plasma to be active only against the patient's platelet and have no effect on donor platelets. An enzyme-linked immunosorbin assay (ELISA) test has been developed to test for binding to the heparin-platelet factor IV complex and may prove useful in evaluating these patients.[61]

Other clotting factors are usually normal. The fibrinogen is normal, fibrin split products can be mildly elevated but not in the range seen with intravascular coagulation; and the prothrombin time is normal or slightly prolonged. All patients have a marked reduction in platelet count of less than 100 000 mm³ or a 50% decrease from admission level. In our series, the platelet count averaged 37 500 with a range of 6000–73 000.

The patients with arterial thromboses often present with unique angiographic findings. These lesions consist of broad-based isolated lobulated excrescences that produce a variable amount of narrowing of the arterial lumen. Usually these findings have an abrupt appearance with prominent luminal contour deformities in arterial segments that are otherwise normal. This distribution of disease is unusual and distinct from findings commonly seen with atherosclerosis. These changes occur in both the suprarenal as well as the infrarenal portion of the abdominal aorta and represent adherent mural thrombi composed of aggregates of platelets and fibrin incorporating varying amounts of leukocytes and erythrocytes. Also platelet aggregating tests should be performed on any patient in whom recurrent pulmonary embolism developed while receiving adequate heparin therapy.

Treatment

When heparin-induced thrombocytopenia is diagnosed, the heparin treatment should be reversed immediately with protamine, and dextran 40 should be administered for its anti-aggregating and rheologic effects. We also begin warfarin therapy and continue it for several months. In patients with arterial occlusive manifestations of heparin-induced thrombosis, we recommend long-term warfarin therapy because of the possibility of coexisting latent venous occlusive disease.

The response of the platelet count to discontinuation of heparin therapy is usually prompt, often resulting in a thrombocytosis of 500 000–600 000 platelets/mm³ in several days. In our experience, the use of dextran 40 facilitated the rebound in the platelet count, most likely because of its antiaggregating effect on the platelet.[60]

Coagulation tests distinguish heparin-induced platelet aggregation from other clotting disorders. The fibrinogen level and prothrombin time are usually normal. The fibrin split products level and prothrombin time are normal or slightly elevated. The sole patient in our series with a noticeably elevated fibrin split products level was the initial patient, in whom the diagnosis was not made ante mortem. The heparin therapy was not stopped, and prior to her death caused by an intracerebral haemorrhage, she had massive venous thrombosis involving both upper and lower extremities that resulted in the elevated fibrin split products level. Early identification of the complication is necessary to minimize the catastrophic complications of major limb amputation and death.

This experience suggests that it is imperative that all patients who are receiving heparin therapy have serial platelet counts done from the 4th day onward. It is our policy to perform platelet counts every other day starting on the 4th day of heparin therapy. If a thrombocytopenia develops, platelet aggregation studies should be performed immediately. With early recognition, the mortality and the morbidity of this syndrome can be minimized. Morbidity rates reported in the literature vary from 22% to 61% and mortality rates from 12% to 33%.[62,63]

STRATEGIES FOR PATIENTS WITH HEPARIN-INDUCED PLATELET AGGREGATION

Patients who require re-exposure to heparin for other vascular or cardiac procedures require special management. Patients who develop heparin-induced platelet aggregation usually have their aggregation tests revert to normal within a 6-week to 3-month time period. It is preferable to delay the vascular or cardiac procedure until these tests revert to normal. We test the patient at 6 weeks, then every 2 weeks thereafter to determine when their platelet-aggregation tests are negative. When they are negative, they are then brought into the hospital. Cardiac catheterization or angiography is done as required without the use of heparin flush solutions. This is extremely important since even small amounts of heparin in the flush solutions can stimulate the development of the heparin-induced antiplatelet antibodies. The patient then has the vascular or cardiac procedure done with the usual administration of heparin. At the conclusion of the procedure, all heparin is reversed with protamine and care is taken during the postoperative period to ensure the patient does not receive heparin inadvertently either through flushing central venous catheters, or arterial lines. By using this procedure, we have not had any difficulty with re-exposure to heparin.

However, for those patients who require an additional vascular or cardiac procedure and cannot wait until the heparin-induced platelet aggregation tests are negative, a different strategy is necessary. In patients requiring procedures that can be done without the use of heparin, such as resection of abdominal aortic aneurysms, heparin is not used. However, in patients that require complex lower extremity revascularization or cardiopulmonary bypass, some sort of anticoagulation is necessary. There are basically two approaches to this. The approach favoured by Silver and his group consists of giving the patients aspirin and Persantin, and using heparin for the operative procedure, as is customary.[64] In addition to the aspirin and Persantin we prefer to also use low-molecular weight dextran, which in addition to its rheologic properties, coats the platelets and interferes with platelet adhesion. In some patients, however, as noted by Kappa and his group, the administration of aspirin had no effect on the heparin-induced platelet aggregation tests.[65] Makhoul *et al.* noted that aspirin abolished the aggregation in nine of 16 patients with heparin-induced platelet aggregation, and only decreased the aggregation in the remaining seven, suggesting that aspirin is not able to reverse the abnormal aggregation in all patients.[66] Because of these reports, our procedure is to place patients who require re-exposure to heparin on aspirin and Persantin for several days prior to the operative procedure.[67] On the day of operation, the platelet aggregation tests are performed with the addition of heparin. If the addition of heparin causes abnormal platelet aggregation, we then use iloprost to prevent heparin-induced platelet aggregation during the procedure. The use of iloprost can be complicated, particularly since it is a very potent vasodilator, and it often needs to be accompanied by rather large doses of α-adrenergic agents to support the blood pressure.

Sobel *et al.* reported an alternate technique of having patients on coumadin anticoagulation combined with dextran as a means of preventing intraoperative thrombosis during reconstruction.[68] This is a reasonable alternative for peripheral vascular reconstructions, but is not possible for cardiopulmonary bypass. In the future, different substances may be available to allow for adequate anticoagulation. Makhoul noted *in vitro* that heparinoids did not cause platelet aggregation in patients with heparin-induced platelet aggregation.[66] It is essential to perform *in vitro* aggregation tests prior to use, since the reactivity to these new heparins and heparin substitutes ranges from 19.6% to 60.8%.[69] These new anticoagulant agents are being developed in Europe and may in the future be available for anticoagulation in this country.

Cole *et al.* have reported the use of ancrod, which is made from the venom of the Malaysian pit viper as an anticoagulant in patients who have heparin-induced platelet aggregation.[70] Ancrod acts enzymatically on the fibrinogen molecule to form a product that cannot be clotted by physiologic thrombin. At the present time this medication is in the investigational phase, and may be cleared by the FDA in the not too distant future.

ANTIPHOSPHOLIPID ANTIBODIES

Lupus anticoagulants are IgG or IgM antibodies which are directed against phospholipids that participate in coagulation disorders, and are found in 16–33% of the patients who have lupus erythematosus, but are also found in a variety of other disorders, including normal individuals.[71–73] These antibodies belong to a family of anti-phospholipid antibodies, which were initially detected by their effect *in vitro* on the prolongation of plasma coagulation times. Most commonly, there is a prolongation of activated partial thromboplastin time, and in some patients also a prolongation of prothrombin time. There have only been rare reports of bleeding tendencies related to the demonstration of a lupus anticoagulant, however in the last decade there have been increasing reports of abnormal thrombosis in both the arterial and venous system, spontaneous abortion secondary to placental thrombosis, cerebrovascular accidents, and thrombocytopenia. Lupus anticoagulants also cause false-positive tests for syphilis. On occasion, lupus anticoagulant can occur after administration of phenothiazines, procainamide, and penicillin, following viral infections in children, and in patients with acquired immune deficiency syndrome (AIDS) suffering from *Pneumocystitis carinii* pneumonia.

Clinical syndrome

Recurrent thromboses have been reported in about one-third of patients with lupus anticoagulant.[74] These consist of both venous thromboses, most commonly involving the lower extremities, and are the most common manifestation. Patients may develop evidence of pulmonary hypertension due to recurrent pulmonary emboli or intra-pulmonary thrombosis. Repeated strokes have been reported in 15–55% of the patients. Obstetric complications have been reported in 25–35% of the women with lupus anticoagulant, and consists of spontaneous abortions, intrauterine growth retardation, and fetal death, all occurring in the second and third trimester.[71,72,73] Ahn, in a study of patients undergoing surgery who had a lupus anticoagulant noted that nine of 18 vascular procedures were complicated by thrombosis.[75] Seven of these patients suffered multiple postoperative thrombotic complications, resulting in amputation in three.

The mechanism of action of lupus anticoagulants is not known. Several theories have been suggested including an inhibitory activity on prostacyclin (PGI_2) which is a potent *in vivo* inhibitor of platelet aggregation. IgG fractions with lupus anticoagulant activity have been shown experimentally to block the production of PGI_2 in rat aortic endothelial cells.[76] Other investigators suggest that the lupus anticoagulant inhibits protein C activation, which is important in preventing thrombosis. Tsakiris *et al.* feel that the inhibition of the catalytic activity of thrombomodulin might be explained by the direct attachment of lupus anticoagulant to thrombomodulin or to adjacent phospholipids of the cell membrane, preventing thrombin and/or protein C from binding to thrombomodulin.[77]

Diagnosis

Often the only indication that a patient has lupus anticoagulant is an abnormally prolonged activated partial thromboplastin time. On occasion, patients can also have a prolonged prothrombin time. Diagnosis of the presence of antiphospholipid antibodies (lupus anticoagulants) can be made by demonstration of a prolongation of the coagulation times which do not correct with the addition of normal plasma. The platelet neutralization assay utilized the antiphospholipid antibodies ability to inhibit platelet binding to collagen as evidence of their presence in a patient's plasma. Reactivity of a patient's plasma with cardiolipin by an ELISA assay is also a useful screening test; however, it is not a specific test and may be confirmed by one of the above mentioned assays. An abnormal rabbit brain neutralization procedure and an ELISA for the presence of anticardiolipin antibodies can more precisely identify the lupus anticoagulant.[75]

Treatment

Because the precise mechanism of action of lupus anticoagulant causing intravascular thrombosis is not known, the treatment has varied from antiplatelet medications with aspirin and dipyridamole, anticoagulation with coumadin and heparin, and the administration of steroids. The reason for the antiplatelet medication is that some authors feel that the lupus anticoagulant causes a decrease in the availability of arachidonic acid, which is necessary for the synthesis of prostacyclin inhibitor and platelet aggregation in vessel walls. In obstetric patients it has been reported that steroid and aspirin are effective in preventing spontaneous abortion. Prednisone has been shown to suppress production and/or the activity of lupus anticoagulant, as measured by lessened prolongation of the activated partial thromboplastin time. Until more information is available, we prefer to have patients on antiplatelet medications prior to procedures, using both aspirin and Persantin. We use dextran routinely in all vascular reconstructions, and have the patients on perioperative heparin. Postoperatively the heparin is converted to coumadin.

ACTIVATED PROTEIN C RESISTANCE

The thrombomodulin/protein C anticoagulant pathway is an essential anticoagulant system. As thrombin is generated at sites of vascular injury it activates and aggregates platelets and clots fibrinogen. It also binds to the endothelial membrane protein thrombomodulin. Upon binding to thrombomodulin, thrombin takes on anticoagulant properties by activating protein C. The activated protein C (APC) cleaves and inactivates factor Va and VIIIa in the presence of protein S. This endothelial base anticoagulant system allows blood to clot while maintaining intravascular fluidity. Defects in this anticoagulant pathway can provoke thrombosis, and indeed protein C and protein S deficiencies which were discussed previously are associated with an increased risk of thrombosis in heterozygous patients. To date prothrombotic mutations have not been found in thrombomodulin or thrombin. A family history of thrombotic events is frequently obtained in young adults with venous thrombosis, however, the inherited deficiencies in the anticoagulant protein such as protein C and protein S are found in only a small proportion of patients, approximately 5%.[78] This suggests the presence of another genetic defect that predisposes these patients to thrombosis. Work done by Svensson and Dahlbäck, has revealed a high prevalence of activated protein C resistance among young persons with a history of venous thrombosis.[78] Dahlbäck originally postulated that a defect in the protein C pathway interferes with the anticoagulant action of APC. He devised an assay to test this possibility in which the clotting time of blood is measured in the presence and absence of exogenous APC. In the normal response the clotting time is prolonged in the presence of APC because of the inactivation of factors Va and VIIIa. A defect is detected as a failure of prolongation of the clotting time resulting from resistance to added APC. Dahlbäck showed that this test detects an autosomal dominant trait associated with thrombosis. Further work done by Bertina and his group[79] have demonstrated that the phenotype of APC resistance is associated with a heterozygosis of hemozygous single point mutation in the factor V gene which predicts the synthesis of a factor V molecule that is not properly inactivated by APC (factor V Leiden).[78] Other data confirming these results were published by Zoller *et al.* who studied 50 Swedish families with inherited APC resistance.[80] They found that the specific point mutation in the factor V gene was present in 47 of 50 families. In their study by age 33 years, 20% of the heterozygous and 40% of the homozygous patients had had manifestations of venous thrombosis.

The laboratory diagnosis is made by measuring the responsiveness of plasma to APC as the ratio of two activated partial thromboplastin times, one in the presence of APC and one in its absence. The APC sensitivity ratio is normalized to the ratio obtained with a reference plasma. Resistance to APC is defined by an APC sensitivity ratio of <0.84. A more recent way of identifying this factor V resistance to activated protein C is by direct assay for the factor V molecule which is resistant to inactivation by APC (factor V Leiden). The question arises as to what can be done about these point mutations which cause factor V to be resistant to activated protein C. It is clear that this is a major risk factor for thromboembolic disease, however, the majority of patients with these mutant proteins will not suffer thrombosis. The risks of lifelong anticoagulation therapy in an asymptomatic patient must be weighed against the benefit of preventing infrequent although devastating thrombotic attacks. At this point, it would be a logical course of action to treat those patients who have already suffered thrombotic attacks with long-term warfarin therapy.

GUIDELINES FOR IDENTIFYING HYPERCOAGULABLE PATIENTS

A good patient history remains the most important means of identifying patients with potential hypercoagulable disorders. Patients should be asked about previously unexplained thromboses in themselves or family members.   Patients with hypercoagulable syndromes will often report episodes of thrombophlebitis as a young adult. Of particular importance are those episodes of thrombophlebitis that do not have any contributing factors for their development, e.g. long leg fractures, or prolonged immobilization or bed rest due to illness. It becomes even more significant in patients with recurrent episodes of thrombophlebitis. Likewise, a history of arterial thrombosis, especially if it occurs at a young age is an indicator of a coagulation disorder.[67] Eldrup-Jorgensen found a 30% incidence of coagulation abnormalities in patients younger than 51 years undergoing vascular reconstruction.[81] Abnormal clotting factors noted consisted of protein S deficiency, protein C deficiency, presence of lupus-like anticoagulants, and plasminogen deficiency. The incidence of arterial graft thrombosis in their group of hypercoagulable patients was 20% at 30 days, which is markedly increased from what one would expect from this type of vascular reconstruction.

Clinical presentation

With experience one has a feeling for what reconstructions should work and some expectations of the types of problems that occur. Likewise, one develops a feel for what are typical presentations of atherosclerotic occlusive disease. When unusual or unexplained thrombosis is identified, for example a thrombosed suprarenal aorta, upper extremity thrombosis, or total tibial artery occlusion in a patient who is neither diabetic nor has any evidence of any atherosclerotic occlusive disease elsewhere, the surgeon should look for hypercoagulable disorders as the cause. Unusual X-ray findings, in particular occlusions seen in young patients or in one extremity when the other extremity has no evidence of any disease should trigger an investigation into the coagulation system.

The role of screening vascular surgery patients for hypercoagulable states is difficult to ascertain. Donaldson et al. found an overall incidence of 9.5% of patients undergoing a variety of vascular surgery procedures having abnormal tests indicating potential hypercoagulability.[82] The three most common entities these patients demonstrated were heparin-induced platelet aggregation, lupus anticoagulants, and protein C deficiency. The incidence of infrainguinal graft occlusion within 30 days was 27% among those patients who were in the hypercoagulable group, compared with 1.6% in those patients who were not. At present we do not screen routinely for the wide variety of hypercoagulable states. We depend on the history and clinical evaluation to identify those patients who may be hypercoagulable. This is probably more cost-effective and efficient in terms of evaluating these patients.

The most difficult time for a vascular surgeon is dealing with unexplained thrombosis intraoperatively. Often, this occurs during late evening or at night when support from the coagulation laboratory is often not available. The first step if indeed heparin has been given is to see if there is any clotting in the operative field which would indicate an antithrombin III deficiency, since antithrombin III is essential for the anticoagulant effect of heparin. The anaesthesiologist should then test the heparin affect, either by doing partial thromboplastin time or one of the other variety of tests to measure heparin anticoagulation. The next step is to obtain a platelet count. If it is higher than 100 000 and the activated and clotting time is not prolonged, the problem is presumed to be the antithrombin system. The patient is then given two units of fresh frozen plasma, and continued with two units every 12 hours for 5 days. The antithrombin III deficiency is then confirmed usually the next day on blood drawn prior to the administration of any fresh frozen plasma. Patients with antithrombin III deficiency are maintained on long-term warfarin therapy. If the platelet count is less than 100 000, we presume the patient has developed heparin-induced platelet aggregation. Certainly the patient's history should be carefully examined to try and document the administration of heparin at some time in the past. At this time we start dextran, 50 cc bolus, and then run it at 25 ml/h. The heparin is reversed with protamine, and the platelet aggregation abnormality confirmed in the morning. Warfarin treatment is continued for 3 weeks to 6 months.

If the platelet count is greater than 100 000 and the ACT is prolonged we presume the patient has some other sort of hypercoagulable state which includes fibrinolytic abnormalities as well as potential problems with protein C, protein S, or lupus-type anticoagulants. In these patients, we institute continuous heparin therapy both intraoperatively and postoperatively, and give the patient two units of fresh frozen plasma. Fresh frozen plasma is shotgun therapy for a wide variety of coagulation abnormalities.

In the operating room, prior to the institution of any therapy, blood should be drawn for coagulation tests, realizing that many of these tests are quite involved such as plasminogen electrophoresis, protein C, protein S, and determinations of lupus anticoagulants, taking sometimes days to a week at some centres. However, if the blood is properly handled, spun down and frozen, the tests can be done routinely. Our policy is to repeat in 5 days all tests which are abnormal. One of the problems in diagnosing accurately coagulation abnormalities is that in the process of clotting, clotting factors can be consumed and abnormalities may be the result of clotting and not the cause of it. All factors which remain abnormal in the 5–7 day period are repeated at 1 month. Patients who then have persistently abnormal values are labelled truly hypercoagulable patients.

McDaniel et al. have noted the change in coagulation factors with operation.[83] They noted that antithrombin III levels fell on the 3rd postoperative day and subsequently returned to normal by 1 week postoperatively. Antithrombin III declined from a mean preoperative level of 110 to 71% on the 3rd postoperative day. This value returned to normal by the 7th postoperative day, when it was 95% of normal activity. All of this demonstrates the dynamic aspect of the clotting system, and points out the danger of attaching significance to just one isolated laboratory finding. Most patients who sustain complications due to hypercoagulable states are placed on coumadin in the perioperative and postoperative period. In patients with heparin-induced platelet aggregation, this can usually be stopped in 3 months, however, we have recommended prolonged administration in patients with protein C and S deficiency, antithrombin III deficiency and plasminogen abnormalities because of the risk of recurrent thrombosis.

REFERENCES

1. Seegers WH: Antithrombin III: Theory and clinical applications. *Am J Clin Pathol* **69:** 367–374, 1978
2. Egeberg O: Inherited antithrombin deficiency causing thrombophilia. *Thromb Diath Haemorrh* **13:** 516–530, 1965
3. Brozovic M, Stirling Y, Hamlyn AN: Thrombotic tendency and probable antithrombin III deficiency. *Thromb Haemost* **39:** 778–779, 1978
4. Mackie M, Bennett B, Ogston D, Douglas AS: Familial thrombosis: Inherited deficiency of antithrombin III. *Br Med J* **1:** 136–138, 1978
5. Marciniak E, Farley CH, DeSimone PA: Familial thrombosis due to antithrombin III deficiency. *Blood* **43:** 219–231, 1974
6. Sorensen PJ, Dyerburg J, Stotterson E, Jensen MK: Familial functional antithrombin III deficiency. *Scand J Haematol* **24:** 105–109, 1980
7. Collen D, Schetz J, DeCock F et al.: Metabolism of antithrombin III (heparin cofactor) in man: Effects of venous thrombosis and of heparin administration. *Eur J Clin Invest* **7:** 27–35, 1977
8. Degaard OR, Abildgaard U: Antithrombin III: Critical review of assay methods. Significance or variations in health and disease. *Haemostasis* **7:** 127–134, 1978
9. Chan V, Chan TK, Wong V et al.: The determination of antithrombin III by radioimmunoassay and its clinical application. *Br J Haematol* **41:** 563–572, 1979
10. Sas G, Blasko G, Banghogyi D et al.: Abnormal antithrombin III (antithrombin Budapest) as a cause of familial thrombophilia. *Thromb Diath Haemorrh* **32:** 105-115, 1974
11. Flinn WR, McDaniel MD, Yao JST et al.: Antithrombin III deficiency as a reflection of

dynamic protein metabolism in patients undergoing vascular reconstruction. *J Vasc Surg* **1**: 888–895, 1984

12. Towne JB, Bernhard VM, Hussey C, Garancis JC: Antithrombin deficiency – A cause of unexplained thrombosis in vascular surgery. *Surgery* **89**: 735–742, 1981

13. Lynch DM, Leff LK, Howe SE: Preoperative AT-III values and clinical postoperative thrombosis: A comparison of three antithrombin III assays. *Thromb Haemost (Stuttgart)* **52**: 42–44, 1984

14. Sagar S, Stamatakis JD, Thomas DP, Kakkar VV: Oral contraceptives, antithrombin III activity, and postoperative deep vein thrombosis. *Lancet* **i**: 509–511, 1976

15. Conrad J, Lecompte T, Horellou MH *et al.*: Antithrombin III in patients treated with subcutaneous or intravenous heparin. *Thromb Res* **22**: 507–511, 1981

16. Tengborn L, Bergqvist D: Surgery in patients with congenital antithrombin III deficiency. *Acta Chir Scand* **154**: 179–188, 1988

17. Salem HH, Mitchell CA, Firkin BG: Current views on the pathophysiology and investigations of thrombotic disorders. *Am J Haematol* **25**: 463–474, 1987

18. Towne JB: Hypercoagulable states. *Sem Vasc Surg* **1**: 201–215, 1988

19. Wiman B, Ljungberg B, Chmielewska J *et al.*: The role of the fibrinolytic system in deep vein thrombosis. *J Lab Clin Med* **105**: 265–270, 1985

20. Castellino FJ, Powell JR: Human plasminogen. *Meth Enzymol* **80**: 365-378, 1981

21. Aoki N, Moroi M, Sakata Y *et al.*: Abnormal plasminogen: A hereditary molecular abnormality found in patients with recurrent thrombosis. *J Clin Invest* **61**: 1186–1195, 1978

22. Kazama M, Tohura C, Suzuki Z *et al.*: Abnormal plasminogen – A cause of recurrent thrombosis. *Thromb Res* **21**: 517–522, 1981

23. Soria J, Soria C, Bertrand O *et al.*: Plasminogen Paris I: Congenital abnormal plasminogen and its incidence in thrombosis. *Thromb Res* **32**: 229–238, 1983

24. Scharrer IM, Wohl RC, Hach V *et al.*: Investigation of a congenital abnormal plasminogen, Frankfurt I, and its relationship to thrombosis. *Thromb Haemostas* **55**: 396–401, 1986

25. Liu Y, Lyons RM, McDonagh J: Plasminogen San Antonio: An abnormal plasminogen with a more cathodic migration, decreased activation, and associated thrombosis. *Thromb Haemostas* **59**: 49–53, 1988

26. Towne JB, Bandyk DF, Hussey CV, Tollack VT: Abnormal plasminogen: A genetically determined cause of hypercoagulability. *J Vasc Surg* **1**: 896–902, 1984

27. Ikemoto S, Sakata Y, Aoki N: Genetic polymorphism of human plasminogen in a human population. *Hum Hered* **32**: 296–297, 1982

28. Towne JB, Hussey CV, Bandyk DF: Abnormalities of the fibrinolytic system as a cause of upper extremity ischemia. *J Vasc Surg* **7**: 660–666, 1988

29. Wiman B: The role of the fibrinolytic system in thrombotic disease. *Acta Med Scand* **715**: (Suppl) 169–171, 1986

30. Hamsten A, Wiman B, deFaire, U, Blomback M: Increased plasma levels of a rapid inhibitor of tissue plasminogen activator in young survivors of myocardial infarction. *N Engl J Med* **313**: 1557–1563, 1985

31. Wiman B, Ljungberg B, Chmielewska J *et al.*: The role of the fibrinolytic system in deep venous thrombosis. *J Lab Clin Med* **105**: 265–270, 1985

32. Wiman B, Chmielewska J, Ranby M: Inactivation of tissue plasminogen activator in plasma. *J Biol Chem* **259**: 3644–3647, 1984

33. Marlar RA: Protein C in thromboembolic disease. *Semin Throm Haemost* **11**: 387–393, 1985

34. Clouse LH, Comp PC: The regulation of hemostasis: The protein C system. *N Engl J Med* **314**: 1298–1303, 1986

35. Stenflo J: Structure and function of protein C. *Semin Thromb Haemost* **10**: 109–121, 1984

36. Kazmier FJ: Thromboembolism, coumarin necrosis, and protein C. *Mayo Clin Proc* **60**: 673–674, 1985

37. Peterson CE, Kwaan HC: Current concepts of warfarin therapy. *Arch Int Med* **146**: 581–584, 1986

38. Branson HE, Kate J, Marble R, Griffin JH: Inherited protein C deficiency and coumarin-responsive chronic relapsing purpura fulminans in a newborn infant. *Lancet* **ii**: 1165–1168, 1983

39. Salem HH, Mitchell CH, Firkin BG: Current views on the pathophysiology and investigations of thrombotic disorders. *Am J Haematol* **25**: 463–474, 1987

40. Broekmans AW, Veltkamp JJ, Bertina RM: Congenital protein C deficiency and venous thromboembolism: A study of three Dutch families. *N Engl J Med* **390**: 340–344, 1983

41. Griffen JG, Evatt B, Zimmerman TS *et al.*: Deficiency of protein C in congenital thrombotic disease. *J Clin Invest* **68**: 1370–1373, 1981

42. Tollefson DFJ, Friedman KD, Marlar RA *et al.*: Protein C deficiency: A cause of unusual or unexplained thrombosis. *Arch Surg* **123**: 881–884, 1988

43. Green D, Ganger DR, Blei At: Protein C deficiency in splanchnic venous thrombosis. *Am J Med* **82**: 1171–1173, 1987

44. Coller BS, Owen J, Jesty J *et al.*: Deficiency of plasma protein S, protein C, or antithrombin III and arterial thrombosis. *Atherosclerosis* **7**: 456–462, 1987

45. Nelson ME, Talbot JF, Preston FE: Recurrent multiple-branch retinal arteriolar occlusions in a patient with Protein C deficiency. *Graefe Arch Ophth* **227**: 443–447, 1989

46. Comp PC, Esmon CT: Recurrent venous thromboembolism in patients with a partial deficiency of protein S. *N Engl J Med* **311**: 1526–1528, 1984

47. Schwarz HP, Fischer M, Hopmeier P *et al.*: Plasma protein S deficiency in familial thrombotic disease. *Blood* **64**: 1297–1300, 1984

48. Rodgers GM, Shuman MA: Congenital thrombotic disorders. *Am J Haematol* **21**: 419–430, 1986

49. Clark DA, Williams WL, Marlar RA: Mesenteric vein thrombosis associated with a familial deficiency of free Protein S. *Arch Pathol Lab Med* **115**: 617–619, 1991

50. Babcock RB, Dumper CW, Scharfman WB: Heparin-induced immune thrombocytopenia. *N Engl J Med* **295**: 237–241, 1976

51. Baird RA, Convery RF: Arterial thromboembolism in patients receiving systemic heparin therapy. *J Bone Jt Surg* **59**: 1061–1064, 1977

52. Bell WR, Romasulo PA, Alving BM *et al.*: Thrombocytopenia occurring during the administration of heparin. *Ann Intern Med* **87**: 155–160, 1976

53. Fratantoni JC, Pollet R, Gralnick HR: Heparin-induced thrombocytopenia: Confirmation of diagnosis with *in vitro* methods. *Blood* **45**: 395-401, 1975

54. Nelson JC, Lerner RG, Goldstein R *et al.*: Heparin-induced thrombocytopenia. *Arch Intern Med* **138**: 548–552, 1978

55. Rhodes GR, Dixon RH, Silver D: Heparin-induced thrombocytopenia. *Ann Surg* **186**: 752–758, 1977

56. Adams JG Jr, Humphrey LJ, Zang X, Silver D: Do patients with the heparin-induced thrombocytopenia syndrome have heparin specific antibodies? *J Vasc Surg* **21**: 247–253, 1995

57. Kapsch DN, Adelstein EH, Rhodes GR *et al.*: Heparin-induced thrombocytopenia, thrombosis, and hemorrhage. *Surgery* **86**: 148–154, 1979

58. Laster J, Silver D: Heparin coated catheters and heparin-induced thrombocytopenia. *J Vasc Surg* **7**: 667–672, 1988

59. Spadone D, Clark F, James E *et al.*: Heparin-induced thrombocytopenia in the newborn. *J Vasc Surg* 1997 (in press)

60. Towne JB, Bernhard VM, Hussey C *et al.*: White clot syndrome. *Arch Surg* **114**: 372–377, 1979

61. Amirol J, Bridey F, Wolt M, et al: Antibodies to macromolecular platelet factor IV heparin complexes in heparin-induced thrombocytopenia: A study of 44 cases. *Thromb Hemost* **73**: 21–28, 1995

62. Silver D, Kapsch DN, Tsoi EKM: Heparin-induced thrombocytopenia, thrombosis, and hemorrhage. *Ann Surg* **198**: 301–406, 1983

63. Laster J, Cikrit D, Walker N *et al.*: The heparin-induced thrombocytopenia syndrome: An update. *Surgery* **102**: 763–770, 1987

64. Laster J, Elfrink R, Silver D: Re-exposure to heparin of patients with heparin-associated antibodies. *J Vasc Surg* **9**: 677–682, 1989

65. Kappa JR, Fisher CA, Berkowitz HD *et al.*: Heparin-induced platelet activation in sixteen surgical patients: Diagnosis and management. *J Vasc Surg* **5**: 101–109, 1987

66. Makhoul RG, Greenberg CS, McCann RL: Heparin-associated thrombocytopenia and thrombosis: A serious clinical problem and potential solution. *J Vasc Surg* **4**: 522–528, 1986

67. Towne JB: Hypercoagulable states and unexplained vascular thrombosis. In: Bernhard VM, Towne JB (Eds) *Complications in Vascular Surgery* 3rd edn. St Louis, MO: Quality Medical Publishing, 1991

68. Sobel M, Adelman B, Szaboles S *et al.*: Surgical management of heparin-associated thrombocytopenia. *J Vasc Surg* **8**: 395-401, 1988

69. Kikta MJ, Keller MP, Humphrey PW, Silver D: Can low molecular weight heparins and heparinoids be safely given to patients with heparin induced thrombocytopenia syndrome? *Surgery* **114**: 705–710, 1993

70. Cole CW, Fournier LM, Bormanis J: Heparin-associated thrombocytopenia and thrombosis: Optimal therapy with ancrod. *Can J Surg* **33**: 207, 1990

71. Espinoza LR, Hartmann RC: Significance of the lupus anticoagulant. *Am J Haematol* **22**: 331–337, 1986

72. Tabechnik-Schor NF, Lipton SA: Association of lupus-like anticoagulant and nonvasculitic cerebral infarction. *Arch Neurol* **43**: 851–852, 1986

73. Shi W, Krilis SA, Chong BH *et al.*: Prevalence of lupus anticoagulant and anticardiolipin antibodies in a health population. *Aust N Z J Med* **20**: 231–236, 1990

74. Dührsen U, Brittinger G: Lupus anticoagulant associated syndrome in benign and malignant systemic disease. *Klin Wachensh* **65**: 818–822, 1987

75. Ahn SS, Kalunian K. Rosove M, Moore WS: Postoperative thrombotic complications in patients with the lupus anticoagulant: Increased risk after vascular procedure. *J Vasc Surg* **7**: 749–756, 1988

76. Greenfield LJ: Lupus-like anticoagulants and thrombosis. *J Vasc Surg* **7**: 818–819, 1988

77. Tsakiris DA, Settas L, Makris PE, Marbet GA: Lupus anticoagulant-antiphospholipid antibodies and thrombophilia: Relation to protein C-protein S-thrombomodulin. *J Rheumatol* **17**: 785–789, 1990

78. Svensson PJ, Dahlbäck B: Resistance to activated protein C as a basis for venous thrombosis. *N Engl J Med* 330: **8**: 517-521, 1994

79. Bertina RM, Koeleman BP, Kosta *et al.*: Mutation in blood coagulation factor V associated with resistance to activated protein C. *Nature* **369**: 64, 1994

80. Zoller B, Svensson PJ, Xuhaua H, Dahlbäck B: Identification of the same factor V gene mutation in 47 out of 50 thrombosis-prone families with inherited resistance to activated protein C. *J Clin Invest* **94**: 2521, 1994

81. Eldrup-Jorgensen J, Flanigan DP, Brace L *et al.*: Hypercoagulable states and lower limb ischemia in young adults. *J Vasc Surg* **9**: 334–341, 1989

82. Donaldson MC, Weinberg DS, Belkin M *et al.*: Screening for hypercoagulable states in a vascular surgery practice: A preliminary study. *J Vasc Surg* **11**: 825-831, 1990

83. McDaniel MD, Pearce WH, Yao JST *et al.*: Sequential changes in coagulation and platelet function following femoro-tibial bypass. *J Vasc Surg* **1**: 261-8, 1984

VENOUS ULCER

The Role of Leukocytes in Venous Ulceration

P. D. Coleridge Smith

INTRODUCTION

Venous diseases cost the healthcare systems of Western countries large sums every year. Venous ulceration becomes more prevalent with advancing age and as the average age of populations increases more patients will require treatment. This chronic relapsing condition is estimated to have a prevalence of 0.2% in Western countries.[1] This may be an underestimate since many patients treat their own ulcers. In the UK venous ulcers are treated in the community by general practitioners and community nurses. Between 10 and 30% of nursing time may be occupied with the dressing of leg ulcers.[2] The cost of this is massive, amounting to £2000–£4000 per year for each of the 150 000–200 000 patients with leg ulcers. In the UK it is estimated that £600–£800 million (US$ 1 billion) is spent on this condition per annum – about 2% of the healthcare budget.

LARGE VESSEL PHYSIOLOGY

Ambulatory venous hypertension is a constant pathological feature in venous disease. This arises because of damage to the venous valves in the lower limb either from a previous deep vein thrombosis or by primary valve failure,[3] a poorly understood process in which venous valves fail to maintain their competence without previous venous thrombosis. In either instance, blood is permitted to flow in the reverse direction, and the pumping efficiency of the musculovenous pumps of the lower limb is impaired. Pressure in the superficial veins of the leg does not fall during exercise and this is the source of damage to the skin microcirculation.

The clinical syndrome that is produced by long-standing ambulatory venous hypertension includes haemosiderin deposition in the skin resulting in brown pigmentation near the ankle. Palpable induration and scarring of the skin – usually referred to as lipodermatosclerosis – may also develop and reflects a more severe stage of tissue injury, affecting both the skin and subcutaneous tissues. This often progresses to venous ulceration with skin loss in the region proximal to the medial or lateral malleolus. Nicolaides *et al.* have shown that the higher the venous pressure during walking, the higher the incidence of ulceration.[4] Patients with haemosiderosis, lipodermatosclerosis or ulceration of the leg due to venous disease are said to have chronic venous insufficiency (CVI).

THE MICROCIRCULATION

Browse and Burnand proposed a theory suggesting that pericapillary fibrin cuffs act as a barrier to diffusion of oxygen and other small molecules. They demonstrated the presence of fibrin cuffs histologically surrounding skin capillaries in the cutaneous lesions produced by ambulatory venous hypertension. This hypothesis saw the explanation as a simple gas transfer problem, although little data was available at that time to support this proposal.[5]

A number of authors have subsequently assessed transcutaneous oxygen tension, as an indicator of oxygen delivery to skin.[6-8] In this test a polarographic electrode covered with a gas permeable membrane (a Clark electrode) is applied to the skin and heated to 43°C. This causes vasodilatation in the skin and increases the amount of oxygen reaching the skin surface. These measurements show reduced trans-cutaneous oxygen tension in the skin of patients with venous disease who have liposclerotic skin change. However, the vasodilatory response of skin damaged by venous disease is reduced compared with normal skin and the reduced oxygen tension measurements at the skin surface may merely represent an attenuated hyperaemic response to heating.[9]

Objective assessments of gas transfer using either xenon clearance[10] or oxygen return time following a period of ischaemia[11] show no evidence of a gas transfer problem. Calculations based on a theoretical model of gas diffusion undertaken by Michel suggest that the composition of the fibrin cuff (99% water) would be unlikely to impair the diffusion of small molecules.[12] He also deduced that oedema of the tissues, often seen in patients with venous disease, would not influence tissue oxygenation, a conclusion that has received experimental support.[13] Subsequently direct needle electrode measurements have been made in liposclerotic skin, and these show a moderate reduction in tissue oxygenation, but insufficient to result in skin necrosis.[14]

ACTIVE MODEL OF VENOUS ULCERATION

In 1987 Moyses et al.[15] noted that leukocyte sequestration occurred in the lower limb of normal subjects when experimental venous hypertension was produced over a 40-minute period. His volunteers sat without moving on a bicycle saddle, raising the venous pressure in the superficial veins of the lower limb to 80–100 mmHg. Blood samples were taken from the long saphenous vein at the ankle. Thomas et al.[16] repeated this experiment, comparing patients with chronic venous disease and skin changes, including ulceration, to control subjects with normal lower limb veins. In this study the patients sat on a hospital bed with the legs dependent, resulting in a venous pressures of about 60 mmHg. He observed a difference in white cell trapping between the two groups. Patients trapped 30% of white cells after 60 minutes of sitting, whilst control subjects trapped only 7% (Fig. 1). After return to the lying position efflux of white cells from the limb was also observed.

Subsequently Vanscheidt investigated the extent of leukocyte sequestration in patients with venous disease when the upper limb was subjected to venous

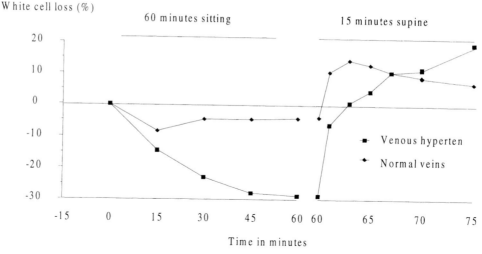

Fig. 1.   White cell trapping in patients compared with controls. Redrawn from ref. 16.

hypertension produced by a arm cuff inflated to a pressure between diastolic and systolic blood pressure.[17] He showed more white cell trapping in the upper limb by patients with venous disease compared with controls (venous disease: 18%, control: 13%).

At the same time Coleridge Smith *et al.* had conducted some capillary microscopy studies which suggested that venous hypertension reduced the number of visible capillaries in the skin of patients with venous disease. These synthesis of these data was a hypothesis that suggested that the 'trapped' white cells were responsible for endothelial injury, which cumulated to produce microcirculatory damage in patients with long-standing ambulatory venous hypertension.[18] This suggestion included the mechanisms known to be responsible for critical ischaemia. We suggested that venous hypertension and the fall in blood flow which occurs in the lower limb on standing favours adhesion of leukocytes to the microcirculatory endothelium.

Capillary microscopy of lower limb skin capillaries during venous hypertension shows that they dilate and that there is a considerable reduction in flow velocity. These factors reduce the shear rate in the microcirculation. A reduction in shear rate favours neutrophil adhesion[19] which probably occurs in the post-capillary venule (Fig. 2). The leukocyte adhesion detected by Moyses in control subjects is probably a physiological phenomenon that does not normally persist for any length of time. Venous pressure in the lower limb falls rapidly on walking, so that venous hypertension is not normally present in the leg. In patients with chronic venous disease who have ambulatory venous hypertension, leukocyte trapping may be more persistent. It was proposed that the trapped leukocytes become activated releasing free radicals and proteolytic enzymes resulting in endothelial injury (Figs 3, 4). It was suggested that over a long period this might lead to cumulative damage in the microcirculation.

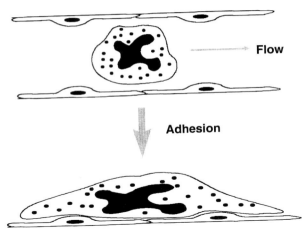

Fig. 2.   Leukocyte adhesion to endothelium is favoured by new flow rates.

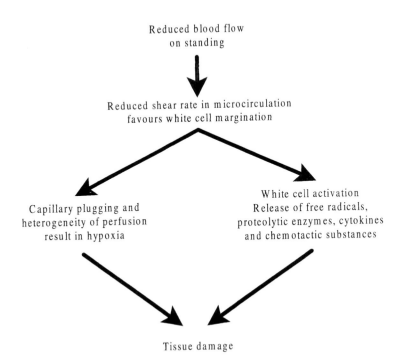

Fig. 3.   White cell trapping hypothesis, indicating the mechanisms that were originally proposed.

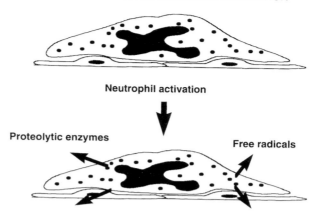

Fig. 4. Leukocyte activation appear to occur following endothelial adhesion of neutrophils.

The effect of venous hypertension has subsequently been studied in our laboratory using a series of markers of leukocyte activation. Control subjects exposed to lower limb venous hypertension produced by standing were studied by taking blood samples from the hand and the leg veins. Degranulation of neutrophils was studied by measuring plasma levels of neutrophil elastase (a primary neutrophil granule enzyme) and lactoferrin (a secondary neutrophil granule enzyme). After a 30-minute period of experimental venous hypertension, a rise in plasma lactoferrin concentration was observed in both the blood taken from the foot and from the arm.[20] When venous hypertension was produced by inflation of a cuff around one lower limb, a rise in lactoferrin was only observed in that limb.

The adhesion of leukocytes to endothelium is a complex process requiring a series of surface ligands on the leukocytes and adhesion molecules on the endothelium (Fig. 5). Adhesion of neutrophils and monocytes is currently regarded as a two-stage process. Initially these cells roll along the endothelium, binding in a loose manner using a ligand on the leukocytes known as CD62L or L-selectin (Fig. 6). When binding occurs a fragment of L-selectin is released into the plasma (soluble L-selectin) and can be detected by an ELISA. Subsequently, firm binding of neutrophils and monocytes occurs using CD11b/CD18 ligands which link to endothelial ICAM (Fig. 7).

Expression of the surface neutrophil ligand, CD11b, has been investigated in our laboratory as a marker of neutrophil activation. The experiment was repeated as before on control subjects. Blood was taken from a dorsal foot vein. CD11b expression was assessed by fluorescent-labelled monoclonal antibody used to label neutrophils in whole blood which were counted using flow cytometry. During the period of ambulatory venous hypertension in control subjects no rise in CD11b expression was seen in the lower limb blood.[21] Following return to the supine position, when neutrophils might be expected to leave the lower limb, according to the studies of Thomas et al.,[16] increased levels of CD11b were observed (Fig. 8). This indicates that neutrophils were upregulated by their period of adhesion to normal

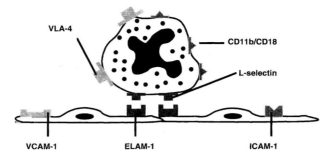

Fig. 5.   A complex series of surface ligands are present on leukocytes which facilitate interaction with the endothelium.

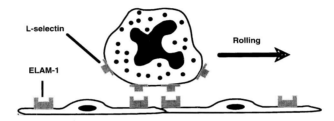

Fig. 6.   The initial stage of neutrophil adhesion to endothelium is 'rolling' which is mediated by L-selectin on the surface of neutrophils.

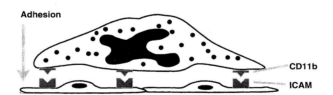

Fig. 7.   Firm adhesion of neutrophils and monocytes to endothelium is mediated by CD11b/CD18 on the surface of these cells.

endothelium. An increased white cell:red cell ratio was also observed during this phase confirming white cell egress from the lower limb.

This study has also been conducted in patients with venous disease, including only subjects with unulcerated skin to avoid the possibility that the inflammatory processes involved in the ulcer may result in upregulation of inflammatory mediators in a way unrelated to the development of the ulcer. Two groups of patients were studied: one group with uncomplicated varicose veins and one with skin changes (lipodermatosclerosis) attributable to venous disease. The adhesion of neutrophils and monocytes to endothelium was investigated by measuring the plasma soluble L-selectin levels using an ELISA. It was found that the concentration

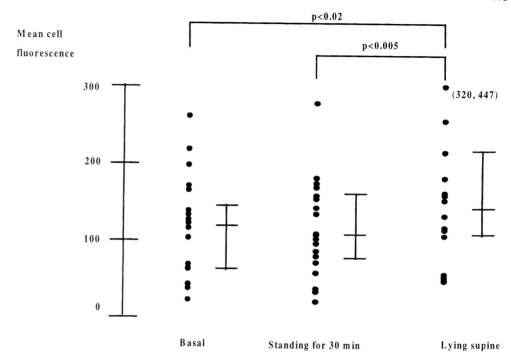

Fig. 8.   Neutrophil CD11b expression measured by flow cytometry in volunteers before and 10 minutes after a period of ambulatory venous hypertension produced by standing. Increased CD11b expression is noted on return to the supine position during the period of in leukocyte efflux. Error bars show the median and inter-quartile range of data. Statistical significance was tested by the Mann-Whitney U test.

of soluble L-selectin rose during venous hypertension, confirming that endothelial : leukocyte binding had occurred. There was no major difference in magnitude between the two groups of patients.

Firm binding of neutrophils and monocytes is reflected in the peripheral blood by a fall in the cells expressing most CD11b. Just such a fall was seen in the blood taken from the leg in both groups of patients. On return to the supine position we had expected to see an egress of leukocytes expressing more CD11b in these patients, but this was not observed, in contrast to the studies on control subjects. In the time-scale of this experiment (up to 10 minutes following venous hypertension), the more activated neutrophils and monocytes remained bound to the endothelium of the lower limb.

Plasma lactoferrin and elastase have been assessed in groups of patients with active venous disease to determine whether they exhibit increased neutrophil degranulation. Blood was taken from the arm veins (not the lower limb veins) of three groups of patients with venous disease: varicose veins, liposclerotic skin change and active venous ulceration.[22,23] In all samples, the levels of lactoferrin and elastase were higher in the patients than the age and sex-matched control groups

(Fig. 8). However, it was found that the highest levels of plasma lactoferrin were present in patients with active varicose veins. Subsequently blood was taken from the arms of patients for measurement of neutrophil CD11b expression. This was elevated in patients with varicose veins, but depressed in patients with lipodermatosclerosis.[24] The explanation may be that the more active leukocytes are attracted to the region of the inflammatory process and do not circulate in the peripheral blood. Alternatively, such patients may have high circulating levels of neutrophil inhibitors.

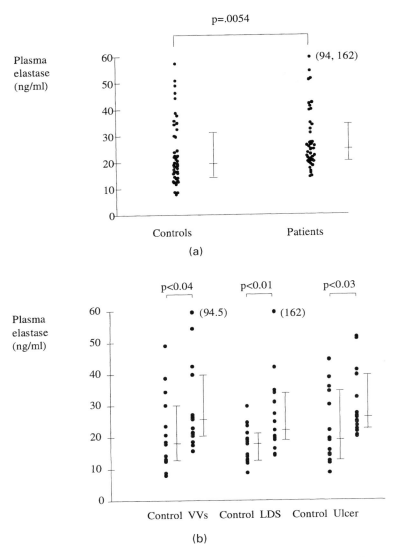

Fig. 9a, b.   Results of plasma neutrophil elastase measurements in patients and control subjects.

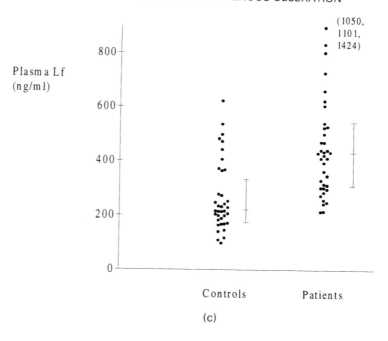

(c)

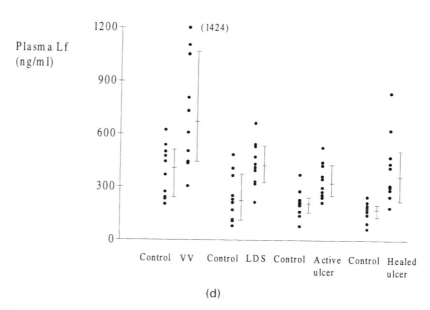

(d)

Fig. 9c, d.   Results of plasma neutrophil lactoferrin measurements in patients and control subjects. Error bars show the median and inter-quartile range of data. Statistical significance was tested by the Mann-Whitney U test.

The microcirculation of the skin has been investigated by histology[25] and by capillary microscopy.[26] Both methods demonstrate capillary proliferation in patients with CVI – vastly more capillaries are visible by both techniques. However, capillary microscopy shows that these probably arise from a single capillary loop and appear like a glomerulus, rather than an increase in the numbers of capillaries. Recent immunohistochemical investigations have shown that the pericapillary cuff contains far more than fibrin. The capillary endothelium is perturbed, expressing increased amounts of factor VIII related antigen[27,28] and adhesion molecules, especially ICAM-1, ELAM-1 may be slightly upregulated but VCAM appears to be normal in patients without venous ulceration. Perturbed endothelium is more likely to attract the adhesion of leukocytes. The presence of the peri-capillary fibrin cuff has been confirmed, but it also contains collagen IV, laminin, fibronectin and tenascin.[29] A strong leukocyte infiltration has been measured in patients with venous disease.[30] These cells are macrophages and T lymphocytes.[27] The cytokines involved include interleukins IL-1α and IL-1β. Tumour necrosis factor (TNF)-α was not detected in these histological sections. The presence of the perivascular fibrin cuff (with other components) is a reflection of the inflammatory process and is seen in other chronic inflammatory conditions. In patients with venous disease increased plasma D-dimer levels have been observed suggesting enhanced deposition of fibrin.[31] The perturbed state of the endothelium allows the passage of large molecules though the endothelium permitting their perivascular accumulation and explains the presence of the fibrin cuff.

In recent studies undertaken in the Department of Surgery, University College London, measurements of plasma levels of endothelial adhesion molecules have been performed along with von Willebrand factor. These may reflect endothelial injury in the circulation. Patients with chronic venous disease (a group with uncomplicated varicose veins and a group with skin changes) were again studied and compared with normal controls. The concentration of soluble VCAM (vascular cell adhesion molecule) was elevated in both patient groups compared with control subjects, and was highest in the group with skin changes. Smaller elevations of von Willebrand factor, soluble ICAM and e-selectin were also observed. All subjects were then exposed to venous hypertension for 30 minutes using the protocol described in earlier sections. Further rises of soluble adhesion molecules were noted, of which the rise in sVCAM was the most marked, and was greatest in the patients with skin changes attributable to venous disease. These elevations of soluble endothelial adhesion molecules probably reflect endothelial injury in response to short-term experimental venous hypertension, which occurs both in control subjects and patients with venous disease.

The vascular proliferation seen in the skin of patients with venous disease has been known for many years[32] but has not been explained. In recent years many angiogenic factors have been recognized which stimulate the growth of blood vessels. In a further study conducted in the Department of Surgery of University College, London, immunohistochemistry was used to evaluate the presence of a number of such factors in the skin of patients with venous disease.[33] Skin biopsies were taken at the time of surgery for varicose veins from the legs of patients with and without skin changes as well as of breast skin in patients without clinical evidence of venous disease, for use as a control. Histology demonstrated no evidence of upregulation of transforming growth factor-β (TGF-β) in the skin of patients with venous disease. In contrast, there was some increase in platelet derived growth factor, subtype BB (PDGF-BB) in patients with venous disease. This was found in the capillary wall in vessels of the dermal papillae. There was also considerable upregulation of the production of vascular endothelial growth factor (VEGF) in the epidermis of patients with venous disease, most marked in those with skin changes. It seems likely that VEGF may account for at least some of the vascular proliferation seen in the skin of patients with venous disease. This growth factor is also responsible for increased vascular permeability to large molecules, a feature of the skin microangiopathy that has been reported from capillary microscopy studies.[26] The mechanism of stimulation of epidermal VEGF production is unclear at present.

Interpretation of data from existing studies

The studies conducted in our laboratory and those of the other small bands of researchers interested in this field have shown probable mechanisms by which endothelial injury is initiated in patients with venous disease, but so far have failed to demonstrate why some patients develop skin changes and others do not.

Endothelial adhesion is a normal physiological activity of neutrophils and monocytes. During venous hypertension the fall in blood flow to the lower limb and increase in diameter of capillaries results in a fall in the shear rate in cutaneous capillaries. This favours leukocyte adhesion, which may be observed, even in control subjects, but is of greater magnitude in patients, presumably due to the modifications that take place in the endothelium in chronic venous disease.

The indicators of leukocyte-endothelial interaction show that this occurs during short-term venous hypertension (within 30 minutes) and that during this period neutrophil degranulation may be detected, releasing primary and secondary granule enzymes into the region of the endothelium. At the same time an increase in von Willebrand factor and soluble endothelial adhesion molecules can be found in the leg blood. These arguments apply to control subject as well as to patients, although the magnitude of change is always greater in the patients rather than the control subjects. In fact it is most unusual for a subject with normal veins to experience venous hypertension for a 30-minute period. Small movements of the calf result in rapid reduction of lower limb venous pressure in a normal subject, so the circumstances of our experiment are not usually experienced by people with normal lower limb veins. However, the experiments do show that when the venous system becomes deranged, endothelial injury my be the result. We have also observed the egress of activated leukocytes from the lower limbs of control subjects following venous hypertension. In patients with venous disease, these cells appear to remain in the lower limb, perhaps attached to the abnormal endothelium.

The chronic changes seen in liposclerotic skin may be the response to sustained, low grade assault upon the endothelium by neutrophils and monocytes over many months or years. The perivascular infiltration of vessels in the papillary dermis by macrophages and T lymphocytes may simply be a tissue response to the chronic inflammatory processes referred to above. The vascular proliferation seen in this condition is also observed in patients with skin conditions such as psoriasis. A consistent pathological feature in patients at risk of venous ulceration is the development of vascular proliferation in the skin, and liposclerotic skin change. Whether this is simply an associated phenomenon or crucial to subsequent ulceration remains unclear at present.

The progression from the chronic skin damage to actual ulceration also remains difficult to understand. Whilst many skin conditions are associated with inflammatory changes, few result in chronic non-healing skin ulceration. This is clearly the cumulation of long-term skin injury attributable to all the processes which I have described above. The progress from the chronic inflammatory state to ulceration is difficult to investigate and there is no animal model. A possible answer is that an initiating stimulus causes massive activation of the perivascular macrophages resulting in extensive tissue and blood vessel destruction. This may be a spontaneous event such as thrombosis of one of the capillary loops, which has been observed using capillary microscopy.[34] Alternatively minor trauma to the region may set in motion the series of events which leads to ulcer formation.

A view which seems to be presented on wound healing platforms is that venous ulcers fail to heal because of faulty wound healing processes. This may be true, but it has long been known that rapid venous ulcer healing can be achieved if the precipitating factor (venous hypertension) can be corrected by a varicose vein operation. The ulcer heals within a week or two and in many cases the skin may return to normal. We therefore believe that the main reason that a venous ulcer fails to heal is that the factors producing it are still present.

The data collected in the studies of neutrophil, monocyte and endothelial cell activity have so far failed to identify major differences between those patients who develop skin changes and are at risk of ulceration and those who do not. Clearly a fairly limited range of processes has been studied so far, and many areas have been left untouched. We have concentrated on the processes which may cause damage, and have so far neglected the defence or response mechanism. Neither have inhibitors of leukocyte activation been studied. Searching each of these areas will take a little time and require differing techniques. Unfortunately few other authors have published research in this area, although increasing interest has been shown in Germany in recent years.

CONCLUSIONS

Many aspects of the pathophysiology of venous disease remain to be clarified, particularly the initial phases of microcirculatory injury which ultimately result in leg ulceration. Leukocyte activation occurs after short periods of venous hypertension, even in control subjects, and is probably one of the factors that causes endothelial damage to cutaneous capillaries if it continues over many months or years. This might eventually be the target of pharmacological treatment.

REFERENCES

1. Callam MJ, Ruckley CV, Harper DR, Dale JJ: Chronic ulceration of the leg: extent of the problem and provision of care. *Br Med J* **290**: 1855–1856, 1985

2. Bosanquet N: Costs of venous ulcers: from maintenance therapy to investment programmes. *Phlebology* Suppl 1: 44–46, 1992

3. Killewich LA, Martin R, Cramer M *et al.*: An objective assessment of the physiologic changes in the post-thrombotic syndrome. *Arch Surg* **120**: 424–426, 1985

4. Nicolaides AN, Zukowski A, Lewis R *et al.*: Venous pressure measurements in venous problems. In: Bergan JJ, Yao JST (Eds) *Surgery of the Veins* pp. 111–118. Orlando: Grune and Stratton, 1985

5. Browse NL, Burnand KG: The cause of venous ulceration. *Lancet* **ii**: 243–245, 1982

6. Stacey MC, Burnand KG, Layer GT, Pattison M: Transcutaneous oxygen tensions as a prognostic indicator and measure of treatment of recurrent ulcer. *Br J Surg* **74**: 545, 1987

7. Clyne CAC, Ramsden WH, Chant ADB, Wenster JHH: Oxygen tension in the skin of the gaiter area of limbs with venous ulceration. *Br J Surg* **72**: 644–647, 1985

8. Moosa HH, Falanga V, Steed-DL *et al.*: Oxygen diffusion in chronic venous ulceration. *J Cardiovasc Surg Torino* **28**: 464–467, 1987

9. Cheatle TR, Stibe ECL, Shami SK *et al.*: Vasodilatory capacity of the skin in venous disease and its relationship to transcutaneous oxygen tension. *Br J Surg* **78**: 607–610, 1990

10. Cheatle TR, McMullin GM, Farrah J *et al.*: Three tests of microcirculatory function in the evaluation of treatment for chronic venous insufficiency. *Phlebology* **5**: 165–172, 1990

11. Stibe E, Cheatle TR, Coleridge Smith PD, Scurr JH: Liposclerotic skin: a diffusion block or a perfusion problem? *Phlebology* **5**: 231–236, 1990

12. Michel CC: Oxygen diffusion in oedematous tissue and through pericapillary cuffs. *Phlebology* **5**: 223–230, 1990

13. Nemeth AJ, Falanga V, Alstadt SP, Eaglstein WH: Ulcerated edematous limbs: effect of edema removal on transcutaneous oxygen measurements. *J Am Acad Dermatol* **20**: 191–197, 1989

14. Schmeller W, Roszinski S, Tronnier M, Gmelin E: Combined morphological and physiological examinations in lipodermatosclerosis. In: Raymond-Martimbeau, Prescott R, Zummo M (Eds) *Phlebologie '92* pp. 172–174. Paris: John Libbey, Eurotext, 1992

15. Moyses C, Cederholm-Williams SA, Michel CC: Haemoconcentration and the accumulation of white cells in the feet during venous stasis. *Int J Microcirc Clin Exp* **5**: 311–320, 1987

16. Thomas PRS, Nash GB, Dormandy JA: White cell accumulation in the dependent legs of patients with ambulatory venous hypertension: a possible mechanism for trophic changes in the skin. *Br Med J* **296**: 1693–1695, 1988

17. Vanscheidt W, Kresse O, Hach-Wunderle V *et al.*: Leg ulcer patients: no decreased fibrinolytic response but white cell trapping after venous occlusion of the upper limb. *Phlebology* **7**: 92–96, 1992

18. Coleridge Smith PD, Thomas P, Scurr JH, Dormandy JA: Causes of venous ulceration: a new hypothesis. *Br Med J* **296**: 1726–1728, 1988

19. Schmid-Schoenbein GW, Fung YC, Zweifach BW: Vascular endothelium-leukocyte interaction; sticking shear force in venules. *Circ Res* **36**: 173–184, 1975

20. Shields DA, Andaz S, Abeysinghe RD *et al.*: Neutrophil activation in experimental ambulatory venous hypertension. *Phlebology* **9**: 119–124, 1994

21. Shields D, Andaz SK, Timothy-Antoine CA *et al.*: CD11b/CD18 as a marker of neutrophil adhesion in experimental ambulatory venous hypertension. In: Negus D, Jantet G, Coleridge Smith PD (Eds) *Phlebology '95* pp. 108–109. *Phlebology* (Suppl. 1): 1995

22. Shields DA, Andaz S, Abeysinghe RD *et al.*: Plasma lactoferrin as a marker of white cell degranulation in venous disease. *Phlebology* **9**: 55–58, 1994

23. Shields DA, Andaz SK, Sarin S *et al.*: Plasma elastase in venous disease. *Br J Surg* **81**: 1496–1499, 1994

24. Shields D, Saharay M, Timothy-Antoine CA *et al.*: Neutrophil CD11b expression in patients with venous disease. In: Negus D, Jantet G, Coleridge Smith PD (Eds) *Phlebology '95* pp. 109–109. *Phlebology* (Suppl. 1): 1995

25. Burnand KG, Whimster I, Naidoo A, Browse NL: Pericapillary fibrin in the ulcer bearing skin of the leg: the cause of lipodermatosclerosis and venous ulceration. *Br Med J* **285**: 1071–1072, 1982

26. Haselbach P, Vollenweider U, Moneta G, Bollinger A: Microangiopathy in severe chronic venous insufficiency evaluated by fluorescence video-microscopy. *Phlebology* **1:** 159–169, 1986

27. Wilkinson LS, Bunker C, Edwards JC *et al.*: Leukocytes: their role in the etiopathogenesis of skin damage in venous disease. *J Vasc Surg* **17:** 669–675, 1993

28. Veraart JC, Verhaegh ME, Neumann HA *et al.*: Adhesion molecule expression in venous leg ulcers. *Vasa* **22:** 213–218, 1993

29. Herrick SE, Sloan P, McGurk M *et al.*: Sequential changes in histologic pattern and extracellular matrix deposition during the healing of chronic venous ulcers. *Am J Pathol* **141:** 1085–1095, 1992

30. Scott HJ, McMullin GM, Coleridge Smith PD, Scurr JH: A histological study into white blood cells and their association with lipodermatosclerosis and ulceration. *Br J Surg* **78:** 210–211, 1990

31. Falanga V, Kruskal J, Franks JJ: Fibrin- and fibrinogen-related antigens in patients with venous disease and venous ulceration. *Arch Dermatol* **127:** 75–78, 1991

32. Burnand KG, Whimster I, Clemenson G *et al.*: The relationship between the number of capillaries in the skin of the venous ulcer-bearing area of the lower leg and the fall in foot vein pressure during exercise. *Br J Surg* **68:** 297–300, 1981

33. Pardoe HD: The expression of angiogenic growth factors in the skin of patients with chronic venous disease of the lower limb. MSc Thesis, University College London, September 1996

34. Franzeck UK, Speiser D, Haselbach P, Bollinger A: Morphologic and dynamic microvascular abnormalities in chronic venous incompetence In: Davy A, Stemmer R (Eds) *Phlebologie 1989* pp. 104–107. John Libbey, Eurotext, Paris: 1989

Management of Venous Ulceration

Stephen D. Blair

INTRODUCTION

Venous ulcers have troubled man through the centuries and it has been known for several hundred years that the way to heal ulcers is through compression. *Wiseman's Medical Textbook* of 1676 illustrates various methods of applying compression to heal venous ulcers. These were gradually modified and in the 1850s Unna developed a non-compliant plaster-type dressing which is still widely used in the USA. Since then the number of treatments has multiplied to the extent that an audit of a district in England carried out in 1995 revealed 143 different dressings, bandages and topical preparations being applied in various combinations to a total of 587 patients.[1] It is, therefore, perhaps not surprising that the care of patients with chronic leg ulcers is estimated to cost around £400 000 000 annually in the UK[2] and consumes approximately 2% of the total healthcare budget in the European Communities.[3] The healing rate using this vast array of treatments is consistently in the range of 20–28% healed within 12 weeks.

Against this depressing background there has been much research showing the effective development of reliable compression bandaging which has greatly improved healing rates. However, the implementation of this research worldwide has been slow and patchy. In the UK the majority of patients with ulcers continue to be looked after by district nurses without proper assessment or effective treatment of the ulcer. This chapter, therefore, summarizes the research into effective assessment and treatment of ulcers and the structures required to administer it.

NATIONAL HEALTH SERVICE EXECUTIVE (NHSE) GUIDELINES FOR THE MANAGEMENT OF LEG ULCERS

In August 1994 a comprehensive literature research and review of all published data on leg ulcers was collated and used as a basis for a national consensus conference held in September 1994 in Liverpool and involving all healthcare professionals. From this, guidelines were drawn up and then implemented in a pilot site which was the Wirral peninsular, south of Liverpool which has the benefit of a very localized population of 360 000 which could be comprehensively studied.

EPIDEMIOLOGY

Population studies have shown a presence of chronic leg ulceration of 0.1–0.3%. On the Wirral, 622 ulcers were identified in 515 patients giving a point prevalence of

0.142. The mean age of these patients was 79 with 88% being over 65 years; 37% of ulcers were larger than 10 cm²; 21% were bilateral and the median duration of current ulceration was 12 months (inter quartile range 4–30 months); 58% of these ulcers were recurrent.

These figures are comparable with other epidemiological studies. In the Scottish Lothian study the prevalence over 3 months was 0.16%.[4] In Perth, Western Australia, epidemiological studies showed 76% of ulcers being recurrent with 47% of patients having had ulcer disease for more than 5 years and 90% of patients being over 60 years old.[5]

The healing rate on the Wirral prior to introducing the NHSE guidelines was 24.8% in 12 weeks. Over the same period, 22% of ulcers had either not changed in size or had grown larger. These figures are very similar to those in Stockport and Trafford[1] where 24.6% were healed within 12 weeks and 20% showed an increase in ulcer area. In the Lothian study only 50% of ulcers were healed at 9 months and 20% had failed to heal after 2 years.[6]

In epidemiological studies it is difficult to know how accurate is the assessment of aetiology. On the Wirral, in the absence of universal use of Doppler ultrasound, 57% of uclers were thought to be venous, 11% arterial, 10% mixed and 20% unknown with only 1% being diabetic or rheumatoid-associated. In studies where formal venous assessment is possible using non-invasive methods, over 80% of patients can be demonstrated to have venous disease.[7] In reality ulcers often are multifactorial with venous insufficiency being compounded by immobility and, therefore, failure to use the calf muscle pump, ankle oedema associated with cardiac failure, obesity and systemic diseases. More than one aetiological factor was present in 33% of the patients in the Perth study.[7]

In the Lothian leg ulcer study using Doppler ultrasound, 21% of patients had evidence of impaired arterial circulation with an ankle brachial pressure index (ABPI) of less than 0.8 which matches the age/sex match population but has important implications for the use of compression as a treatment modality.[8]

ASSESSMENT OF ULCERS

Simply looking at an ulcer will not necessarily tell you what the aetiology is. It is simplistic to think that lateral ulcers are arterial; frequently venous ulcers have no visible varicose veins and venous ulcers that have been complicated by infection may look punched out, even though there is no arterial element (Fig. 1).

A full history and examination of the legs is therefore necessary with particular attention to any venous disease, previous deep venous thrombosis, history of claudication or arterial disease and assessment of non-venous causes such as diabetes mellitus and rheumatoid arthritis. On examination, particular attention should be paid to signs of skin disease such as psoriasis and eczema which may be venous or non-venous in origin and the presence of malignant changes such as melanoma or squamous cell carcinoma. Venous assessment should include standing the patient up to look for varicose veins, lipodermatosclerosis and evidence of phlebitis. Arterial assessment will include palpating pulses, looking for ischaemic changes and most importantly, measuring the ABPI with Doppler ultrasound.

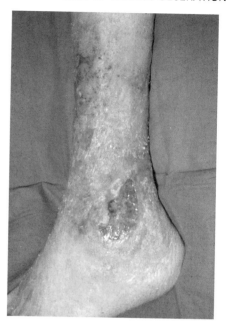

Fig. 1. A lateral venous ulcer in a patient with no arterial disease is best treated with multilayer compression bandaging.

Routine bacterial swabbing is *unnecessary* unless there is clinically active infection with evidence of cellulitis. It is possible to grow bacteria from all leg ulcers and their presence does not delay healing unless cellulitis develops. In fact, topical antibiotics may delay healing. In a prospective randomized trial comparing topical Flamazine with simple non-adherent dressings, both under a standard four-layer compression bandage, the healing rate for Flamazine was 63% compared with 77% for non-adherent dressings and 15% of the Flamazine group developed skin sensitivity to the topical antibiotic.[9]

As it has been established that compression therapy is the best way to treat venous ulcers, the most important aspect of the assessment is to exclude malignant and arterial ulcers. Compression bandaging can be applied to any leg with an ABPI of more than 0.8 and the NHS consensus conference guidelines suggest that anyone with an ABPI of less than 0.8 should be referred for vascular assessment, and in cases of ABPI less than 0.5, for an urgent appointment with the vascular surgeon.

A full venous assessment on all patients presenting with a venous ulcer is probably really only of academic interest. On the Wirral 62% of patients were over 75 years of age and 49% were housebound. Patients making up this significant part of the population with leg ulcers are, therefore, unlikely to want venous surgery, even if a full venous assessment shows that surgery would reduce recurrence. Therefore, in our practice, full venous assessment is reserved for those patients who might be suitable for surgery. The assessment includes simple Doppler insonation of the long and short saphenous veins to detect superficial venous incompetence and this is used in combination with photoplethysmography (PPG) to assess whether there is a functional improvement in venous return with tourniquets. If, with this simple screening process, patients are thought to have a correctable superficial venous disease, they then undergo colour duplex scanning of superficial veins prior to surgery[23] (Fig. 2).

Those patients with arterial disease will undergo standard assessment with colour duplex scanning and arteriography as appropriate.

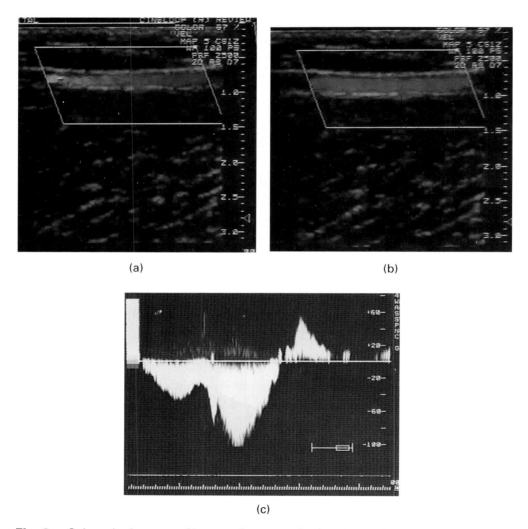

(a)   (b)

(c)

Fig. 2.   Colour duplex scan of long saphenous vein showing (a) flow towards the heart; (b) reflux towards the ground; and (c) the Doppler wave form in the vein on calf compression and then reflux back down the vein.

TREATMENT

Cleansing

Cleansing of the leg ulcer should be kept as simple as possible. Strict asepsis is unnecessary but a clean technique aimed at preventing cross-infection is important. Antiseptics are not advisable and are generally unnecessary and the cleansing should not involve scrubbing the wound with gauze or cotton wool as this will remove granulation tissue and early epithelializing tissue. Ideally the leg should be soaked in a bucket lined with a plastic bag using warm tap water and then dabbing the leg dry. This enables superficial desquamated skin to be washed off without traumatizing the healing ulcer. Scabs should be removed with forceps as compression on top of them can lead to further ulceration and necrotic and devitalized tissue should be removed by sharp debridement using a scalpel. Chemical debridement is not recommended as there is no evidence that it enhances healing and there is some evidence that it may have deleterious effects on cells in the healing wound (Fig. 3).

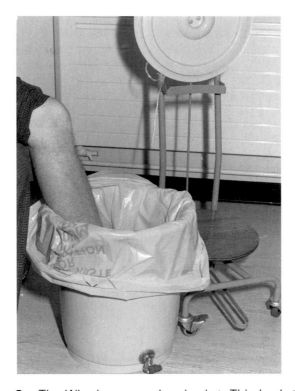

Fig. 3. The Wirral venous ulcer bucket. This bucket on wheels enables a patient leg to be soaked inside a plastic bag. When the patient has finished, the bag is torn and the bucket emptied by a tap. The nurses do not need to lift heavy buckets and risk back injuries and spillage. Cross-infection between patients is prevented.

Dressings and topical preparations

In the Stockport and Trafford study[1] a total of 113 different dressings and topical preparations were being applied. On the Wirral this was somewhat less as only 39 different agents were used. The array of different treatments being applied by district nurses indicates that it does not really matter what you put on an ulcer, it is not going to change the healing rate since healing is achieved with compression. It is, therefore, logical to use the most simple dressing which does not adhere and is cheap. Ideally it should enable exudate to go through it so that the surrounding skin does not become macerated. This increases the comfort to the patient and by being non-adherent, enables easy removal. There are very few trials with standardized compression over different dressings or topical preparations but a number of trials used them with control subjects where the healing rate was of the order of 25%. In one prospective randomized trial there were three arms – one using a hydrocolloid dressing, one using Flamazine and one using a non-adherent dressing (NA) (Johnson and Johnson). Overlying these, a standard four-layer compression bandage was applied. In the Flamazine group 63% healed in 12 weeks, with hydrocolloid dressings 73% healed and with non-adherent dressings 77% healed within 12 weeks.[9]

The one exception to this rule is where there is active venous eczema separate from the area of ulceration and a moderately potent steroid ointment such as clobetasone butyrate 0.05% may be of use. However, this should not be applied to the ulcer directly and should be withdrawn as soon as the eczema has settled.

If the skin of the leg is just dry without evidence of any eczema, a simple emollient to soothe and hydrate the skin such as arachis oil is useful.

Compression therapy

Compression therapy is the most important element in treating venous leg ulcers and the consensus conference concluded that graduated multilayer compression systems capable of sustaining compression for at least a week should be available to all patients with venous leg ulceration. The essential components of a graduated multilayer compression system are that it should provide adequate padding to relieve pressure over bony high points such as the tibia and the malleoli and also provide an absorptive area for the exudate from the ulcer. Compression should be adequate, in the region of 40 mmHg at the ankle and be achieved through the elasticity of the bandages rather than the strength of the bandager in order to have a reproducible amount of pressure applied. The compression system should be able to stay in place for at least a week without slippage or reduced compression.

The original multilayer compression system known as the four-layer bandage was developed at Charing Cross Hospital and consists of a first layer of Velband (Johnson and Johnson) which is a cotton wool layer. This was then smoothed over with a crepe bandage and compression applied with a stretchy Elset bandage (Seton). The final and fourth layer was Coband (3M) which is a self-adherent but non-sticky bandage. Using this system in outpatients 148 chronic ulcers with a mean ulcer area of 15.4 cm^2 were treated for a 12-week period, at the end of which 74% of ulcers were healed.[10] (Fig. 4).

This system which produced a mean pressure at the ankle of 42 mmHg on

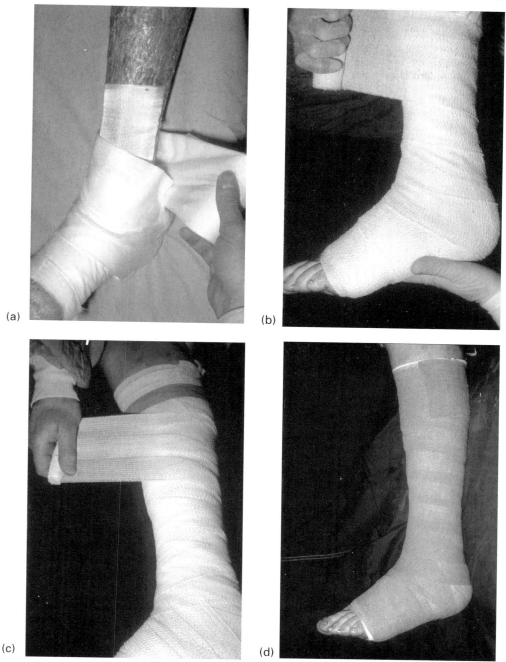

Fig. 4. Four-layer bandage. (a) A wool bandage over a simple non-adherent dressing (Johnson and Johnson). This protects bony high points from excess pressure; (b) A crepe bandage to provide a smooth base for pressure to be applied. (c) Compression bandage applied at mid-stretch with two-thirds overlap in a figure of 8. (d) Self-adherent bandage which is not sticky but prevents bandage slipping down or becoming loose for over a week.

application, falling to 37 mmHg at the end of 1 week was applicable to average ankles with a circumference of 18–25 cm. However, for people with very small ankles identical bandaging will produce too high a pressure and for larger ankles too small a pressure is achieved. In response to this, a single pack four-layer bandage is now available under the trade name of Profore (Smith and Nephew) and these are graded for ankle circumference so that the appropriate bandages can be applied.

These initial results were then used to provide a community-based study in Riverside, London where in 2 years 550 venous ulcers were treated. There were no exclusions and a 2% non-compliance rate. By 12 weeks 69% of venous ulcers had completely healed and 83% had healed by 24 weeks. Patients with an ABPI between 0.5 and 0.8 were treated with reduced compression and they still achieved a 56% healing rate at 12 weeks and a 75% healing rate at 24 weeks.[11]

In a separate study comparing two adjacent health authorities at Stockport and Trafford, the healing rate of venous ulcers was increased in 3 months from 26% to 42% in Stockport, whereas in Trafford, where four-layer bandages were not introduced, the healing rate changed from 23% to 20% over a similar period. However, where the four-layer bandage was introduced through clinics as opposed to being administered at the patient's home, the healing rate was 65% in 3 months.[1]

Similarly, on the Wirral, the introduction of four-layer bandaging as part of the guidelines which were implemented has resulted in an improved healing rate of 47% at 12 weeks and 82% at 24 weeks across the whole community. The healing rate is better in specific community ulcer clinics and this could either be because totally immobile patients who are unable to get to clinics may have a poorer healing rate, or that the expertise developed within a clinic means that more effective consistent treatment is applied leading to a higher healing rate. It is also pertinent to note that the healing rate achieved in Riverside improved over their 2-year study period. The healing rate in the first 3 months was 55%. A year later their 3-month healing rate had risen to 86%. This indicates that introducing an effective venous ulcer treatment takes longer to heal large chronic ulcers but that over time as they are removed from the population, the healing rate improves. This is further supported by the progressive fall in prevalence of venous ulcers in Riverside of 20% per annum – in 1988 the number of patients suffering from venous ulcers was 475 and by 1993 this was reduced to 144.[12]

The effectiveness of four-layer bandaging has been confirmed in a prospective randomized trial in Edinburgh where 200 ulcers were randomized to either four-layer bandage or a new Granuflex single-layer compression bandage which had been shown to produce 40 mmHg pressure at the ankle. At 24 weeks 69% of the four-layer bandage group had healed which was significantly more than the 49% treated with Granuflex compression bandage p<.003.[13]

Other compression systems

On the Wirral 33 different types of bandages and compression devices were being used in different combinations and yet a full review of the literature revealed very few studies with large enough numbers to make any significant conclusions. Indeed, the majority of bandages being used are not reported in the literature as a treatment for venous ulcers. A variety of different paste bandages are available. These have frequently been used in control groups and have consistently performed less well than high compression bandaging with healing rates of 20–28%.

Short stretch bandages are used more in Europe and again research evidence of their benefit is limited. One such bandage is Rosidal K which healed 71% of 26 ulcers over 12 weeks. However, the bandages have to be changed up to three times a week because they do not maintain their pressure as the oedema in the leg goes down. With such small numbers it is impossible to say if this is a meaningful result using statistical power analysis. Any prospective randomized trial needs to have a minimum of 200 patients in order to show a 15% difference between two treatment groups.[14]

Two prospective randomized trials of single-layer short stretch bandage vs four-layer bandage have been attempted. One trial had to be abandoned as more than 30% of the short stretch group found they could not keep their bandage from falling off and the remaining patients in that group, having seen the results of other patients in the clinic, withdrew their informed consent. In the other trial additional layers were added to keep the single layer up.

Finally, a three-layer bandage system has been described made up of wool, Tensopress and then shaped Tubigrip. Of 65 patients treated with this, 12% were withdrawn due to bandage slippage leaving an overall 48% healing rate in 12 weeks. Again the number of patients involved make it impossible to know how effective this really is[15] (Table 1).

Table 1. Trials involving more than 100 patients with venous ulcers

Reference	No. of ulcers	Bandage	Healed at 12 weeks (%)	Healed at 24 weeks (%)
10	148	Four-layer	74	
11	550	Four-layer	68	82
15	65	Three-layer Tensopress	48	
	67	Three-layer Tensoplus Forte	28	
13	100	Four-layer		69
	100	Single-layer		49 p = 0.003
1	252	Nurses choice	26	
	233	Four-layer	42 p <0.001	
	416	Nurses choice	21	
Wirral	622	Nurses choice	24	
	209	Four-layer	47 p <0.001	82

Pain management

All patients with leg ulcers experience a varying amount of pain. Pain may relate to underlying pathology such as arterial disease or acute infection, in which case the underlying cause needs to be actively treated. However, uncomplicated venous ulcers can also be very painful, particularly where they are large. Adequate opioid analgesia may be required in order to make patients pain-free and, therefore, able to walk around and use their calf muscle pumps to increase the healing rate.

Prevention of recurrence of ulceration

A highly selected group of fit patients with superficial venous disease are suitable for corrective venous surgery and this does reduce the recurrence rate. However, the mainstay of prevention in the majority of people will be compression stockings being worn below the knee.[16,17] A Class II compression stocking providing pressure of between 18 and 24 mmHg is used normally as this is not too difficult to get on as long as the patient does not suffer from arthritis and have difficulty in bending fingers and knees.[18]

Two drugs have been tried to reduce the incidence of recurrence. Oxerutins and Oxpentifylline. Neither of these drugs in prospective randomized trials against placebo showed benefit for the active drug.[13,19]

HOW TO IMPLEMENT A COMMUNITY VENOUS ULCER PROGRAMME

There are three models which have now been tried and the main difference relates to the geography of the area being cared for.

Community ulcer clinics

This system is most applicable to city areas where there are short distances to be travelled and where communications are good. In Riverside District in London six community ulcer clinics were established and a modified ambulance was used to collect patients from their homes if they were unable to get to the clinic on their own. This was outside of the normal ambulance service and reduced waiting times for patients before and after clinics. This system means that relatively few nurses had to be fully trained in the management of venous ulcers. It is easy logistically to make sure that the necessary bandages are together and that the basic cleaning equipment and space to do bandaging is available. This system has the advantage of a small group of nurses becoming highly skilled in the management of venous ulcers and its complications. It significantly reduces the nursing time involved in looking after these patients as if the nurse goes to the patient, there is normally at least 30 minutes travelling time between patients. Furthermore, when dressing large and difficult ulcers which require two nurses at the same time, much time and effort is saved by having them in the clinic rather than travelling separately to patients' homes. The clinics have had the unexpected benefit of significantly improving the quality of life of these patients as many of them have not been outdoors or met other people for a long time. They have felt isolated and not realised that others are suffering from the same condition. Their quality of life has been improved by meeting fellow sufferers over a cup of tea and making friends. In the Wirral study, it would have been possible for 80% of patients to have been able to be treated in this type of clinic and yet before the start of the pilot study, 80% of patients were treated in isolation at home.

The community ulcer clinics have been highly efficient and as reported earlier, once established, have achieved a healing rate of 86% over 12 weeks. They have also led to significant reduction in the prevalence of venous ulcers. In addition the team of nurses in the clinics can continue to keep up their expertise.

Universal training

District nurses are not trained to treat venous ulcers and therefore a programme to train all district nurses can be set up. On the Wirral peninsular 120 nurses underwent a 2-day training course on bandage technique and ulcer care. In addition, there are six locality venous ulcer nurses who have undergone a 2-week ENB training course so they can provide back-up for the individual nurses. Unfortunately, there are still problems. Training is expensive to set up, with costs in the region of £30 000. A large number of Dopplers also need to be purchased so that they are accessible to all district nurses in their venous assessments. There are logistic problems when treating patients in their own homes, particularly the soaking of legs to remove desquamated skin to keep ulcers clean as many homes are not suitable for the carrying of large buckets of water around. Treatment of ulcers continues to be a very time consuming, particularly when more than one nurse is required.Even with the implementation of four-layer bandaging, and the reduction of the average twice weekly visits by nurses to a single visit each week, the total nursing time did not fall significantly. As mentioned earlier in Stockport, although the overall healing rate following implementation of four-layer bandaging increased from 26% to 42%, this was not as high as the 65% healing rate among those treated in a clinic. Therefore, we propose that where it is physically possible, ulcer clinics should be established so that the best practice and the highest healing rates can be achieved.

Cascade system

In rural areas such as Scotland, it is not possible easily to set up community ulcer clinics as patients may be many miles apart in remote areas. On the other hand, as illustrated on the Wirral, training all district nurses to treat venous ulcers can be quite an expensive undertaking. The proposed implementation in Scotland, therefore, of four-layer bandaging will start with specialist nurses undergoing a full 2-week ENB training course. These nurses will then cascade information down to nurses in rural areas and will train and oversee them applying bandages once the initial assessment has been made of patients suitability.

Training

Within each district there needs to be a number of nurses with a specialist interest in venous ulcers who have undergone a 2-week course to fully understand the aetiology and management of ulcers and their complications. However, for other nurses involved in treating ulcers under their supervision, a much briefer training is required and there are good training packages now available with videos, etc, which enable people to be trained in good bandage technique, Doppler assessment of arterial pressures, and the basics of wound care management. It should be pointed out that the majority of venous ulcers in the UK are, in fact, treated by nurses. On the Wirral, the treatment of venous ulcers was originally provided for 10% of patients through the hospital and 0.5% by the GP. Therefore, 90% were treated by practice nurses and district nurses and they were the principal people choosing treatments, with General Practitioners instigating treatment in only 12% of cases. This is particularly worrying as the district nurses maintained that their total training on venous ulcers both in their primary and district nurse training added up to a total of 1 hour. When they were asked where they got their information about wound care products, 55% took their advice from a colleague and 24% took their advice from pharmaceutical representatives; only 14% would consult a doctor.

COSTS

The costs of venous ulcers have been fairly thoroughly investigated and can be broken down into the costs of materials needed and the associated costs of nursing care and hospital admissions. In Stockport and Trafford a full investigation of all ulcers being treated over a 3-month period showed that the average annual cost for a patient with an active leg ulcer was £2356. The weekly cost of materials was £10.28 in Stockport, £9.07 in Trafford £8.47 on the Wirral and £9.67 in Riverside per patient per week. It is interesting how close these figures are to one another across the country although all these figures are more expensive than Profore four-layer bandage, which at the time of these studies cost about £5.50 per patient per week.

In Riverside between 1989 and 1991, while the healing rate improved from 22% to 68%, the total National Health Service cost fell from £433 600 to £169 000. In the Stockport and Trafford study in 1993/1994, the healing rate improved from 26% to 42% and the costs dropped from £409 991 to £253 371 in Stockport, whereas in the adjacent district of Trafford where four-layer bandaging was not introduced, the healing rate went from 23% to 20% and the costs went from £556 039 up to £673 318. On the Wirral, the annual saving in material costs alone was £72 843 for one year.[2, 20–21, 22]

CONCLUSION

Following proper assessment of leg ulcers the majority of venous ulcers can be rapidly healed using a four-layer bandage with up to 86% being healed within 3 months. This has resulted in a real fall in prevalence of ulcers of 20% per year. While time needs to be invested to set up an effective venous ulcer service, the cost savings are high. However, implementation of a venous ulcer programme is difficult as the nurses who carry out treatment do not have the political muscle to instigate a new integrated treatment for venous ulcers. Vascular surgeons should take up the challenge of introducing a comprehensive ulcer service to benefit patients and ensure that they receive appropriate referrals.

REFERENCES

1. Simon DA, Freak L, Kinsella A et al.: Community leg ulcer clinics: a comparative study in two health authorities. Br Med J 312: 1648–1651, 1996
2. Bosanquet N: Costs of venous ulcers: from maintenance therapy to investment programmes. Phlebology 7 (Suppl 1): 44–46, 1992

3. Laing W: *Chronic Venous Ulcers of the Leg*. London: Office of Health Economics, 1992
4. Cornwall JV, Dore CJ, Lewis JD: Leg ulcers: epidemiology and aetiology. *Br J Surg* **73:** 693–696, 1996
5. Baker SR, Stacey MC, Jopp-McKay AG, *et al.*: Epidemiology of chronic venous ulcers. *Br J Surg* **78:** 864–867, 1991
6. Callam NJ, Harper DR, Dale JJ, Ruckley CV: Chronic ulcer of the leg: clinical history. *Br Med J* **294:** 1389–1391, 1987
7. Baker SR, Stacey MC, Singh G *et al.*: Aetiology of chronic leg ulcers. *Eur J Vasc Surg* **6:** 245–251, 1992
8. Fowkes FGR, Callam NJ: Is arterial disease a risk factor for chronic leg ulceration? *Phlebology* **9:** 87–90, 1994
9. Blair SD, Backhouse CM, McCollum CN: Do dressings affect the healing of chronic venous ulcers? *Phlebology* **3:** 129–134, 1988
10. Blair SD, Backhouse CM, McCollum CN, *et al.*: Sustained compression and healing of chronic venous ulcers. *Br Med J* **297:** 1159–1161, 1988
11. Moffatt CJ, Franks PJ, Greenhalgh RM, McCollum CN, *et al.*: Community clinics for leg ulcers and impact on healing. *Br Med J* **305:** 1389–1392, 1992
12. Moffatt CJ, Franks PJ, Greenhalgh RM: Community leg ulcer clinics: a four-year review. *Proceedings 3rd European Conference on Advances in Wound Management, Oct 19–22 1993*. London: MacMillan Magazines, 1994
13. Nelson EA, Harper DR, Ruckley CV, *et al.*: Single layer versus four layer bandaging in the treatment of venous ulcers; A randomised controlled trial. *Br J Surg* **83:** 563, 1996
14. Charles, H: Compression healing of venous ulcers. *Nursing Times* **3:** 52, 1992
15. Callam NJ, Harper DR, Dale JJ, *et al.*: Lothian and Forth Valley leg ulcer healing trial, Part 1: Elastic versus non-elastic bandaging in the treatment of chronic leg ulceration. *Phlebology* **7:** 136–41, 1992
16. Gillies TE, Ruckey CV: Does Surgery Play Any Part in the Management of Venous Ulcers? Greenhalgh RM, Fowkes FGR (Eds) *Trials and Tribulations of Vascular Surgery* pp. 411–422. London: WB Saunders, 1995
17. Negus D, Friedgood A: The effective management of venous ulceration. *Br J Surg* **70:** 623, 1983
18. Moffatt CJ: Recurrence of leg ulcers within a community ulcer service. *J Wound Care*; **4:** 57–61, 1995
19. Wright DDI, Blair SD, McCollum CN, *et al.*: Oxerutins in the prevention of recurrence in chronic venous ulceration: Randomised controlled trial. *Br J Surg* **78:** 1269–1270, 1991
20. Tighe M, Greaney MG, Blair SD: What is the price of not having guidelines for the management of venous ulcers? *Br J Surg* **83** (Suppl) 50: 1996
21. Bosanquet N, Franks P, Moffatt C, *et al.*: Community leg ulcer clinics: cost effectiveness. *Health Trends* **24:** 146–148, 1993
22. Freak L, Simon D, Kinsella A, McCollum CN: Leg ulcer care: An audit of cost effectiveness. *Health Trends* **27:** 133–136, 1995
23. Grabs AJ, Wakely MC, Nyamekye I *et al.*: Colour duplex ultrasonography in the rational management of chronic venous leg ulcers. *Br J Surg* **83:** 1380–1382, 1996

The Unhealed Venous Ulcer

C. V. Ruckley and A. W. Bradbury

INTRODUCTION

One could be forgiven for concluding, on perusal of the recent literature, that the vascular surgeon has largely overcome the difficulties associated with the treatment of chronic leg ulceration. Epidemiological studies have defined the scale and nature of the disease;[1-4] effective bandaging systems and dressings have been developed and successfully evaluated in clinical trials;[5] and panels of experts have published consensus statements[6] and National Guidelines.[7] Armed with hand-held Doppler ultrasound devices. evidence-based protocols and treatment algorithms,[8] an evangelical army of hospital trained nurse specialists will take their skills into the community, and lo, leg ulcers will surely be a thing of the past?

Of course the reality of the situation is quite different. While improvements in community leg ulcer services have been shown to impact positively on healing rates,[9,10] there remains a significant proportion of patients whose ulcers either cannot be healed or cannot be prevented from recurring. Such patients suffer long-term morbidity,[11] are a source of disappointment and frustration for their attendants, and represent a major financial burden on health and social services.[12] Furthermore, given that the prevalence of leg ulceration peaks in the eighth decade of life, and that the elderly population will continue to grow well into the next millennium, the clinical problems posed by the intractable leg ulcer are likely to increase.

It is also our perception that the nature of chronic leg ulceration changes with age. As mobility, healing and nutritional status decline,[13] and the prevalence of arterial disease rises,[14] the proportion of chronic leg ulcers which are 'purely venous', and therefore readily amenable to standard compression therapy, diminishes. As a result, having 'cured' the 'easy' ulcers, we sense that we are now increasingly faced with a population of frail, elderly patients with complex ulcers and an accumulation of adverse risk factors.[15]

Many questions relating to these patients remain unanswered. For example, how does one define the intractable ulcer and what are its characteristics? Can we predict at the outset which ulcers will be resistant to community-based treatment so that increasingly scarce hospital resources can be targeted at those patients most likely to benefit? Does surgery, and in particular the new technique of subfascial perforating vein ligation (SEPS) have anything to offer? The aim of this paper is to address some of these questions through analysis of the epidemiological and clinical studies undertaken by the Lothian and Forth Valley Leg Ulcer Group and through a preliminary audit of the Edinburgh Royal Infirmary Leg Ulcer Clinic between 1984 and 1995.

EPIDEMIOLOGICAL STUDIES

How should ulcer healing be defined?

Re-epithelialization would seem the most obvious endpoint for any wound-healing regimen, but in chronic leg ulceration this is all too often a transient phenomenon with early recurrence being the rule rather than the exception. Thus, while the duration of a single ulcer episode can usually be measured in months, the duration of ulcer disease is usually measured in years or even decades. It could be argued, therefore, that sustained healing is the only worthy endpoint of any treatment programme.

Callam identified 1477 patients with chronic leg ulceration of whom 600 (827 legs) were entered into a cross-sectional cohort study.[16] Of these, 22% had first developed ulceration before the age of 40 years; 66% had suffered multiple recurrences extending over a period of 5 years or more; 50% had an ulcer history dating back more than 10 years; and 33% had never healed their first ulcers – most of which had been present for more than a year and a fifth for more than 5 years. Baker found that the longest time an ulcer had remained unhealed was 26 weeks in 60% of their 259 patients, and 2 years in 23%.[2] Ulcer history dated back more than 5 years in 47%, and more than 10 years in 34%. Recurrent ulceration affected more than 75% of the population with 28% reporting more than 10 episodes. Similarly, both Cornwall[17] and Nelzen[18] found that 50% of ulcers had been present for more than 12 months.

CLINICAL TRIALS

What healing rates can be expected from medical management?

Trial protocols, by virtue of their inclusion and exclusion criteria, inevitably result in the selection of patients likely to exhibit better overall responses to treatment than can be expected in the generality of the disease population.

In a study of 56 patients, the Charing Cross group reported complete healing of ulceration in 75–78% of patients at 12 weeks using multilayer compression therapy.[19] Excellent though these results are, it must be remembered that this still leaves the 25% of patients who did not heal their ulcer, that the ulcers were small ($< 10 \text{ cm}^2$), and that ulcers of non-venous aetiology were excluded.

We have conducted a number of randomized controlled clinical trials in this area under the auspices of the Lothian and Forth Valley leg ulcer group. In none of these have we observed healing rates that approach those cited above. For example, in a trial of therapeutic ultrasound and standard compression treatment versus standard compression alone, although healing rates were 20% higher with ultrasound, less than 60% of patients were healed at 12 weeks.[20] In a trial of elastic compression versus limited stretch compression healing rates were 54% and 28% respectively at 12 weeks;[21] and in a comparison of a non-adherent knitted viscose versus hydrocolloid dressing healing rates were 35% and 47% respectively.[22] Where single layer compression has been compared with multilayer compression in a trial of 200 patients with chronic venous ulceration, healing rates at 24 weeks of 49% and 69% respectively have been obtained.[23,24] In a randomized, double-blind controlled trial of placebo versus oxipentifylline in the treatment of venous ulceration, although healing rates were significantly better in the treated group, 34% of patients still remained unhealed at 24 weeks.[25]

Healing rates in ulcers where there is an arterial component, as demonstrated by an ankle brachial pressure index (ABPI) of less than 0.8, are even more disappointing. In a randomized, double-blind, controlled trial of placebo versus oxipentifylline in the treatment of 41 such ulcers, only 1 of 19 (5%) untreated and 7 of 32 (32%) treated ulcers were healed at 24 weeks.[26] In a study comparing non-adherent with hydrocolloid dressing in mixed arteriovenous ulcers the trial had to be stopped after 22 patients because of 100% withdrawal from the non-adherent group due to pain, and 33% withdrawal from the hydrocolloid group due to skin maceration, cellulitis or ulcer deterioration.[27]

In summary therefore, despite the favourable effect of selecting suitable patients for clinical trials, and the close attention of hospital-based leg ulcer nurse specialists, we still fail to heal 30–40% of venous ulcers, and perhaps 50–60% of mixed arteriovenous ulcers over a 6-month period. The situation is likely to be worse than this in the community. For example, in the Edinburgh studies only 50% of leg ulcers were healed after 9 months of community nursing care; and in Newcastle 50% of ulcers remained unhealed at 6 months.[28]

Can medical therapy prevent recurrence?

Once an ulcer is healed what can be done to prevent recurrence? In a 5-year follow-up of 300 consecutive patients with healed venous ulcers, subjects were randomized to either Class 2 or Class 3 graduated compression.[29] Patients were closely supervised by leg ulcer nurses throughout the follow-up period. Compression hosiery was carefully fitted and renewed 6 monthly. In the Class 2 and Class 3 groups compliance rates were 89% and 75%, and recurrence rates 32% and 21% respectively. Recurrence was significantly more frequent in the non-compliant patients. Thus one-fifth to one-third of patients suffer recurrence of venous ulcer with conservative treatment even when closely supervised and supported.[30]

Is there a role for surgery?

Forty-three patients undergoing superficial varicose vein surgery plus open perforating vein ligation (Linton's procedure) were followed for a median of 66 (range 18–44) months. Of these, nine developed recurrence and this was strongly associated with the presence of popliteal vein incompetence as shown by colour flow duplex ultrasound.[31] In another study of 53 patients undergoing Linton's procedure, with or without saphenous surgery, the recurrence rate was 23% and the median time to recurrence was 48 (range 10–72) months.[32] In neither study was there a control group for comparison and, indeed, to our knowledge there has never been a prospective randomized controlled trial of best medical therapy versus best medical therapy plus surgery in this condition. Nevertheless, many experts in the field extol the benefits of correcting saphenous[33,34] and perforator[35] incompetence in these patients. This topic has been reviewed previously in more detail and it is concluded that, while surgery probably does play a beneficial role in some cases, there is an urgent need for controlled trials in this area.[36]

AUDIT OF AN OUTPATIENT LEG ULCER CLINIC

In order to obtain a 'warts and all' picture of what can be achieved in a hospital-based leg ulcer clinic we have audited the work carried out in the Edinburgh Royal Infirmary between 1 January 1984 and 31 December 1995; a 12-year period. Patient demographic and outcome data are recorded on a standard proforma at the time of initial assessment, during subsequent treatment, and then entered into a computerized database. A preliminary analysis of these data has identified a total of 914 new patients with unilateral ulceration who, at the time of writing, had completed their first treatment episode at the clinic. There were 307 men (median age 61, range 17–86 years) and 607 women (median age 72, range 27–97 years, p < 0.01 Mann–Whitney U-test). The aetiology of the ulcer was predominantly venous in 675 (74%), predominantly arterial in 40 (4.5%)%, and mixed arteriovenous in 83 patients (9%). There has been a steady increase in the number of new patients attending the clinic each year (Fig. 1). There has also been a significant change in the aetiology of ulcers. For example, in the period 1984–1986, 286 of 367 (78%) ulcers were predominantly venous, whereas in the period 1990–1995 this had fallen to 387 of 547 (71%, p < 0.02 by Fisher's exact test, FET). At the same time there was an increase in

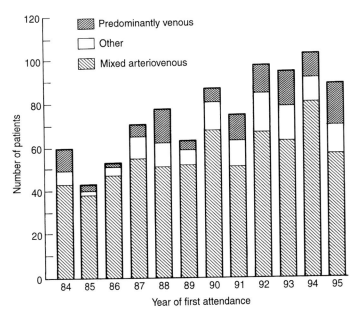

Fig. 1.   Chronic leg ulcers by year of first presentation to the leg ulcer clinic and aetiology.

the proportion of patients with an arterial component to their ulceration, and an increase in those ulcers that possessed non-arterial, non-venous factors. For example, there was significant increase in the proportion of patients who were diabetic (12/367, 3%, vs 50/547, 9%, p < 0.001, FET) and who had clinical and/or serological evidence of rheumatoid disease (17/367, 5%, vs 44/547, 8%, p = 0.05, FET). A total of 196 patients (21%) had a history of ulceration dating back more than 10 years and 71 patients (8%) more than 25 years. The median number of episodes of previous ulceration was 3 (range 1–14) and 116 patients (13%) reported more than 10 previous episodes. The median duration of current ulceration was 6 months (range 1–408 months). Complete healing while still attending the leg ulcer clinic was reported in 578 (63%) ulcers. Patients with non-healing ulcers were more likely to be female, to have had their current ulcer for longer, and to have an arterial component to their ulceration (Table 1, Fig. 2). Total duration of ulcer disease, number of previous episodes, and age did not appear to significantly affect healing.

Table 1 Characteristics of patients with non-healing and healing leg ulcers

Parameter	Healed n = 578 (63%)	Unhealed n = 336 (36%)	p value
Age (mean, years)	64.5	66.5	NS
Male patients	209 (36%)	98 (29%)	< 0.05[b]
Male age (mean, years)	60	61	NS
Female patients	369 (64%)	238 (71%)	< 0.05[b]
Female age (mean years)	72	73	NS
Duration current ulcer in months (mean, median and range)	11, 5, 1-280	25, 9, 3-408	< 0.05[c]
Time since first ulcer in months[a] (mean, median and range)	150, 84, 2-840	150, 120, 4-720	NS
Previous episodes[a] (mean, median and range)	3.5, 3, 1-9	3.5, 4, 1-14	NS
Aetiology			
Venous	488 (84.5%)	187 (56%)	< 0.05[b]
Arterial	8 (1.5%)	32 (9.5%)	
Arteriovenous	41 (7%)	42 (12.5%)	
Other	41 (7%)	75 (22.5%)	
Presence of diabetes	27 (5%)	35 (10.5%)	< 0.05[b]
Presence of rheumatoid disease	28 (5%)	33 (10%)	< 0.05[b]

[a] Data are based on those patients with recurrent ulceration; [b] Fisher's exact test; [c] Mann-Whitney U-test; NS = not significant.

PATTERNS OF VENOUS REFLUX AND DELAYED HEALING

In all, 155 patients with chronic venous ulceration underwent duplex ultra-sonography prior to 6 months of compression therapy in our leg ulcer clinic.[37] At 24 weeks, 104 (67%) ulcers had healed. There was no significant difference in the pattern

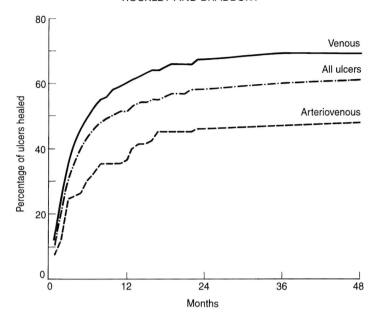

Fig. 2.   The effect of ulcer aetiology on healing.

of deep and superficial venous reflux between the healed and non-healed group except at the popliteal segment (Table 2). In healed legs, 39 (38%) scans indicated competence of the above-knee popliteal vein (PV) compared with 5 (10%) scans in the non-healing group (p < 0.001 by χ^2 test). Similarly, 44 (43%) scans showed below-knee PV competence in the healed group compared with only five (10%) scans performed in leg remaining ulcerated (p < 0.001 by χ^2 test). Four of 42 (10%) patients with competent, and 45 of 103 (44%) patients with incompetent, above- and below-knee PV failed to heal (sensitivity 40%, specificity 90%, positive predictive value 40%, negative predictive value 90%). Therefore PV incompetence appears to exert a strong negative impact on the ability of standard compression to heal venous leg ulceration.

In another study, we identified 54 patients from the large leg ulcer population described above who possessed the following characteristics: current ulceration confined to one leg; no current or previous ulceration in the contralateral leg; not diabetic; ankle brachial pressure index (ABPI) of > 0.8 in both legs; no clinical evidence of significant lower limb arterial disease; no clinical or serological evidence of connective tissue disorder; no previous major venous surgery in either leg; and no evidence of a malignant aetiology.[38] Application of these strict criteria clearly excluded the vast majority of patients but did define a population of patients whose ulcer would almost certainly be diagnosed as one of 'pure' venous aetiology by the great majority of clinicians. In addition, by excluding patients who had undergone major venous surgery, it is also a population that has not been tampered with surgically.

Table 2. Relationship between deep and superficial venous reflux and healing of chronic venous ulceration

Venous segment	No reflux	No reflux healed	Reflux	Reflux healed	p value
Long saphenous origin	24	18	108	70	0.47
Long saphenous mid-thigh	21	17	116	75	0.23
Short saphenous origin	35	28	110	69	0.09
Common femoral	25	21	127	80	0.072
Superficial femoral	53	35	98	65	0.89
Above-knee popliteal	44	39	110	64	0.001
Below-knee popliteal	49	44	105	59	0.001
Posterior tibial	52	36	79	51	0.72
Peroneal	54	37	53	34	0.78

Colour flow duplex ultrasonography of the deep and superficial venous systems of both legs was performed by a single consultant radiologist. Reflux was considered pathological if reverse flow exceeded 0.5 seconds. There was no significant difference between ulcerated and non-ulcerated legs with respect to the pattern of venous reflux except in the popliteal and tibial veins (Table 3). Thus, 42 ulcerated legs had proximal (above-knee) popliteal vein reflux compared with 30 non-ulcerated legs (p = 0.034, χ^2 = 4.53). Similarly, 39 ulcerated legs had distal (below-knee) popliteal vein reflux

Table 3. Patterns of venous reflux in ulcerated and non-ulcerated legs

Venous segment	Ulcerated leg			Non-ulcerated leg			p value[a]
	Reflux	No reflux	Not seen	Reflux	No reflux	Not seen	
Common femoral	45	8	1	42	12	–	NS
Superficial femoral (proximal)	30	23	1	26	28	–	NS
Superficial femoral (distal)	27	24	3	23	29	2	NS
Proximal popliteal	42	12	–	31	23	0	0.034
Distal popliteal	39	15	–	26	27	1	0.024
Posterior tibial	27	17	10	16	31	7	0.016
Anterior tibial	9	33	12	2	42	10	0.044
Peroneal	19	19	16	10	28	16	NS
Long saphenous (origin)	37	6	11	36	8	10	NS
Long saphenous (mid-thigh)	41	6	7	37	9	8	NS
Short saphenous (origin)	41	12	1	33	17	4	NS

[a] Statistical analysis takes into account informative scans only

compared with 26 non-ulcerated legs (p = 0.024, χ^2 = 5.09). The popliteal vein was visualized in all ulcerated legs and in all but one non-ulcerated leg. The proportion of uninformative scans was much higher when examining the crural veins making differences between ulcerated and non-ulcerated legs more difficult to interpret. Nevertheless, ulcerated legs were also significantly more likely to have venous reflux in the posterior tibial (27/44 vs 16/47 informative scans, p = 0.016, χ^2 = 5.75) and anterior tibial (9/42 vs 2/44 informative scans, p = 0.044, χ^2 = 4.08) veins than legs unaffected by chronic venous insufficiency.

For the individual patient there may be additional factors, perhaps at a microvascular level, which determine whether a particular pattern and severity of reflux leads to ulceration.[39,40] However, as we have no clear understanding of what these additional factors might be, or how to influence them, the surgeon must adopt a pragmatic approach. When contemplating surgery it would seem reasonable to advocate correction of that reflux which is present in the ulcerated but not present in the unaffected limb. In a minority of patients this entails superficial venous surgery alone and is straightforward. However, the present data confirm the results of earlier studies[41] that have demonstrated the importance of the popliteal vein in maintaining the clinical and haemodynamic normality of the calf.

CONCLUSIONS

Non-surgical therapy

A review of the available literature indicates that there is a substantial, but largely unpublicized, failure of non-surgical therapy in patients with chronic leg ulceration. Even in the most favourable circumstances where patients with small, pure venous ulcers are entered into trials conducted by interested groups, and cared for by specialist leg ulcer nurses, over one-third of patients fail to heal and the same proportion again suffer a recurrence of their ulcer within a few months or years. The results of epidemiological studies suggest that the overall picture is far worse than that painted by even this depressing scenario; and probably reflects the true situation in most communities. There is an urgent need for the principles of ulcer assessment and compression therapy to be exported from the hospital clinic, through community link nurses, to the generality of district nurses who, on average, spend one-third of their time dressing leg ulcers and yet may never have received any specialist training in this condition. It is astounding how may patients with chronic venous leg ulceration still attend our clinic having never received compression therapy, while at the same time we still see patients with arterial disease who have sustained tissue loss due to inappropriate bandaging.[42]

Surgical therapy

There is a natural reluctance to operate on elderly patients with open wounds especially since surgery has never been shown in a controlled trial to alter the natural history of venous ulceration. Nevertheless, excellent healing rates have been described following saphenous surgery in the absence of deep venous disease.[33]

Although, in our experience, only a small minority of venous ulcers are due to isolated superficial reflux, it is likely that saphenous surgery, perhaps together aggressive skin grafting, could be more widely used than it is at present. In patients with deep venous disease the situation is much less clear and heated debate continues over the role of deep venous reconstruction and endoscopic perforator division in this group of patients.[43] In patients with mixed arterial and venous ulcers, attention should be directed to the arterial component first and an aggressive approach to angiography, angioplasty and open surgery is appropriate.

Future studies

Three main areas can be identified where further studies are required if the current management of chronic leg ulceration is to be improved:

1. studies examining the effect of evidence-based treatment regimens and guidelines on healing rates achieved in the community;
2. studies aimed at identifying those patients with intractable ulcers who would most benefit from increasingly scarce hospital-based therapy;
3. therapeutic trials looking at the effect of best medical treatment, with and without various surgical interventions, on healing and recurrence rates.

These studies must include quality of life and health economic analyses so that purchasers can be persuaded to buy those treatments which are most effective. As such treatments will undoubtedly reduce the current wastage of resources on unproved, expensive, and ineffective therapy, it should also be possible to persuade the purchasers that funding research is in their own best interests.

REFERENCES

1. Callam MJ, Ruckley CV, Harper DR, Dale JJ: Chronic ulceration of the leg: extent of the problem and provision of care. *Br Med J* **290:** 1855–1856, 1985
2. Baker SR, Stacey MC, Jopp-McKay AG *et al.*: Epidemiology of chronic venous ulceration. *Br J Surg* **78:** 864–867, 1991
3. Nelzen O, Bergqvist D, Lindhagen A: Leg ulcer aetiology – a cross-sectional population survey. *J Vasc Surg* **14:** 557–564, 1991
4. Fowkes FGR: Epidemiology of chronic venous insufficiency. *Phlebology* **11:** 2–5, 1996
5. Moffatt CJ, Franks PJ, Oldroyd MI, Greenhalgh RM: Randomised trial of occlusive dressing in the treatment of chronic non-healing leg ulcers. *Phlebology* **7:** 105–107, 1992
6. Alexander House Group: Consensus paper on venous leg ulcers. *Phlebology* **7:** 48–58, 1992
7. Douglas WS, Simpson NB: Guidleines for the namagment of chronic venous leg ulceration. Report of a multidisciplinary workshop. *Br J Dermatol* **132:** 446–452, 1995
8. Nelson EA, Ruckley CV, Dale JJ, Morison M: The managment of leg ulcers. *J Wound Care* **5:** 73–76, 1996
9. Jopp-McKay AG, Stacey MC, Rohr JB *et al.*: Out-patient treatment of chronic venous ulcers in a specialised clinic. *Aust J Dermatol* **32:** 143–149, 1991
10. Moffatt CJ, Frank PJ, Oldroyd M *et al.*: Community clinics for leg ulcers and impact on healing. *Br Med J* **305:** 1389–1392, 1992
11. Callam MJ, Harper DR, Dale JJ, Ruckley CV: Chronic leg ulceration: socio-economic aspects. *Scot Med J* **33:** 358–360, 1988
12. Laing W: *Chronic Venous Diseases of the Leg.* London: Office of Health Economics, 1992

13. Lewis BK, Hitchings H, Bale S, Harding KG: Nutritional status of elderly patients with venous ulceration of the leg – report of a pilot study. *J Hum Nutr Diet* **6**: 509–515, 1993

14. Callam MJ: Arterial disease in chronic leg ulceration: an underestimated hazard? Lothian and Forth Valley leg ulcer study. *Br Med J* **294**: 929–931, 1987

15. McRorie ER, Jobanputra P, Ruckley CV, Nuki G: Leg ulceration in rheumatoid arthritis. *Br J Rheumatol* **33**: 1078–1084, 1994

16. Callam MJ, Harper DR, Dale JJ, Ruckley CV: Chronic ulcer of the leg: clinical history. *Br Med J* **294**: 1389–1391, 1987

17. Cornwall JV, Dore CJ, Lewis JD: Leg ulcers: epidemiology and aetiology. *Br J Surg* **73**: 693–696, 1986

18. Nelzen O, Bergqvist D, Lindhagen A: Venous and non-venous leg ulcers: clinical history and appearance in a population study. *Br J Surg* **81**: 182–187, 1994

19. Backhouse CM, Blair SD, Walton J, McCollum A: A controlled trial of occlusive dressings in the healing of chronic venous ulcers. *Br J Surg* **74**: 626–627, 1987

20. Callam MJ, Harper DR, Dale JJ *et al.*: A controlled trial of weekly ultrasound therapy in chronic leg ulceration. *Lancet* **i**: 204–206, 1987

21. Callam MJ, Harper DR, Dale JJ *et al.*: Lothian and Forth Valley leg ulcer healing trial, part 1: elastic versus non-elastic bandaging in the treatment of chronic leg ulceration. *Phlebology* **7**: 136–141, 1992

22. Callam MJ, Harper DR, Dale JJ *et al.*: Lothian and Forth Valley leg ulcer healing trial, part 2: Knitted viscose dressing versus a hydrocellular dressing in the treatment of chronic leg ulceration. *Phlebology* **7**: 142–145, 1992

23. Nelson EA, Harper DR, Ruckley CV *et al.*: A randomised trial of single layer and multi-layer bandages in the treatment of chronic venous ulceration. *Phlebology* Suppl 1 852, 1995

24. Nelson EA, Harper DR, Ruckley CV *et al.*: A randomised trial of single layer and multi-layer bandages in the treatment of chronic venous ulceration. *Phlebology* Suppl 1 915–916, 1995

25. Dale JJ, Ruckley CV, Harper DR *et al.*: A randomised, double-blind, placebo controlled trial of oxipentifylline in the treatment of venous leg ulcers. *Phlebology* Suppl 1 917–918, 1995

26. Prescott RJ, Ruckley CV, Harper DR *et al.*: Results of a randomised, double-blind, placebo controlled trial of oxipentifylline in the treatment of arterial leg ulcers. *Phlebology* Suppl1 938, 1995

27. Gibson B, Harper DR, Nelson EA *et al.*: A comparison of a hydrocolloid and a knitted viscose dressing in the treatment of arterial leg ulcers. *Phlebology* Suppl 1 1071–1072, 1995

28. Lees TA, Lambert D: Prevalence of lower limb ulceration in an urban health district. *Br J Surg* **79**: 1032–1034, 1992

29. Harper DR, Nelson EA, Gibson B *et al.*: A prospective randomised trial of class 2 and class 3 elastic compression in the prevention of venous ulceration. *Phlebology* Suppl 1 872–873, 1995

30. Mayberry JC, Moneta GL, Taylor LM, Porter JM: Fifteen-year results of ambulatory compression therapy for chronic venous ulcers. *Surgery* **109**: 575–581, 1991

31. Bradbury AW, Stonebridge PA, Callam MJ *et al.*: Foot volumetry and duplex ultrasonography after saphenous and subfascial perforating vein ligation for recurrent venous ulceration. *Br J Surg* **80**: 845–848, 1993

32. Bradbury AW, Ruckley CV: Foot volumetry can predict recurrent ulceration after subfascial ligation of perforators and saphenous ligation. *J Vasc Surg* **18**: 789–795, 1993

33. Darke SG, Penfold C: Venous ulceration and saphenous ligation. *Eur J Vasc Surg* **6**: 4–9, 1992

34. Sethia KK, Darke SG: Long saphenous incompetence as a cause of venous ulceration. *Br J Surg* **71**: 754–755, 1984

35. Negus D, Friedgood A: The effective managment of venous ulceration. *Br J Surg* **70**: 623–627, 1991

36. Gillies TG, Ruckley CV: Does surgery play any part in the managment of venous ulcers?

In: Greenhalgh RM, Fowkes FGR (Eds) *Trials and Tribulation of Vascular Surgery* pp. 411–422. London: WB Saunders, 1996

37. Brittenden J, Bradbury AW, Milne AA *et al.*: Popliteal vein reflux demonstrated by duplex ultrasonography is associated with delayed and non-healing of chronic venous ulceration. *Phlebology* Suppl 1 796–798, 1995

38. Bradbury AW, Brittenden J, Allan PL, Ruckley CV: Comparison of venous reflux in the affected and non-affected leg in patients with unilateral venous ulceration. *Br J Surg* **83:** 513–515, 1996

39. Bradbury AW, Murie JA, Ruckley CV: The role of the leucocyte in the pathogenesis of vascular disease. *Br J Surg* **80:** 1503–1512, 1993

40. Coleridge-Smith PD: Venous ulcer. *Br J Surg* **81:** 1404–1405, 1994

41. Burnand KG, O'Donnell TF, Thomas ML, Browse NL: Relation between post-phlebitic changes in the deep veins and the results of surgical treatment of venous ulcers. *Lancet* **ii:** 936–938, 1976

42. Callam MJ, Ruckley CV, Dale JJ, Harper DR: Hazards of compression treatment of the leg: an estimate from Scottish surgeons. *Br Med J* **295:** 1382, 1987

43. Ruckley CV, Makhdoomi KR: The venous perforator. *Br J Surg* **83:** 1492–1493, 1996

LYMPHOEDEMA

Cellulitis, Inflammation with Lymphoedema

K. G. Burnand, C. L. McGuinness, J. W. Quarmby and
Sir Norman Browse

LYMPHOEDEMA

Lymphoedema is defined as an excessive accumulation of interstitial fluid as a result of a deficiency of normal lymphatic clearance. Lymphoedema is usually caused by obstruction or obliteration of lymphatic ducts and it results in impaired transport of autologous and foreign proteins. This causes an increased pool of extravasated plasma proteins with accumulation of recirculating lymphocytes, monocytes and Langerhans' cells. Cytokine production by the parenchymal and immune cells may be responsible for fibroblastic and epithelial cell proliferation which in turn cause sclerotic changes in the skin and subcutaneous tissues[1] (Figs 1a,b).

CELLULITIS

Cellulitis is inflammation which spreads through the subcutaneous or subfascial planes, often as a result of infection with *Streptococcus pyogenes* which has entered the tissue from a wound or accidental minor trauma. Cellulitis may be either acute or chronic in patients with lymphoedema.

ACUTE CELLULITIS/ERYSIPELAS

This is a spreading inflammation of the skin and subcutaneous tissue as a result of infection by *Strep. pyogenes* (*Streptococcus haemolyticus* of Lancefields group A) (Fig. 2).

Source of infection

The cause is usually direct entry of organisms into subcutaneous tissues. This may be from cuts, scratches and insect or animal bites. Diseased skin is another portal of entry and chronic eczema causes lymphoedema while Tinea pedis often develops in patients with lymphoedema. Tinea pedis is very common perhaps because of altered immunity, but in addition, the swollen toes and deep crevices make adequate drying in this area difficult. Patients with ectatic megalymphatics reflux lymph on standing

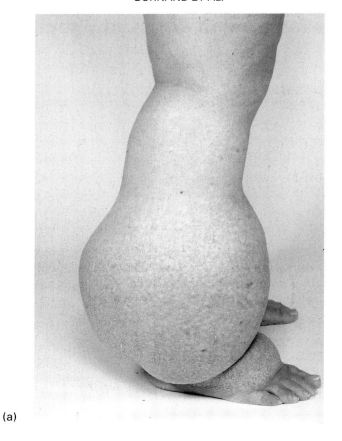

(a)

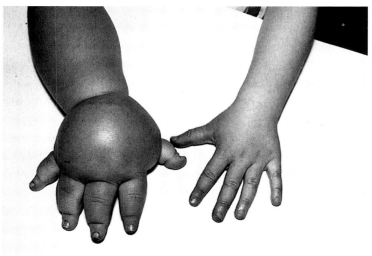

(b)

Fig. 1.   Lower limb lymphoedema (a) and congenital right arm lymphoedema (b).

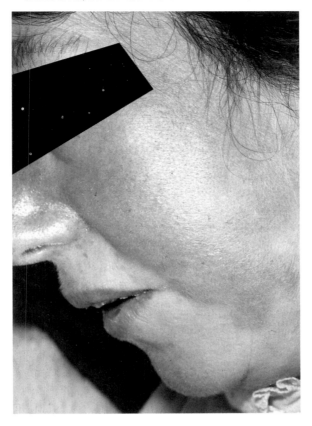

Fig. 2.   Cellulitis of the face with periorbital oedema.

and develop little vesicles within the skin from the increased back-pressure. These vesicles have a very thin epithelial covering and rupture easily following minor trauma, allowing egress of bacteria.

Factors which allow spread and growth of bacteria

Enlarged interstitial space

The interstitial space is normally a small compartment with a negative pressure of −5 mmHg. Any bacteria entering this space are in close proximity to the capillary bed from which escaping polymorphs provide an early defence mechanism. In addition, there is a constant flux and change of fluid which rapidly clears bacteria to the lymphatics which convey the organisms to the local nodes where the immuno-logically competent lymphocytes are situated.

Protein content

In patients with lymphoedema the interstitial compartment is loose with a positive pressure of +1–2 mmHg. The clearance of fluid is slower and the spread of bacteria within the space occurs early as the stagnant interstitial fluid is a nutritive culture medium with a high protein content.

Capillary and lymphatic permeability

Once infection has begun, an inflammatory reaction develops which increases capillary permeability. This in turn results in an increased amount of interstitial fluid, an increased leak of protein, increased tissue pressure and a greater spread of bacteria. There is also a considerable reduction in flow within the draining lymphatics which therefore fail to 'scavenge' bacteria. 'Open' junctions are present between the endothelial cells of lymphatics in inflamed tissue. These spaces allow further protein and fluid leak increasing oedema further.[2,3]

Spread beyond interstitial fluid

Burke showed that the normal lymphatic system is 99% effective in protecting the bloodstream from receiving particulate matter, malignant cells and bacteria from the tissues. The most efficient points of filtration are the initial lymphatics and the first node.[4] Bacteria are quickly removed by normal lymphatics and their localization within lymphatic trunks between the initial lymphatic entry-point and first node may explain the rapid appearance of lymphatic streaks observed in lymphangitis (Fig. 3).

Lymphadenopathy, lymphadenitis and abscess formation in local lymph nodes are common complications of infection. Bacteraemia and septicaemia can result from

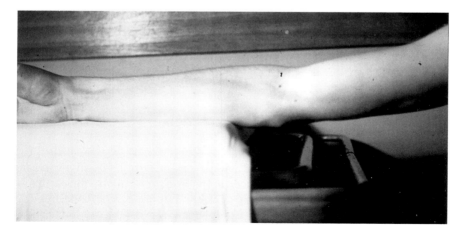

Fig. 3.   Lymphangitis in a patient with sepsis of the hand.

either direct entry of bacteria into capillaries and then to the systemic circulation, or via the lymphatics into the subclavian vein.

Effects of lymphangitis and lymphadenitis

Lymphoedema therefore makes patients more susceptible to infection but lymphangitis may also cause permanent damage to the lymphatics. The damage that follows lymphangitis may cause secondary lymphoedema although lymphangitis is more common in patients who already have lymphoedema. Histological examination of tissue taken from areas with recurrent erysipelas combined with lymphangiography has revealed damaged and in some cases, obliterated lymphatic channels.[1]

Symptoms and signs

The patient may complain of red, hot, tender skin. Streaks of lymphangitis may be visible passing up the limb and large tender nodes may be palpable in the groin or axilla. Patients are usually pyrexial with a tachycardia. Patients with recurrent cellulitis may recognize prodromal symptoms some hours prior to the onset of skin changes. Prodromal symptoms include 'chills' and general malaise.

There may be evidence of an obvious infected wound, bite or sting. All patients should have their interdigital spaces inspected for fungal infection which is a common cause of skin breaches.

DIFFERENTIAL DIAGNOSIS OF CELLULITIS

Many patients with cellulitis and lymphoedema are erroneously diagnosed as having a deep vein thrombosis. Duplex scans show normal deep veins and subsequent isotope lymphography confirms lymphoedema. Acute lipodermatosclerosis can also be mistaken for lymphoedema but there are usually other signs of venous disease. Other conditions that may be misdiagnosed include erythema nodosum, dermatomyositis and dermatitis.

TREATMENT

Patients should be put to bed, the limbs should be elevated and antipyretics given. Intravenous antibiotics should be commenced as soon as possible. Most patients have streptococcal infection which will respond to penicillin if the patient is not sensitive but more broad-spectrum antibiotics such as cephalosporins can be prescribed. Blood-cultures should be taken and any obvious wounds should be swabbed but this will only alter management if the patient fails to respond to the initial antibiotic.

PROPHYLAXIS

There is no evidence that compression or reduction surgery reduces the incidence of cellulitis. Despite this, most clinicians will attempt to limit swelling by conservative measures including bandaging, compression hosiery or mechanical compression devices (e.g. ®Lymphapress).[5,6]

Most patients who have had one attack of cellulitis should be given one course of antibiotics to be started immediately that any prodromal symptom or skin change develops. Long-term low-dose antibiotics can be considered if recurrent infection occurs after eradication of portals of entry e.g. athletes foot.

In patients with skin vesicles and constant lymph leak from fistulae, maceration of the skin may occur and this predisposes to fungal and secondary bacterial infection. A similar problem is seen in patients with deep clefts in verrucous lymphoedema, particularly in the foot and lower leg. In such patients clefts may also be colonized by anaerobic bacteria and offensive leakage may occur (Fig. 4). There are several drugs

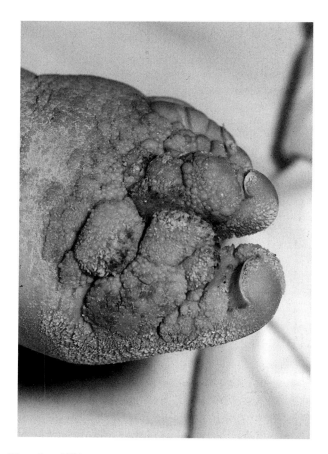

Fig. 4.   Filiform verrucae on a lymphoedematous foot.

which are effective topically against dermatophytes (clotrimazole, tolnaftate and miconazole). Cutaneous candidiasis may be problematic in moist areas and in patients with cutaneous lymph leakage. Nystaform HC ointment (nystatin with vioform and hydrocortisone) is a very effective treatment. Hibiscrub® baths can also be used in patients with repeated infections.

Only a small percentage of patients with lymphoedema require surgery. Many operations have been described and are still used in practice today. These include ligation, lymphovenous anastomosis, mesenteric bridge formation, limb reductions and shaving of verrucae with skin grafting.[7,8] Occasionally, amputation is deemed appropriate (Fig. 5). It is worth reiterating that the only operations which *may* reduce infection are 'drainage' procedures, such as the bridge and lymphovenous anastomosis.

The Casley-Smiths in Australia have championed the use of benzopyrones. These compounds are reported to reduce lymphoedema by increasing proteolysis by tissue

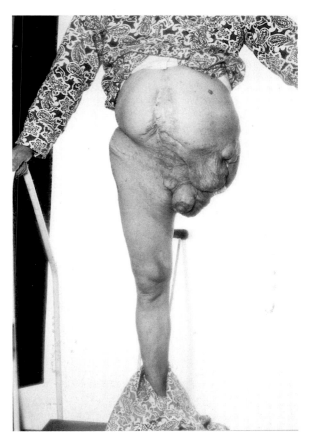

Fig. 5. A patient with severe lymphoedema of the left leg and restriction of mobility eventually treated by disarticulation of the hip.

macrophages.[9] The benzopyrone, 5,6-benzo-α-pyrone has been used orally in randomized double-blind trials in patients with filarial lymphoedema and also patients with primary lymphoedema and other causes of secondary lymphoedema with statistical success.[10,11] However, there remains some scepticism about the use of these drugs in the UK.

Recurrent infection, especially cellulitis is still a severe problem in lymphoedema but may be reduced by the sensible use of the simple measures described above.

REFERENCES

1. Olszewski WL (Ed): *Lymph stasis: Pathophysiology, diagnosis and treatment*. Bocan Rata, FL: CRC Press, 1991
2. Leak LV, Burke JF: Studies on the permeability of lymphatic capillaries during inflammation. *Anat Res* **151**: 489, 1965
3. Viragh P, Papp M, Rusznyak I: The lymphatics in edematous skin. *Acta Morphol Acad Sci Hung* **19**: 203, 1971
4. Burke JF: Lymphatic localisation of malignant and bacterial cells. *Surg Forum* **11**: 36, 1960
5. Zelikovski A, Deutsch A, Reiss R: The sequential pneumatic compression device in surgery for lymphedema of the limbs. *J Cardiovasc Surg* **24**: 122–126, 1983
6. Zelikovski A, Haddad M, Reiss R: The 'Lympha-Press' intermittent sequential pneumatic device for the treatment of lymphoedema: five years of clinical experience. *J Cardiovasc Surg* **27**: 288–290, 1986
7. Kinmonth JB, Hurst PA, Edwards JM, Rutt DL: Relief of lymph obstruction by use of a bridge of mesentery and ileum. *Br J Surg* **65**: 829–833, 1978
8. Gloviczki P, Fisher J, Hollier LH *et al.*: HW Microsurgical lymphovenous anastomosis for treatment of lymphedema: A critical review. *J Vasc Surg* **7**: 647–652, 1988
9. Casley-Smith JR, Casley-Smith JR (Eds): *High-protein Oedemas and the Benzo-pyrones*. Philadelphia: JB Lippincott 1986
10. Casley-Smith JR, Morgan RG, Piller NB: Treatment of lymphedema of the arms and legs with 5,6-benzo-[α]-pyrone. *N Engl J Med* **329**: 1158–1163, 1993
11. Casley-Smith JR, Wang CT, Casley-Smith JR, Zi-hai C: Treatment of filarial lymphoedema and elephantiasis with 5,6-benzo-α-pyrone (coumarin). *Br Med J* **307**: 1037–1041, 1993

Index